Revision Total Hip Arthroplasty

Yixin Zhou
Editor

Revision Total Hip Arthroplasty

Approaches to THA Failure

PMPH PEOPLE'S MEDICAL PUBLISHING HOUSE

Springer

Editor
Yixin Zhou
Department of Adult Joint Reconstructive Surgery
Beijing Jishuitan Hospital, Capital Medical University
Beijing, China

ISBN 978-981-97-9806-3 ISBN 978-981-97-9804-9 (eBook)
https://doi.org/10.1007/978-981-97-9804-9

Jointly published with People's Medical Publishing House, PR of China.

This Springer imprint is published by the registered company Springer Nature Singapore Pte Ltd.
The registered company address is: 152 Beach Road, #21-01/04 Gateway East, Singapore 189721, Singapore

Foreword

For surgical clinicians, taking surgical notes should be an excellent habit. Just like a commander of thousands of troops, a detailed plan is required before a battle, as well as a post-battle review after the event. A piece of homework you should not avoid whether after a bloodless victory without fighting or after an enduring and tough war with lingering fears is to calm your mind, carefully summarize the gains and losses in battle, and figure out how to optimize the process and reduce the cost. Similarly in revision surgery, it is necessary to reflect in peace after an operation as to whether the preoperative plan is comprehensive, the surgical procedure is reasonable, the technical operation is standardized, and whether the trauma of the operation has been minimized. The final question is to ask yourself, "Is this already the best outcome for this patient? If I had to do the operation again, would I be able to do better?" When these thoughts and answers to the questions are condensed and written down, a "surgery note" is created. Summarizing and contemplating one operation earnestly is far more rewarding than operating ten carelessly.

In the early years, when we received intraoperative hand guiding provided by the seniors in the department, we would constantly come across abnormally complicated revision cases with severe bone defect, despite the small number of operations in total. It was demonstrated in exhaustive detail on how to inquire in depth about the patient's medical history and complaints by their bedside, how to conduct physical examination, how to plan the surgical approach by superior physicians, as well as organizing considerable preoperative discussion, analysing the reasons of previous failure mechanism, planning detailed operation procedure, identifying the tools, prosthesis, and allogeneic bone required, and planning postoperative rehabilitation. The skilful exposure, calm judgement, and standardized procedures during the operation, especially the focus on protecting soft tissues and minimizing the trauma to the patients, impressed us young practitioners profoundly. The humanistic care for patients, the rigorous academic attitude, and the pursuit of excellence in surgery of the seniors in the department became the solid foundation for us to continuously progress forwards.

Afterwards, since the increase of complications in hip arthroplasty revision surgery, as well as a continuous improvement in theoretical knowledge and technological level, we gradually realized that as the old saying goes, "just as water retains no constant shape, in warfare there are no constant conditions", big differences always exist between any two revisions. In terms of the reason behind a failure, it could be aseptic loosening, infection, bone fracture around the prosthesis, instability, or metal ions. Each reason of failure means that the concept of revision varies. Based on this fact, this book categorized cases according to different failure mechanisms, aiming to present different preoperative plans and treatment processes for each individual type.

The presentation of each case in this book follows the actual operation procedure, including preoperative planning, intraoperative findings, and postoperative reflections, in which the experience and lessons gained by the surgeons and the description of some operation techniques are also presented. Besides, the concept of reconstruction has altered significantly. Due to the long operation time and high infection rate, previously used common structural bone-grafting and compression bone-grafting have been gradually replaced by the current biological reconstruction methods. These are based on the combination of metal augment and microporous-coated acetabular cups, and the concept of biostem assembling was also introduced for the proximal femur reconstruction. Looking back a decade ago, our team had just accessed these brand-new techniques and tools under the supervision of Professor Zhou Yixin and went through a period of exploring and learning. As a man with a responsible and conscientious attitude, Professor Zhou would take notes of what he experienced and learnt in terms of techniques and operation procedures after each surgery. These materials are the valuable primary sources that contributed to the birth of this book. With the accumulation of more cases and the gradual enrichment of practical experience, certain hip revision theories such as RPC theory of acetabular reconstruction, valid fixation length theory of femoral reconstruction, and SMA principle have been gradually established, so that more advanced and precise work (robot-assisted hip revision surgery) can be successfully carried out at a later stage. Therefore, the publication of this book, as well as years of our progress in hip arthroplasty revision theory and practice, is due to the hard and innovative work of Professor Zhou Yixin over the years.

Practice refines theory, and theory guides practice in turn. At present, the process of hip revision surgery has been optimized, the operation time is largely shortened, and the operational effect is significantly improved. We present it to readers in the form of surgical notes, interspersing relevant theories within clinical practice and sharing some of our thoughts, in order to create a reading experience like discussing the cases face-to-face, in which the readers will enjoy the pleasure brought by the revision surgery with a relaxed mind. In addition, although this book focuses on hip arthroplasty revision, we believe that understanding the different failure mechanisms of hip arthroplasty can provide some insight into how we can best perform primary hip arthroplasty.

We would like to thank all the team members who participated in the surgery. Without them, the success of so many complex revision surgeries would not have been possible. We also appreciate all the colleagues and friends who have worked hard for the successful publication of this book. They provided us with the opportunity to share the fun of our work with peers.

If any flaws in the content or presentation of this book are noticed, we would be more than happy to receive any advice and suggestions from the readers.

Jishuitan Hospital
Beijing, China

Shengjie Guo

Preface

To see a world in a grain of sand, and a heaven in a wild flower.
——William Blake

The writing of this book has lasted for more than a decade when counting from the first note pieces on revision total hip arthroplasty. There has always been some sensational impulse aroused from my heart and mind every time I took notes of what I have seen and comprehended when sitting in the corner of the operation room, every time I filed intraoperative photographs and video records in front of a computer, every time I fix my gaze towards an X-radiography on the negatoscope, and every time I watch the steps and smiles of a patient in a follow-up examination. What is this impulse? Be it the introspection after a failure, the joy after applying a new surgical method, or the epiphany after being puzzled in pondering? Perhaps …… all of them together.

Naturally, writing has become the solid choice to record the experience, expand the understanding, and condense knowledge. Frankly speaking, I have no idea how the printed notes of operations for audience are supposed to be. Nevertheless, I could not help the desire of sharing it with those with the same interest. Hence, I used the operation cases as the main body, outlined the chapters according to the postoperative failure mechanism of hip arthroplasty, and presented our practice and reflection in the revision total hip arthroplasty with narration interspersed with comments.

The Notebook Records the Experience and Perception in Clinical Practice

The content of this book is a faithful record of what was observed, heard, experienced, reflected on, and thought of during clinical practice of revision total hip arthroplasty. Generally, information referred to books, journals, conferences, and the communication with colleagues from other institutions is not included. What was observed, heard, experienced, reflected on, and thought of refer to their respective points, yet all of them covered preoperative, intraoperative, and postoperative (including medium and long-term follow-up examination) stages.

What was observed refers to various clinical and imaging features, intraoperative gross and microscopic pathology features, ionic concentration, and biomarkers.

What was heard refers to the opinions over treatment and knowledge of the conditions towards revision total hip arthroplasty cases provided by surgeons, physicians, plastic surgeons, anaesthetists, pathologists, microbiologists, ICU physicians, rehabilitation physicians, and nurse practitioners within a surgical team.

What was experienced refers more to the notes about immediate intraoperative experience and what surgeons saw that was often written down on any piece of paper available right after taking off their surgical gloves.

What was reflected on and thought of seems to share one meaning, but it is worth explaining as they are distinctive to the author. *What was reflected on* refers to the progress of reflection, any minor ideas and interim understandings. Conversely, *what was thought of* is the most precious part to me, which specifically refers to something that can advance to *thought* based on all that was *observed, heard, experienced, and reflected* on in this book, such as the *ring-point-column (RPC) theory* in acetabular reconstruction, *valid fixation length theory* in femoral reconstruction, and *SMA principle* (i.e., stability, mechanics, and abductor).

The Notebook Records the Process from Perceptual Cognition to Rational Cognition Towards Revision Total Hip Arthroplasty

The establishment of ring-point-column (RPC) theory in acetabular reconstruction is an abstracting and condensing process of the supporting mechanism of various previous reconstruction methods. Freshmen in hip revision always stand in awe of bone defect, and as a result, few do not regard the classification of bone defects as a standard. In fact, it is the bone left on semi-pelvis that determines the reconstruction method. The real importance is to confirm the strength of the remaining bone for mechanical support of the acetabular cup and the vitality of osseointegration.

RPC theory brings us back to the first principle, focusing on the mechanical stability of cup construct (including hemispherical cup and each augment) and the capability of bone ingrowth, regardless of the specific shape and size of the defect. Therefore, RPC is free from the constraints of one or several defect types, and it has the universality of acetabular reconstruction guidance.

Readers will encounter many "conceptual" terms in this book, many of which are created or defined by us. Conceptual terms such as valid fixation length reflect the surgeon's understanding, internalizing, abstracting, and condensing of the observed objective phenomenon in clinical practice.

The Notebook Records the Process of Coming Up with a Series of Innovative Solutions Generated from Practice

On the basis of RPC theory in acetabular reconstruction and valid fixation length theory of femoral prosthesis, we established extending-fixation technique and designed a series of ABM hip arthroplasty revision prostheses, which realized the theories above. We conducted a multi-centre clinical research and have received encouraging results.

Innovative surgical techniques such as endosteal reconstruction (inspired by the construction technology of the Hong Kong-Zhuhai-Macao Bridge) and isthmus plasty, aiming for the reconstruction of severely damaged femoral stump and isthmus, are also presented in this book.

Similarly, in the chapter "Robot-Assisted Hip Arthroplasty Revision", the way in which we expanded the indications of Mako Robot and how to establish the method of intraoperative registration of hip revision, as well as the procedure of robotic revision, is presented for the first time.

In the chapter "Hip Dislocation", I explain how we applied anatomical, kinematic, and kinetic parameters to model construction to optimize each feasible domain and to establish patient-specific functional safety zones.

The innovative work is not fully listed in consideration of the length, though it is clear that we have been working at the forefront in hip arthroplasty revision.

The Notebook Is the Fruit of Collective Intelligence

It is a rather onerous program to carry out hip arthroplasty revision in a large scale. There are a great number of different types of operations under the category of hip arthroplasty revision. They are often in demand due to various failure mechanisms. Even for the same failure mechanism, the approaches to revision often radically differ from one another depending on the stage of the disease and the degree of hip bone and soft tissue damage.

Patients of revision hip arthroplasty tend to be of an advanced age, often with frequent and severe comorbidities, as well as a high risk of complication. Without a highly specialized team and an efficient, precise working mechanism, it would be either an impossible mission to perform hip arthroplasty revision at a large scale or a land of complications in our operating rooms and wards.

Unprecedented challenges constantly lie in the practice of revision hip arthroplasty: large bone defects make it almost impossible to reconstruct, along with metallosis (there is no clue of how to diagnose this and no consensus on the treatment) and recurrent dislocation of unknown reason…

After all, this book wouldn't exist without the trust and cooperation among surgical teams and colleagues from different backgrounds. Neither this book would be published without the curiosity and courage in the bond and mutual affinity among the work partner. Without their help, the hundreds of cases that built up this notebook wouldn't be present anymore.

I sincerely hope that this book will provide aid to all those who work in hip joint diagnosis and treatment. Here, the author is not claiming that revision hip arthroplasty is the "ultimate power" in the hip reconstruction field, as some other surgeries bear similar or even greater practical and educational value. Nevertheless, the various mental activities and teamwork required for revision hip arthroplasty, the comprehension and application of all the exposure and reconstruction techniques, as well as corresponding prosthesis and tools will be an excellent training material for all colleagues in hip surgery to study, understand, and practise complex hip surgery at strategic and tactical level.

I received plenty of encouragement and support from my friends, mostly colleagues, training physicians, and even some of my patients if being honest, during the writing of this book. They reckon that a notebook, different from a textbook, is likely to be closer to clinical practice and better for the presentation of the thinking process. I also consider it as simple as writing straight to the point, which should be easier than an academic literature. Surprisingly, it is not that simple anymore when you pick up your pen, with hundreds and thousands of words pouring in mind, not knowing where to start. As a result, the writing had been started and paused over and over again and was finally completed over many years.

Defects and mistakes could exist to a certain extent in the content, please do not hesitate to point them out. Despite the inevitably monotonous expression, this book represents the passion of the author towards revision hip arthroplasty.

Beijing, China Yixin Zhou

Contents

Editors and Contributors

Editor

Yixin Zhou Department of Adult Joint Reconstructive Surgery, Beijing Jishuitan Hospital, Capital Medical University, Beijing, China

Associate Editors

Hongyi Shao Department of Adult Joint Reconstructive Surgery, Beijing Jishuitan Hospital, Capital Medical University, Beijing, China

Shengjie Guo Department of Adult Joint Reconstructive Surgery, Beijing Jishuitan Hospital, Capital Medical University, Beijing, China

Secretary Editor

Hanlong Zheng Department of Adult Joint Reconstructive Surgery, Beijing Jishuitan Hospital, Capital Medical University, Beijing, China

Contributors

Tao Bian Department of Adult Joint Reconstructive Surgery, Beijing Jishuitan Hospital, Capital Medical University, Beijing, China

Lang Chen Department of Adult Joint Reconstructive Surgery, Beijing Jishuitan Hospital, Capital Medical University, Beijing, China

Xi Chen Department of Adult Joint Reconstructive Surgery, Beijing Jishuitan Hospital, Capital Medical University, Beijing, China

Wang Deng Department of Adult Joint Reconstructive Surgery, Beijing Jishuitan Hospital, Capital Medical University, Beijing, China

Xiao Feng Department of Adult Joint Reconstructive Surgery, Beijing Jishuitan Hospital, Capital Medical University, Beijing, China

Jianming Gu Department of Adult Joint Reconstructive Surgery, Beijing Jishuitan Hospital, Capital Medical University, Beijing, China

Yong Huang Department of Adult Joint Reconstructive Surgery, Beijing Jishuitan Hospital, Capital Medical University, Beijing, China

Zhuyi Ma Department of Adult Joint Reconstructive Surgery, Beijing Jishuitan Hospital, Capital Medical University, Beijing, China

Yang Song Department of Adult Joint Reconstructive Surgery, Beijing Jishuitan Hospital, Capital Medical University, Beijing, China

Hao Tang Department of Adult Joint Reconstructive Surgery, Beijing Jishuitan Hospital, Capital Medical University, Beijing, China

Siyuan Wang Department of Adult Joint Reconstructive Surgery, Beijing Jishuitan Hospital, Capital Medical University, Beijing, China

Dejin Yang Department of Adult Joint Reconstructive Surgery, Beijing Jishuitan Hospital, Capital Medical University, Beijing, China

Xinghua Yin Department of Adult Joint Reconstructive Surgery, Beijing Jishuitan Hospital, Capital Medical University, Beijing, China

Liang Zhang Department of Adult Joint Reconstructive Surgery, Beijing Jishuitan Hospital, Capital Medical University, Beijing, China

Hanlong Zheng Department of Adult Joint Reconstructive Surgery, Beijing Jishuitan Hospital, Capital Medical University, Beijing, China

1 The Concerto of Revision Total Hip Arthroplasty

Dejin Yang

1.1 Introduction

Dejin Yang

Revision total hip arthroplasty is the culmination of hip reconstruction techniques, which is challenging and fascinating. The motivation for our team to devote more than 10 years to this field stems from the impulse of curiosity and challenge on the one hand and its unique attraction on the other. It has brought us relief, a weight off our shoulders, joy after a near-miss, excitement after a whim, comfort after a sudden enlightenment, as well as open-mindedness after experiencing diversity. As it is said, "the infinite scenery lies on the dangerous peak."

Revision total hip arthroplasty is a concerto of classic principles and innovative techniques. It primarily follows the classical principles that cover anatomy, kinematics, biomechanics, pathophysiology, and materials science. The localization and protection of neurovascular structures, the enhancement of joint stability and safe motion range, the optimization of prosthesis stress distribution and load, the consideration of bone vitality and osseointegration potential, and the appropriate application of metal materials and biomaterials, all of which must follow the classic principles without exception. However, revision total hip arthroplasty often encounters unexpected challenges and even dangers that do not often occur in conventional surgeries, requiring adaptability and improvisation to turn the corner. For example, our pioneered femoral reconstruction techniques for type IV bone defect, namely, isthmus plasty and endosteal reconstruction, are innovative techniques that had to be created in extreme cases due to the impossibility of reconstruction via classic methods. As a Chinese adage goes, "The Confucianists of Han Dynasty interpreted the scriptures by deducing them according to the text; people of Jin Dynasty, on the other hand, discarded the scriptures and create their own essays" (refer to *Zhu Zi Yu Lei*, Zhu Xi 1270). For the revision total hip arthroplasty, it is necessary to both interpret the scriptures according to the text and create our own essays.

The concerto of revision total hip arthroplasty is a comprehensive presentation of knowledge, skills, and judgment. The preoperative diagnosis is actually the analysis and verification of the failure mechanism of the index surgery. An in-depth understanding of the risk factors and features of various failure mechanisms, the efficacy of various diagnostic methods, the pros and cons of different prosthesis designs, and different surgical options are all dependent on the knowledge of classic textbooks, thorough reading of literature in this field, and international communication, cross-disciplinary collaborations, and knowledge updates from scientific research. The improvement of basic techniques, such as prosthesis removal, bone defect reconstruction, and soft tissue balance, comes from the deconstruction and restructure of the surgical

D. Yang (✉)
Department of Adult Joint Reconstructive Surgery, Beijing Jishuitan Hospital, Capital Medical University, Beijing, China

Y. Zhou (ed.), *Revision Total Hip Arthroplasty*, https://doi.org/10.1007/978-981-97-9804-9_1

techniques of the index surgery, as well as the reflection and improvement after thousands of routine operations or innovative operations; while some innovative technologies are born from translational research driven by clinical demand. For instance, the piezoelectric ultrasonic osteotome for cement removal, hip revision module in robotic system, ABM (stands for Anatomy, Biology, and Mechanics) revision system based on medical-engineering-industrial joint research, as well as a series of clinically established innovative techniques such as isthmus plasty and endosteal reconstruction, all originated from practical clinical demand. These are revolutionary techniques that were bound to be generated when there was no appropriate solution. Because of the limitations of fundamental principles and surgical trauma in revision surgery, we have to operate while constantly making choices and trade-offs. For example, we will face the choice of when to perform an extended trochanteric osteotomy, when to split the femoral sheath, and when to adopt the regular operation skills every time a well-fixed femoral stem needs to be removed. Being precise and decisive will improve the operation efficiency and avoid complications. We have summarized the rim-point-column strategy (RPC) of acetabular reconstruction and the valid fixation length theory of the femur through practice and research, which are no doubt further guiding strategies for the rational application of knowledge and technology, as well as a sharp tool to boost decision-making ability.

The execution of hip revision necessitates the excellence of operating team's in-house work, which comes from knowledge and skill training for a high-level team. Fighting alone seems courageous but is not ideal in hip revision. Teamwork is necessary in the process of hip revision surgery and perioperative management. In terms of preoperative diagnosis, evaluation, and optimization, a series of specialized teams have been established in authors' institute, such as a periprosthetic infection research team, a surgical team for rheumatology, a metallosis research team, and so on, to carry out relevant work and research in diagnosing failure mechanisms of hip revision and optimization of clinical patient management. The mutual benefit between clinical practice and research not only increases our understanding of artificial joints, but also provides actual clinical solutions, improves the precision and accuracy of diagnosis, and enhances surgical safety. In our clinical team, we have doctors and nurses with relatively fixed cooperative relationships, as well as anesthesiologists, rehabilitation medicine experts, pharmaceutical experts, pathologists, microbiology experts, and supporting experts from outside research institutions, laboratories, and product engineers.

Hip revision without teamwork will not only be short of hands to deal with practical clinical difficulties but also leave the practitioner stranded, forced to cope with various clinical affairs and troubleshooting, risking them of occupational burnout and difficulty in skill improvement and scientific experience accumulation.

Hip revision is the art of *circle in a square*. The square is the principles, while the circle is flexibility and compromise. While sticking to principles and pursuing effectiveness, we have to stay vigilant at all times regarding surgical trauma that may occur in hip revision, even life-threatening dangers to patients. Making adjustments, even compromises, under certain situations is an optional strategy to keep surgical trauma under control and minimize complications. Consider an example of conducting operations for advanced-age patients, we can either retain the prosthesis parts in well-fixed and well-positioned condition or employ the cement-in-cement technique on the remaining cement mantle. It is a necessary skill for hip revision practitioners to develop the habit of maintaining awareness of the overall condition of the patient and the operation room, the integral structure of the operation procedure, and the capability limits of the operation team, as well as controlling the pace throughout the operation. Therefore, *being decisive between circle and square* is a fundamental professional quality required for a hip revision practitioner.

This book presents our journey and achievement in revision total hip arthroplasty in the form of surgical notes. It represents our respect for the fundamental principles, embracement and encouragement of new technology and unremitting pursuit toward a more skillful team and self, without reserving any dilemma or regret. It is revision total hip arthroplasty that provides us with the freedom to be honest and sincere.

2 Aseptic Loosening on the Femoral Side

Shengjie Guo, Yixin Zhou, Yong Huang, Hanlong Zheng, and Wang Deng

2.1 Introduction

Shengjie Guo and Yixin Zhou

Aseptic loosening is one of the main reasons for revision after total hip arthroplasty (THA). Studies have found that the most common indications for revision total hip arthroplasty in the United States include hip instability (22.5%), mechanical loosening (19.7%), and infection (14.8%) [1]. The statistical data of 397 cases of revision total hip arthroplasty from December 2010 to December 2015 in Jishuitan Hospital, Beijing, showed that the most common indications for revision total hip arthroplasty were aseptic loosening (70.3%), osteolysis (14.9%), and infection (13.9%).

If the osseointegration between the prosthesis surface and the host bone is not ideal (for cementless prosthesis), or proper interlocking between the cement and the host bone fails (cement-based prosthesis), aseptic loosening may occur. This is largely associated with the experience and skill of the surgeon, as well as the application of prosthesis with adverse follow-up records.

Revision total hip arthroplasty procedures tend to face all degrees of bone defects or reshape deformities on the acetabular and proximal femur (usually on the proximal femur) [2], such as severe osteolysis due to loosening or wear, stress shielding, multiple previous surgeries, osteoporosis, iatrogenic bone defect caused by original prosthesis removal, or residual bone cement, which is the difficulty in revision and reconstruction. The main goals of revision total hip arthroplasty are to achieve stable fixation of the stem, stability, biomechanically restoring functions, and ultimately realizing long-term prosthesis survival.

The proximal femur can be evaluated in two ways. First is the severity of the bone defect; second is with or without remodeling deformity, such as varus or backward remodeling. Many researchers have proposed different classification systems for femoral bone defects in revision total hip arthroplasty. One that is usually referred to is the Paprosky classification [3]. The Type IV femoral bone defect is particularly difficult to deal with due to the loss of support from the isthmus, which is a significant challenge to achieve the initial stability of the stem. The Paprosky classification of the proximal femur is shown in Fig. 2.1.

The reconstruction strategy for femoral bone defect is determined based on the severity of the bone defect, residual bone mass and quality, and changes in anatomical remodeling. Proximal femur reconstruction aims to achieve the following three goals: (1) initial stability of the stem; (2) restoration of hip biomechanics; and (3) the reconstruction of the abductor.

S. Guo (✉) · Y. Zhou · Y. Huang
H. Zheng · W. Deng
Department of Adult Joint Reconstructive Surgery, Beijing Jishuitan Hospital, Capital Medical University, Beijing, China

Y. Zhou (ed.), *Revision Total Hip Arthroplasty*, https://doi.org/10.1007/978-981-97-9804-9_2

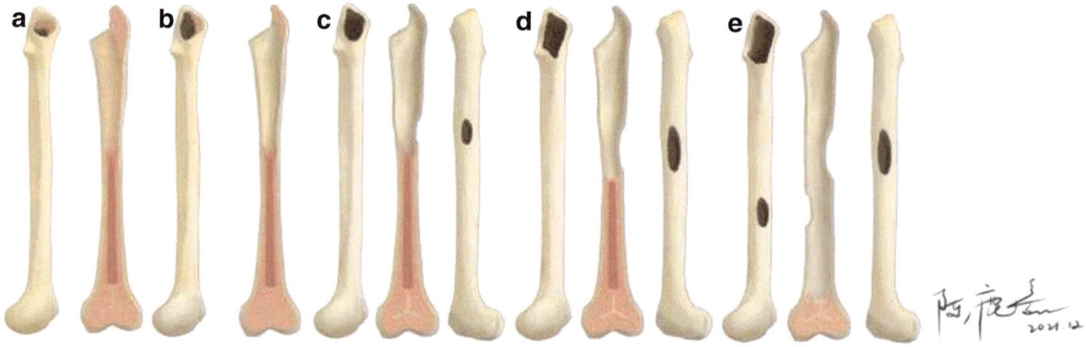

Fig. 2.1 Paprosky classification of proximal femur. (**a**) Type I femoral bone defect: A slight cancellous bone defect of distal femoral metaphysis with the intact cortical bone of the diaphysis; (**b**) Type II femoral bone defect: An extensive cancellous bone defect of distal femoral metaphysis with the intact cortical bone of the diaphysis; (**c**) Type IIIA femoral bone defect: Severe destruction of the distal femoral metaphysis, cannot provide support, but with over 4 cm of intact cortical bone on the diaphysis to provide adequate distal stable fixation; (**d**) Type IIIB femoral bone defect: Severe destruction of distal femoral metaphysis, cannot provide support, with less than 4 cm of intact cortical bone on the diaphysis to provide distal stable fixation; and (**e**) Type IV femoral bone defect: Severe destruction in both distal femoral metaphysis and diaphysis with enlarged femoral medullary cavity, no support from the isthmus of the diaphysis

There are several methods of proximal femur reconstruction in revision total hip arthroplasty, including cement stem fixation, proximal porous-coated non-cement stem fixation, proximal porous-coated modular non-cement stem fixation, fully porous-coated distal-fixed cylindrical vitallium stem, modular or non-modular distal-fixed conical ridged titanium stem, compression bone grafting, allograft prosthesis composite, and proximal femoral replacement [4]. The modular distal-fixed conical ridged titanium stem is commonly used. This type of stem has certain advantages in the reconstruction of hip mechanics, limb length adjustment, and stem subsidence resistance, with ideal long-term follow-up results [5, 6, 7].

The biggest challenge for surgeons is still conditions like Type IV severe bone defects from the Paprosky classification. We summarized two technical methods for reference, namely, isthmusplasty and endosteal reconstruction, specific to such conditions. See Appendix 3 for details.

2.2 Case 1

Yong Huang and Shengjie Guo

2.2.1 Case Summary

Medical History Female, 74-year-old, presented with an intertrochanteric fracture of the left hip caused by a fall 2 years ago. After the injury, the fracture was treated with open reduction and internal fixation (ORIF) with a plate. Postoperative review revealed internal fixation failure. THA was performed in another hospital over 1 year ago. The patient developed left hip pain and limited mobility over 3 months ago.

Physical Examination Claudication; visible incision cicatrix on left hip joint; no swelling or sinus tract; skin temperature was not high; tenderness in left inguinal, hip, greater trochanter and proximal thigh area (+); axial percussion pain (+);

obviously limited mobility; Patrick's sign on the left side (+); Thomas' sign on the left side (+); and Trendelenburg's sign on the left side (+).

Laboratory Examination No abnormality was detected in a routine blood test, erythrocyte sedimentation rate (ESR), and C-reactive protein (CRP).

Radiographic Data Radiographs of first-time proximal femoral plate internal fixation failure and initial total hip arthroplasty (THA); immediate postoperative radiographs are shown in Fig. 2.2; the anterior and lateral radiographs before revision are shown in Fig. 2.3.

2.2.2 Case Analysis and Surgical Planning

1. The reason for the loosening and sinking of the femoral stem after THA was the undersized Wagner stem for the initial replacement. This type of femoral stem could hardly be fixed at both proximal and distal ends. If the distal end was well fixed, the proximal site was likely to be loose at the same time.
2. Femoral medullary cavity factors: The intact femoral isthmus of the distal end of the patient was relatively short; lack of valid fixation length; the medullary cavity was wide; thus, it was hard for the femoral stem to have enough stability within the medullary cavity; and medullary cavity shrinking osteotomy was required to reduce the diameter of the medullary cavity.

2.2.3 Preoperative Planning

1. Extended trochanteric osteotomy (ETO) was decided for the following reasons:
   (a) ETO is suitable for adjusting the lateral cortical deformity and reshaping the medullary cavity; it is a medullary cavity shrinking osteotomy that generates an artificial femoral isthmus and also a type of isthmusplasty.
   (b) Without ETO, the medullary cavity incisional point and the surgical access would be blocked by the trochanter and the prosthesis would be hard to remove. In order to place the non-cement stem into the medullary cavity, the medullary cavity required careful clearing; perforation could have happened to such patients with osteoporosis during the process of filing medullary cavity due to the poor femur quality, with a high risk of torsion fracture, if ETO was not performed.
   (c) Without ETO, the stem was likely to be varus, which was difficult to be well fixed, and may lead to further revision in the future.

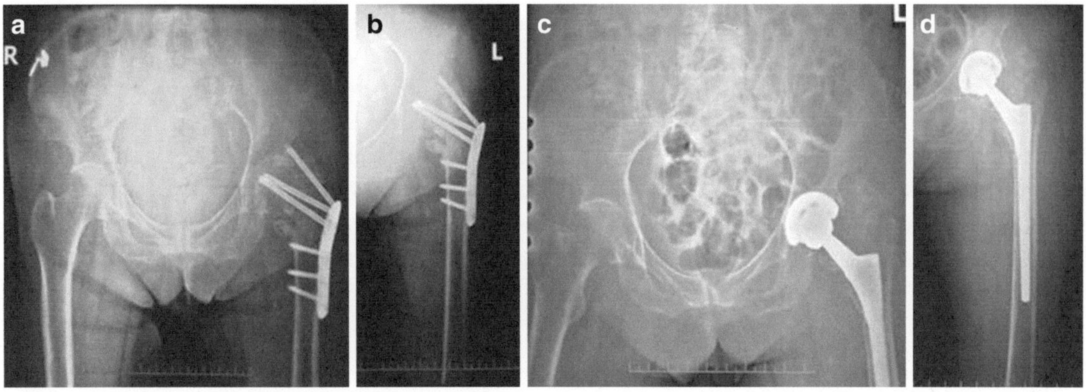

Fig. 2.2 Radiographs of first-time proximal femoral plate internal fixation failure (**a**, **b**) and immediate X-rays after the initial THA (**c**, **d**)

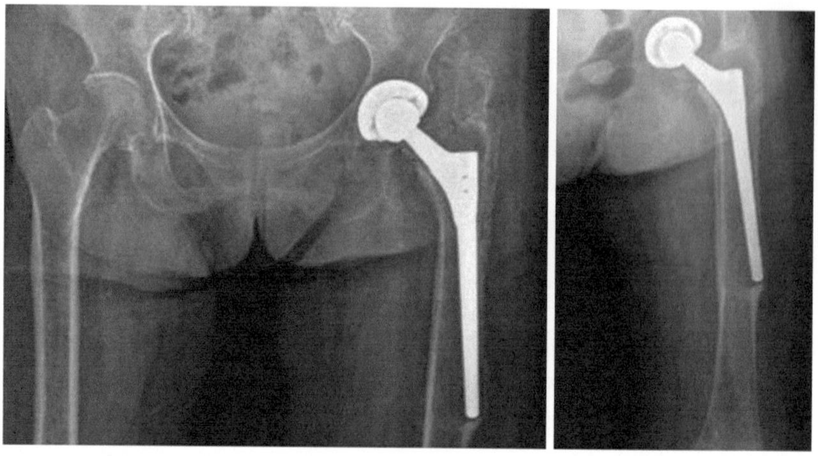

Fig. 2.3 Anterior and lateral X-ray views before revision

(d) ETO enables better visibility of the medullary cavity, thus soft tissues such as pseudomembrane in the medullary cavity could be removed more efficiently, and the sclerotic bone in the medullary cavity could be better treated until the bone matrix seeped with fresh bleeding, so that the bone matrix was refreshed, which would benefit the bone ingrowth of the femoral stem; even the increase in bone mass could be seen in the postoperative follow-up examinations.

2. A tapered, modular, fluted titanium (TMFT) stem with distal fixation was selected, with a thick stem equipped on the distal end.
3. After ETO, the bone block was attached to the shoulder of the proximal femoral stem, which benefited the proximal bone ingrowth of the prosthesis and promoted the long-term fixation of the proximal femoral stem.

2.2.4 Operation Situation

During the operation, ETO was performed according to the preoperative plan. The bone cortex was observed to be thin, the bone quality was poor, and the femoral stem was loose, which was easily retrieved. A titanium cable was applied for cerclage at the distal end of the ETO block and implanted into a TMFT stem of 195 mm × 23 mm at the distal end and 31 + 10 mm at the proximal end. The ETO block was tied and placed to reduce the diameter of the medullary cavity.

2.2.5 Postoperative Outcome

The immediate postoperative X-rays are shown in Fig. 2.4.

2.2.6 Conclusion and Reflection

In this case, the bone quality on the femur was very poor. How can we choose anti-osteoporosis therapy for such patients? Which therapy is appropriate for bone metabolism adjustment? If it is necessary, when do we apply it?

Drugs that inhibit bone turnover may not be appropriate at the early stage of bone ingrowth of prosthesis. Teriparatide might be a good choice if financially allowed. It would certainly be excellent if there were better drugs to increase the patient's bone mass so that future periprosthetic femoral fractures could be avoided.

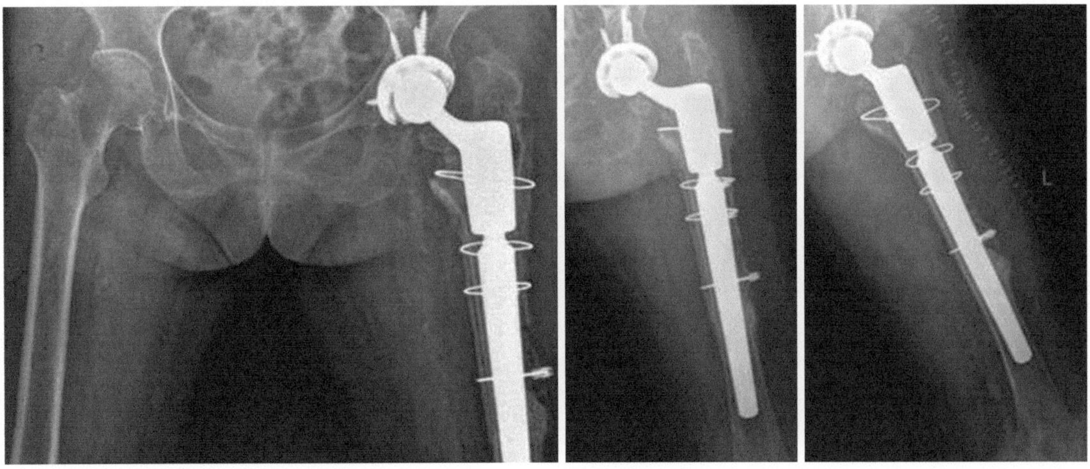

Fig. 2.4 Immediate postoperative X-rays

2.3 Case 2

Hanlong Zheng and Yixin Zhou

2.3.1 Case Summary

Medical History Female, 45-year-old, patient underwent osteosarcoma resection and total hip arthroplasty (left) at a local hospital due to osteosarcoma of the left femur 25 years ago. The osteosarcoma recurred 22 years ago, and the patient underwent osteosarcoma resection for the second time. Before 14 years, the patient underwent revision THA with a tumor prosthesis in another hospital because of aseptic loosening. Recovery was ideal after the operation. In recent 2 years, the left lower extremity of the patient gradually shortened, causing claudication accompanied by hip and knee discomfort. The condition gradually aggravated. Recently, the patient registered in our hospital and completed the relevant examination. The diagnosis was prosthetic loosening following a revision THA, indicating the need for surgical treatment, and the patient was subsequently hospitalized. The patient had been in good health prior to this.

Physical Examination The patient walked into the ward with a crutch. The pelvis was tilted to the left; the left lower limb showed obvious muscle atrophy, shortening, and external rotation; the knee joint was everted, 3 cm shorter than the right lower extremity. There was no redness, swelling, or pigmentation in both hips; multiple surgical incision scars were observed in the left hip, which healed well without redness or swelling. Left hip area and proximal thigh tenderness (±); axial percussion pain (±); left hip joint was mobile; right hip joint mobility was good; mobility of both knees, ankles, and toes was normal. Left hip motion range: flexion 80°, extension 5°, abduction 15°, adduction 0°, internal rotation 10°, and external rotation 10°.

Laboratory Examination Routine blood test, CRP, and ESR were normal.

Radiographic Data Preoperative X-rays are shown in Fig. 2.5.

2.3.2 Preoperative Planning

1. Radiography Illustration: The stem of this tumor prosthesis was significantly loosened; the prosthesis sunk and migrated medially; the distal isthmus disappeared. Condyle penetrates occurred in the medial femur. The medial side of the acetabulum did not appear to be loose; eccentric wear of the acetabular prosthesis could be observed. The greater trochanter was missing.

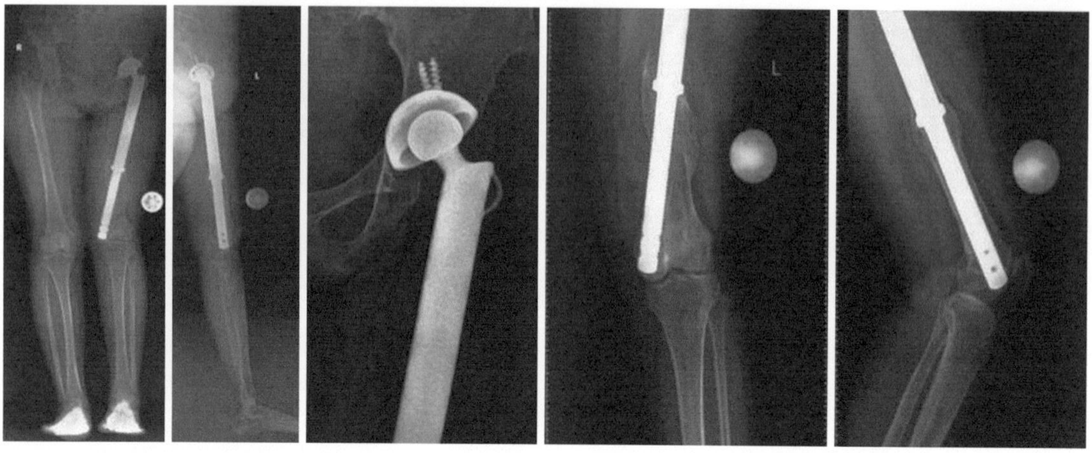

Fig. 2.5 Preoperative radiograph

2. The Reconstitution Strategy: Infection was ruled out first. The biggest difficulty in this case is how to fix the femoral stem, whether to choose tumor prosthesis reconstruction, monoblock, modular stem, or ABM system? Most surgeons would probably consider total femoral replacement as the first choice.

Indeed, the advantage of total femoral replacement was avoiding the femoral side fixation. The distal hinged knee was fixed to the tibia; thus, all stress was concentrated on the tibia–prosthesis interface. Without dispersion over the collateral ligament and capsule on the side of the cruciate ligament, the load of the femoral condyle on the tibia platform was concentrated on the femoral condyle or hinge. Moreover, as the patient was relatively younger, she tended not to undergo total femur replacement, with a strong desire to preserve the knee joint. In addition, several publications have reported high complications and failure rates in cement tumor prosthesis revision. Therefore, tumor prosthesis was a poor choice in terms of fixation, age, and functioning and should be avoided for this patient.

The next question is, without total femur replacement, where would the initial stability of the prosthesis come from? The medullary cavity is small at the top and large at the bottom. Modular stem would allow lower limb length adjustment, but it still cannot achieve the fixation. However, a cement tumor stem would not be possible either because a complete sleeve, cancellous bone, and cement interlock were required. Without a cortical sleeve, the bone cement cannot be pressurized and permeate into the trabecula, with a high risk of failure.

So, what kind of fixation should be adopted? According to the author, the most ideal method was non-cement fixation, achieving long-term stability through osseointegration. Even though bone cement could be fixed in a short time, the sleeve would withstand high torsional force and loosen easily. Therefore, either the cement or non-cement method alone is not feasible in this case. The author once watched the documentary *Hong Kong-Zhuhai-Macao Bridge*. The underwater part of the bridge adopts the endosteal reconstruction technology, in which the tunnel parts were prefabricated and sunk into the sea and then connected underwater. In this case, could we press the porous metal preform into the medullary cavity, fix the distal end through porous metal osseointegration, and fix the prosthesis stem with bone cement? In the long term, this fixation method could be regarded as an irregular THA with porous surface osseointegration. The author's team 3D-printed the distal femur model for the patient before surgery, as shown in Fig. 2.6.

2.3.3 Surgical Procedure and Intraoperative Observation

1. Prosthesis Exposure and Removal: The boundary between the iliotibial band and tensor fasciae latae was cut open and separated

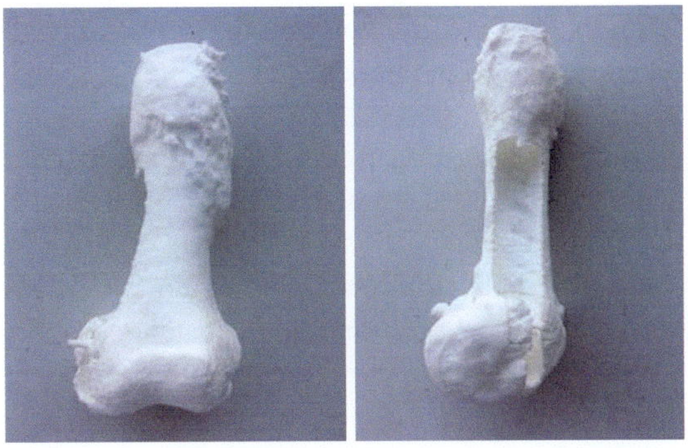

Fig. 2.6 Preoperatively 3D-printed distal femur model

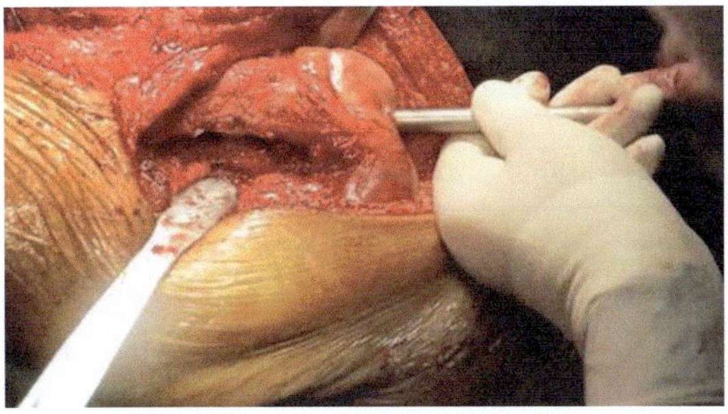

Fig. 2.7 Intraoperative defect of medial condyle of distal femur

using the posterolateral approach for about 25 cm long; cicatrix tissue in severe adhesion was debonded; tissue along the posterior edge of gluteus medius was cut by layer, and the femoral stem and hip joint were exposed. The femoral head was separated and removed. The femoral stem was notably loose, which could rotate and move longitudinally; the acetabular liner was slightly worn; the acetabular prosthesis was slightly inclined backward without significant loosening. The acetabular liner was removed, the screw was taken out, and the acetabular prosthesis was removed.

An incision on the distal, anterolateral thigh of 15 cm long was created and cut by layers. It was observed that the proximal bone had atrophied and thinned, with a bone defect extending from the mid-distal medial femur to the condyle, exposing the prosthesis. Periprosthetic cicatrix was excised, and the complete femoral stem was taken out. It was observed that the medial condyle revealed a cavity defect. Extended the incision to the center of the front knee joint, cut the skin open, reaching about 20 mm deep; the joint capsule was cut open through the medial parapatellar approach, and the canon bone was laterally dislocated; flexing the hip to expose the femoral condyle. The cartilage was intact, and the medial condyle cartilage revealed a focal dimmed color. The granulation tissue in the medullary cavity was cleared.

2. Acetabular Preparation and Prosthesis Placement: The acetabular file was placed at 40° abduction and 10° anteversion, and a 56-mm-diameter Trabecular metal (TM) acetabular prosthesis was used to implant.
3. Preparation and Placement of Femoral Prosthesis: The stump of the femur was exposed (Fig. 2.7), proximal bone was trimmed; one titanium cable was prefixed to prevent bone splitting; suitable-sized bone window was opened up at the defect of the medial condyle; an approximately 8-mm bone channel was opened at intercondylar fossa toward medullary cavity, in order to insert rod and auxiliary tools to revise medullary cavity; bone graft was implanted in the defect of medial condyle, along with cocktail of antibiotics; multiple trabecular metal augment were placed into the medullary cavity through the window. The augments were placed at the defect of the medial femur, wrapped and fixed with two titanium cables, and the conical filling block was placed at the proximal femur. The femoral prosthesis trial was placed, its length and soft tissue tension were adjusted; bone cement was injected into the medullary cavity, and the tumor femoral stem was implanted to maintain a mild eversion position of the femur, so as to reduce the load of the medial condyle and avoid collapse at the medial condyle defect area. The anteversion was adjusted to 15°, and the 36-mm ceramic femoral head was implanted. After reduction, the gluteus medius was fixed to the proximal femoral stem with non-absorbable sutures, and the tightness and motion range of the hip joint and the position were tested satisfying.

2.3.4 Postoperative Condition and Outcome

Clinical function: The affected hip joint was completely painless; the patient could walk with the help of a cane.

Postoperative X-rays at 1 month are shown in Fig. 2.8. Postoperative digital tomosynthesis at 1 month is shown in Fig. 2.9.

2.3.5 Conclusion and Reflection

In this case, the cone technique of knee revision was employed to fill the bone defect at the interface between the residual femur and the prosthesis to prevent the subsidence of the tumor prosthesis. Stem of the prosthesis went through a 3D-printed "ring" at the distal end to prevent rotational instability and lateral stress concentration. The combination of the two techniques above guaranteed the biological stability of the stem. The titanium ring required a good press fit in the medullary cavity. Even without it, cement fixation can provide good rotational and vertical stability. However, the surgeon should try to pursue the stability of press fit. Therefore, for the customization of the distal "ring," it is better to order more than one model from the manufacturer (Fig. 2.10).

If press fit was confirmed distally, and the medial window of the femur was penetrated through by the distal prosthesis stem, the ring could be placed in laterally by opening an appropriately sized hole between the femur condyles and then performing retrograde reaming with a custom holder and reamer. The four rings should line up into a row, with a 3D-printed lateral patch sealing the bone window as an "armor"; the stem entered from the proximal to the distal end.

During this procedure, the femoral stem only penetrated through the two proximal rings, and the distal two rings were missed. However, during the follow-up, we found that the cone performed good osseointegration into the bone, with ingrowth through both proximal rings, and the distal rings were properly filled up in the medullary cavity. There was good osseointegration around the cone and the proximal rings, and no progressive translucent line was observed around the cement. In addition, a bone graft was applied in the medial femoral condyle, and the bone mass was restored to a certain extent. The 3D-printed patch was well integrated with the cortical bone. The stem was slightly valgus, which protected the medial femur to some extent. The patient had no pain in the hip joint and could walk with a walking cane.

In this case, the surgeon could have chosen non-cement fixation, whereas it might not achieve as good osseointegration as the applied one. The fixation method in this case can be regarded as the reconstruction of cancellous

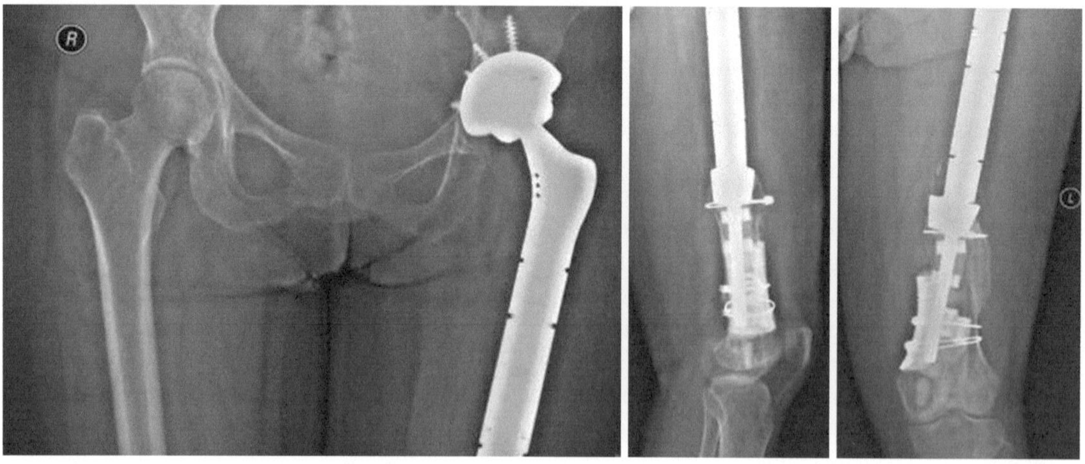

Fig. 2.8 Postoperative X-rays after 1 month

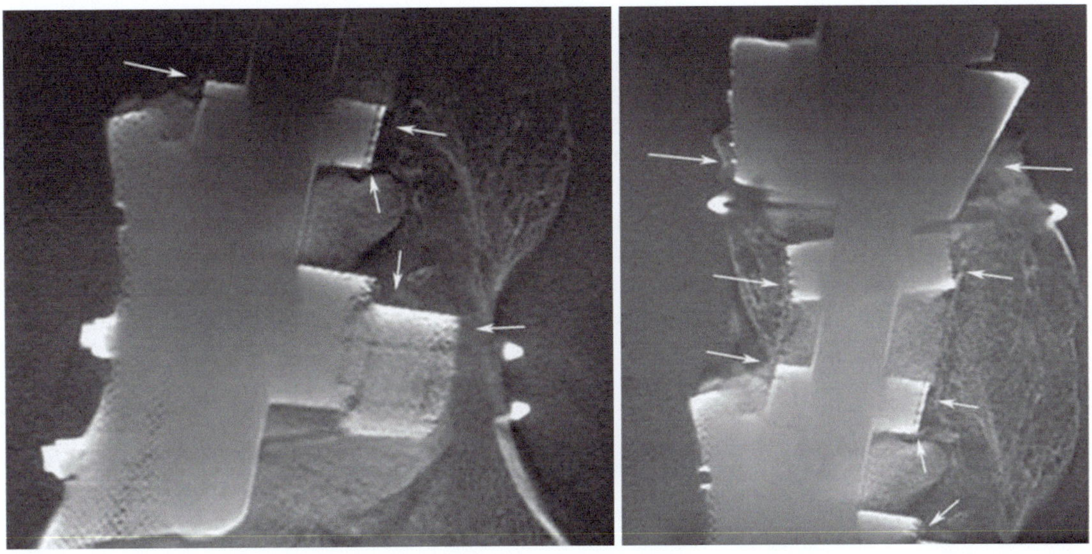

Fig. 2.9 Postoperative digital tomosynthesis after 1 month

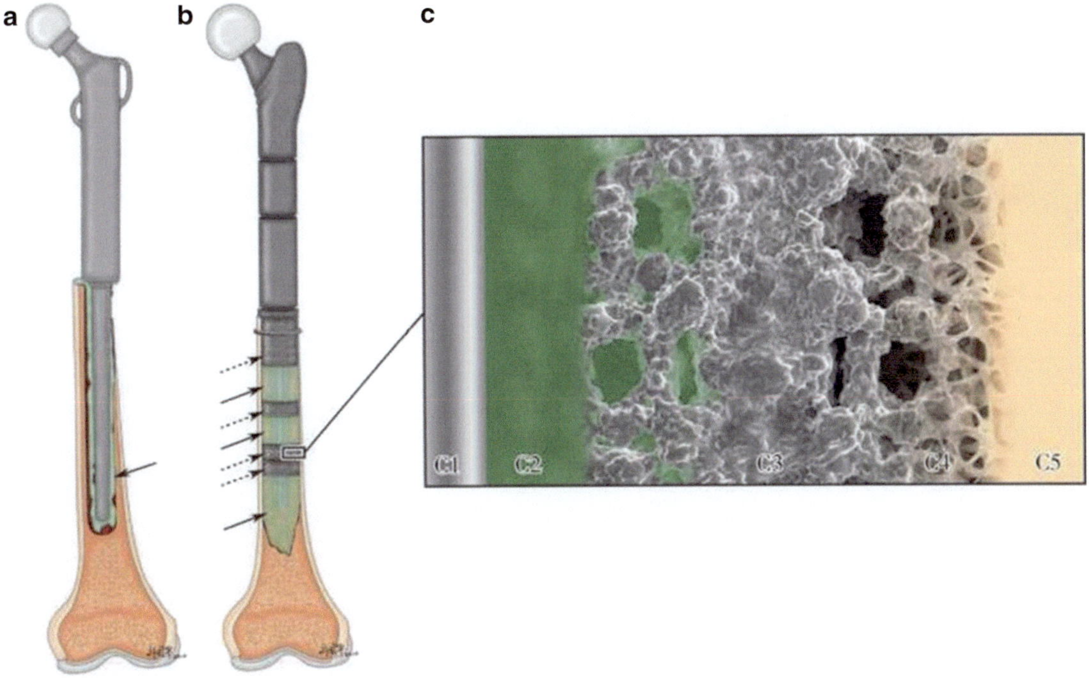

Fig. 2.10 Technical illustration of endosteal reconstruction. (**a**) Type IV femoral bone defect, femoral bone marrow cavity sclerosis, lack of cancellous trabeculae, impossible to achieve cement interlocking fixation. (**b**) Porous titanium ring with bone ingrowth potential made by 3D printing. (**c**) Interface of endosteal reconstruction: C1, prosthesis stem; C2, bone cement; C3, porous metal ring; C4, metal ring and cortical bone interface; C5, cortical bone

bone in the medullary cavity because the metal cancellous bone was customized at the distal end, which provided interlocking. It can also be seen as a deformed uncemented hip joint stem, and a porous metal surface was attached to the surface of the stem via bone cement, or a combined fixation, using cement for initial stability and distal rings for long-term stability. In short, this type of fixation can at least be used as a complement to pure cement/non-cement stem, which simplifies the revision.

After this case, the author's team successively completed several similar tumor prosthesis revisions; the endosteal reconstruction was adopted, and good short-term efficacy was achieved in all of them (Figs. 2.11 and 2.12).

The authors believe that from the perspective of short-term follow-up, the endosteal reconstruction technique can solve the revision problem of tumor prosthesis to some extent, but the fixation efficiency requires a larger sample capacity and longer follow-up to verify.

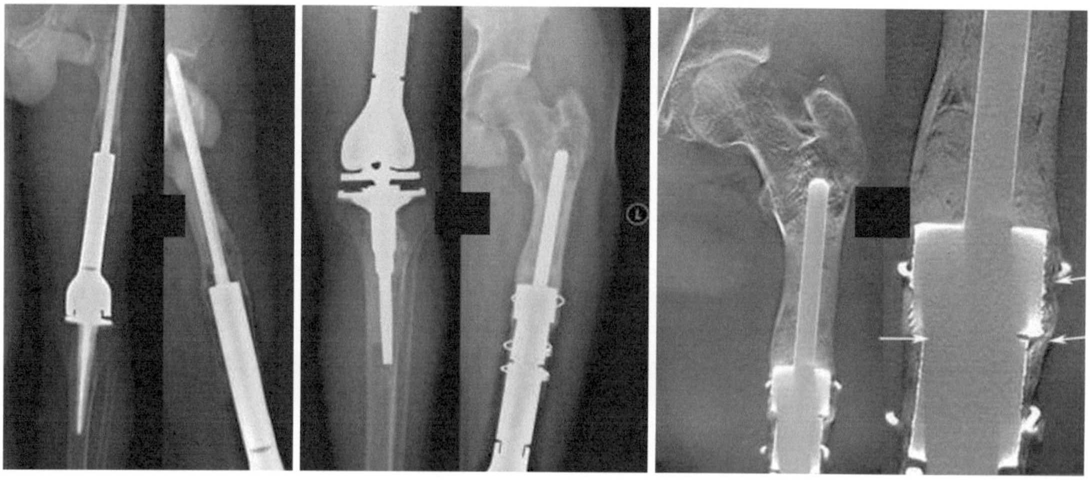

Fig. 2.11 X-rays after endosteal reconstruction revision (1)

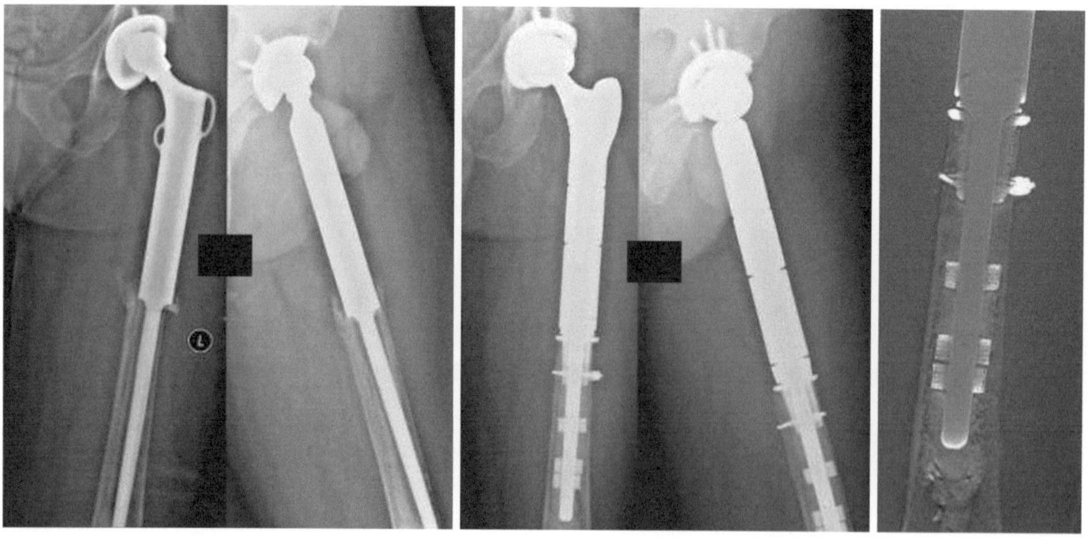

Fig. 2.12 X-rays after endosteal reconstruction revision (2)

2.4 Case 3

Wang Deng and Shengjie Guo

2.4.1 Case Summary

Medical History Female, 51-year-old, patient presented with right hip pain without obvious inducement 35 years ago, which affected daily activity and could be relieved by rest. She had nocturnal pain and limited mobility; "osteomyelitis of the femoral head (right)" was diagnosed locally, and femoral head resection was performed (right). In 2001, a right hip replacement was performed in another hospital. The patient recovered well after surgery. Four months later, the patient presented aggravated pain again, accompanied by limited movement and difficulty in squatting and walking up and down stairs; she could walk for less than 200 m. In our hospital, the patient was diagnosed with periprosthetic infection after right hip replacement by aspiration test, and a spacer was implanted in the right hip. Four months after the surgery, she was taken in as an outpatient for further diagnosis and treatment considering the infection was under control.

Physical Examination Lameness when entering the ward; the pelvis was right inclined; no deformity of the right hip joint; no joint swelling; tenderness in the greater trochanter of the right hip joint (+), axial percussion pain (+), and mildly limited mobility. Patrick's sign on the right (+), Thomas' sign on the right (+), Trendelenburg's sign on the right (+), Allis's sign (+), and Ober's sign on the right (−); no edema in both lower limbs; no hypoesthesia; and the pulse of the bilateral dorsal artery of foot was palpable.

Laboratory Test CRP 2.02 mg/L; ESR 7 mm/h; routine blood test showed no obvious abnormalities.

Radiographic Data Preoperative X-rays of the spacer are shown in Fig. 2.13. X-rays before the second phase of renovation are shown in Fig. 2.14.

2.4.2 Case Analysis

1. According to the history, second-stage revision surgery was planned considering the infection was under control.

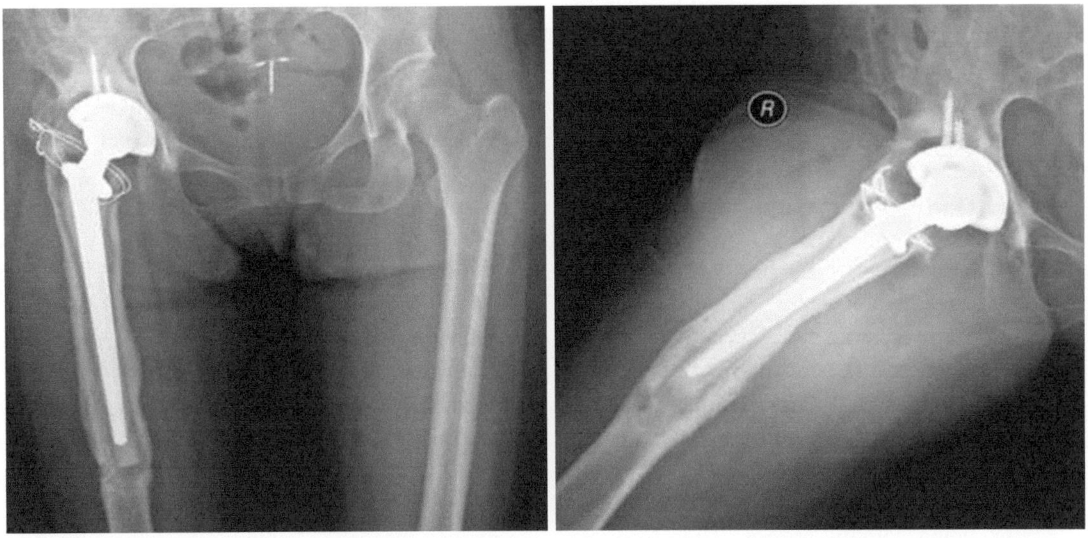

Fig. 2.13 Preoperative X-rays before Stage I revision

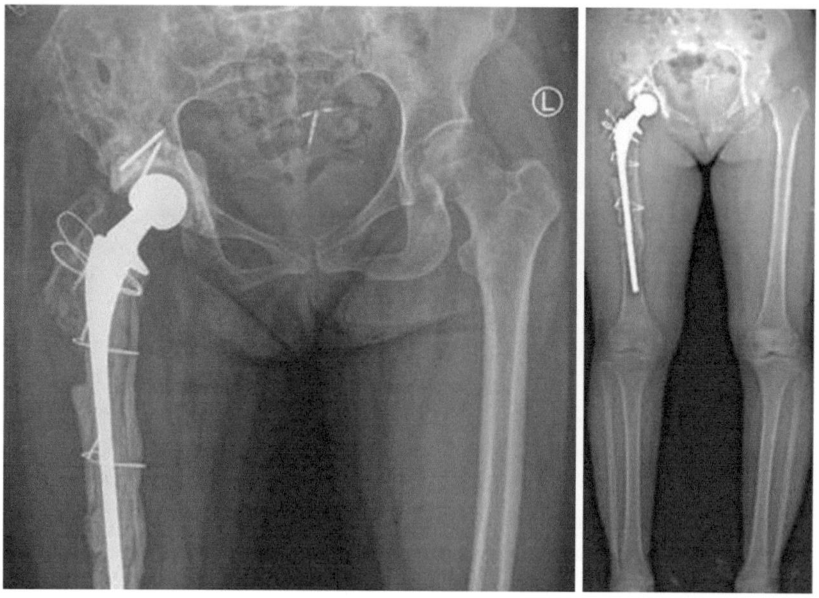

Fig. 2.14 X-ray before Stage II revision

2. Plain X-rays revealed that:
   (a) There was a certain degree of bone defect superior to the acetabulum, and the anterior and posterior columns of the acetabulum, pubic rami, and ischial rami were relatively intact.
   (b) Bone defect was notable on the femoral side, especially on the lateral cortical bone, frequent interruptions were observed. It was worth noting that the isthmus was basically missing, and the greater trochanter was temporarily fixed with wire.

2.4.3 Preoperative Planning

1. From the perspective of the three-point fixation theory, the reconstruction of the acetabular side is not complicated. The lower posterior and anterior points could still provide sufficient support, and augment could be used to reconstruct the upper point.
2. The femur had lost the ability of distal prosthesis fixation due to the lateral isthmus of the femur being largely absent. Therefore, we designed a new procedure to reconstruct the isthmus of the femur, called isthmusplasty. A tongue-shaped bone plate was generated through a U osteotomy in the distal femur, and then the customized isthmusplasty plate was tied and fixed with steel cable. The unique slope of the isthmusplasty plate extruded the tongue-shaped bone plate and reduced the diameter of the medullary cavity, forming a new isthmus with a relatively larger proximal end and a smaller distal end to fix the distal femoral stem.
3. The bone condition of the greater trochanter was poor; thus, the claw plate of the greater trochanter was prepared to restore the alignment of the greater trochanter after the bone cement was removed during the operation.

2.4.4 Operation Situation

1. To thoroughly remove the cement and preserve as much bone mass as possible, extended osteotomy of greater trochanteric was performed to remove the cement and spacer of the femoral prosthesis.
2. Isthmusplasty. According to preoperative planning, the incision was extended distally to expose the distal femur. A U osteotomy was performed on the distal femur with an ultrasonic knife, and the AK B distal femoral isthmusplasty system was employed and fixed with

two cables. The femoral bone marrow cavity was filed to size 17 with a medullary file after size-wise reaming. The press fit and position were satisfying. Intraoperative radiography was performed, and the position was satisfying.

3. The U osteotomy of the distal femur is shown in Fig. 2.15.
4. The acetabulum was exposed, and the spacer and cement were removed. Acetabular files were used from small to large ones to file the acetabulum into 56 mm. An upper posterior bone defect was seen, and 54/15 augment was applied and fixed with two screws. The wound was rinsed, and a 56-mm non-cement Tritanium porous acetabular cup was implanted, with a good press fit, 42° extraversion, and 16° anteversion. Three screws were used for secondary fixation.
5. The femoral bone marrow cavity was rinsed, and RM 195/17 distal body and 21 + 0 proximal body were implanted. The torsion test was negative. A polyethylene liner was implanted, and the 36 + 0 mm ceramic (powder) femoral head prosthesis was inserted. The proximal greater trochanter was fixed with a greater trochanter plate and secured with cable.

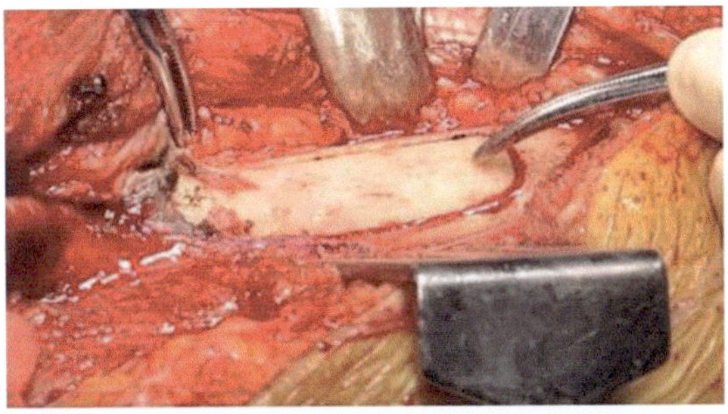

Fig. 2.15 U osteotomy of distal femur

The intraoperative distal femoral isthmusplasty system is shown in Fig. 2.16.

Intraoperative fluoroscopy confirmed a good fit between the distal femur and the isthmusplasty plate, as shown in Fig. 2.17.

2.4.5 Postoperative Condition and Outcome

1. The patient was instructed to walk on crutches 2 weeks after the operation, partial weight bearing at 6 weeks, and complete weight bearing at 3 months.

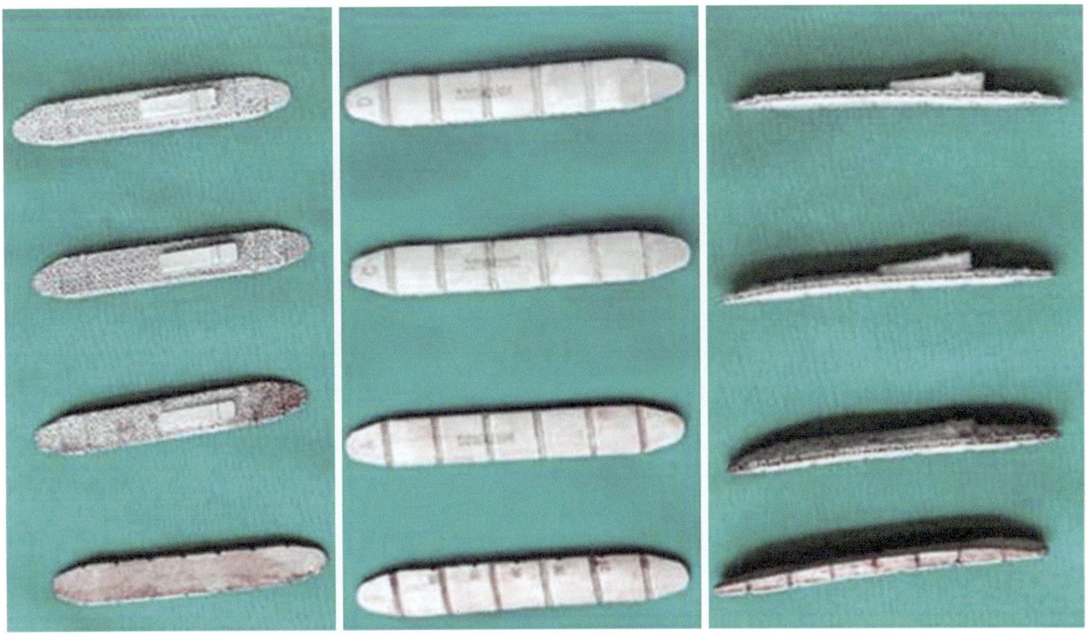

Fig. 2.16 Intraoperative femoral isthmusplasty system

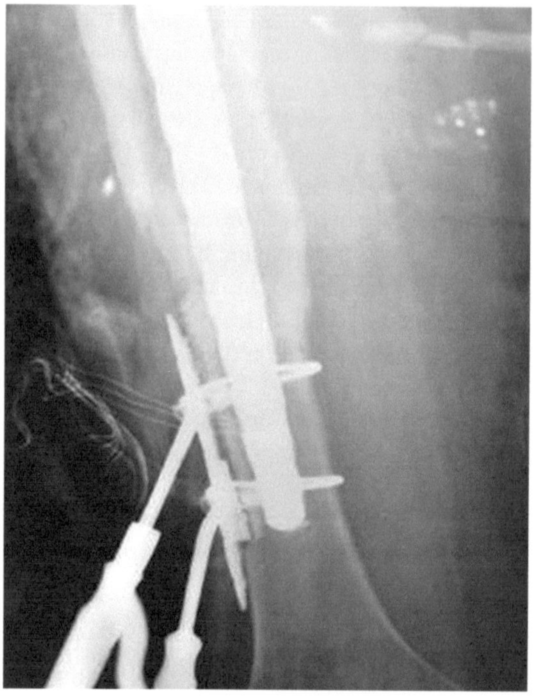

Fig. 2.17 Intraoperative fluoroscopy confirmed a good fit between distal femur and the isthmusplasty plate

2. Postoperative radiographic follow-up:
   (a) Immediate postoperative Anteroposterior (AP) view: A cleft in the anterior cortex was seen (Fig. 2.18).
   (b) Postoperative follow-up after 3 months: The anterior cortical cleft was healed, as shown in Fig. 2.19.
   (c) Postoperative follow-up after 6 months: The cortical step healed well, and the distal taper and isthmus were finely attached; no notable sinkage of the stem (Fig. 2.20).

2.4.6 Conclusion and Reflection

1. Train of thought: It was no doubt a complex revision case, the main difficulty of which is the reconstruction of the femoral side. It should be emphasized that the surgeon must have a clear idea to avoid further failure and guarantee a smooth and safe surgical process in a complex revision. We would like to emphasize the following two points: ① For such a complicated situation on the femoral

Fig. 2.18 Immediate postoperative AP view

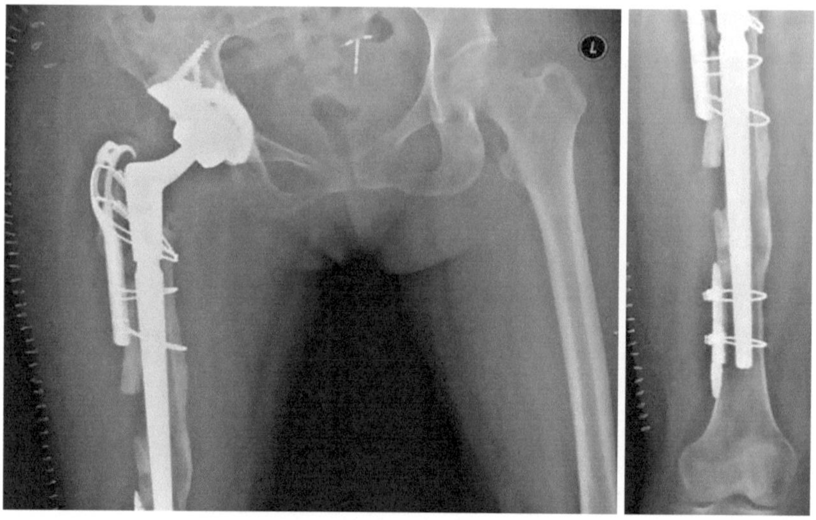

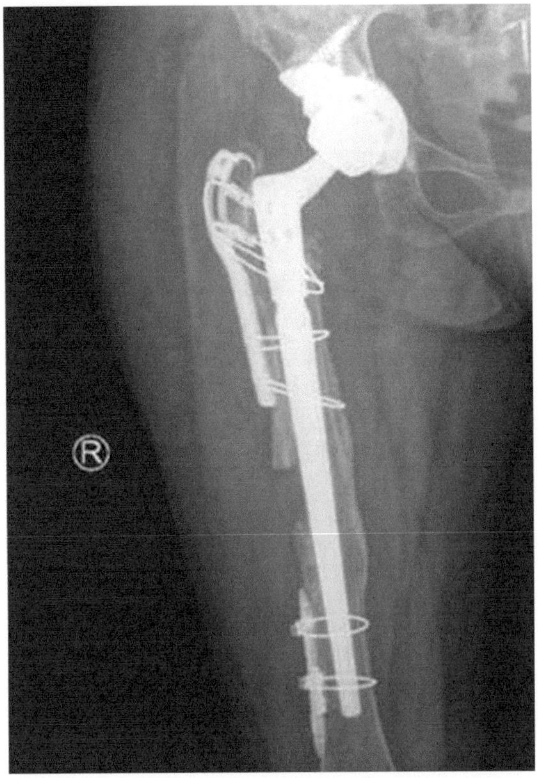

Fig. 2.19 Postoperative follow-up X-ray after 3 months

side, the acetabular reconstruction needed to be fast and simple so that more time could be allocated to the femoral side operation. ② Considering that this was a two-stage revision case, the history of multiple surgeries, the current status of the greater trochanter, and the rotation center and angle of the acetabulum, instead of compromising, the reconstruction of acetabulum should be as good as possible, leaving more possibilities for the femoral side. For optimal acetabular outcome, the surgeon recommends a robot for preoperative design, as well as intraoperative control of the rotation center and the entrance plane. Just as our ring-point-column (RPC) theory of acetabular reconstruction, "Forget bone loss, find bone left and let augment do the rest." The robot, combined with RPC technology, can optimize acetabular reconstruction as much as possible.

2. The principle of SMA (stability, mechanics, abductor): The reconstruction of the femur side should follow the principle of SMA (stability, mechanics, abductor). Stability in SMA refers to good initial stability, optimized medullary mechanics (such as lower

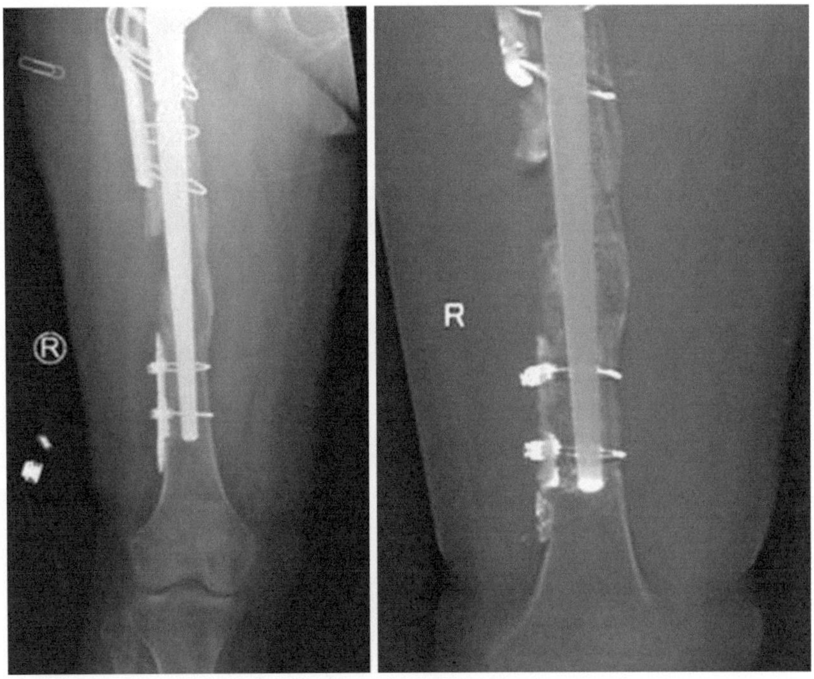

Fig. 2.20 Postoperative follow-up X-rays after 6 months

limb length, femoral antegrade inclination, eccentricity, etc.), and finally the treatment of greater trochanter and abduction device. The SMA principle helps surgeons put their ideas of reconstruction into shape, determine the appropriate prosthesis, and reach ideal postoperative results.

3. For femur reconstruction, we mostly involve complex femur reconstruction cases that require the surgeons' capability to clarify the advantages and disadvantages of common femoral revision prosthesis and the use of techniques. In general, the fixation efficiency of the non-cement prosthesis is relatively unpredictable, whether columnar, cone, or tumor prosthesis is adopted, whereas the long-term results of cement prostheses are usually less ideal. In this case, we chose a non-cement modular fluted tapered stem with comprehensive consideration. The distal end of the stem can guarantee good initial stability and long-term fixation in regular cases. Due to the loss of fixation at the distal end of the distal femoral isthmus in this case, we designed the isthmusplasty to rebuild the isthmus, in order to realize good initial stability and better long-term fixation. It is worth mentioning that the isthmusplasty conducted in this case is not a routine procedure.
4. Isthmusplasty: It means to generate a tongue-shape bone plate in the distal femur via U osteotomy and fix the isthmusplasty plate through the steel cable. A unique slope of the isthmusplasty plate is formed and extrudes the tongue-shaped bone plate to reduce the diameter of the medullary cavity, forming a new isthmus with a relatively larger proximal end and a smaller distal end, so as to fix the distal femoral stem. As a special approach in femoral reconstruction, isthmusplasty is an option to regenerate the initial stability, which is unnecessary for the vast majority of patients of hip revision. It is only suitable for cases where the stem continuously sinks toward the distal end because of the lack of adequate distal fixation during the implant of the test model of the femoral stem (see Accessory Case). Isthmusplasty certainly carries a risk of fracture, which can be somewhat reduced by creating a curved, tongue-shaped bone plate via ultrasonic.

Accessory Case A 58-year-old woman underwent THA for bilateral hip fractures after a car accident 33 years ago, revision right THA 25 years ago due to loosening, and plate fixation for periprosthetic bone fracture 12 years ago.

Preoperative radiography: shown in Fig. 2.21.

After the intraoperative placement of the modular stem prosthesis, the femoral stem continued to sink toward the distal end, and the original proximal body had to be abandoned due to a lack of soft tissue stability. Therefore, we had no choice but to adopt isthmusplasty during the operation. The intraoperative scenograph is shown in Fig. 2.22, and the proximal body prosthesis that had to be abandoned is shown in Fig. 2.23.

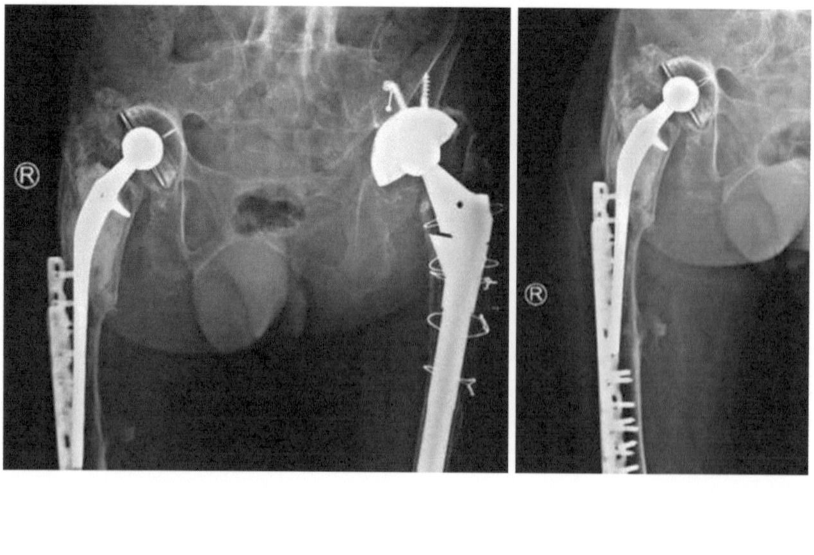

Fig. 2.21 Preoperative radiography

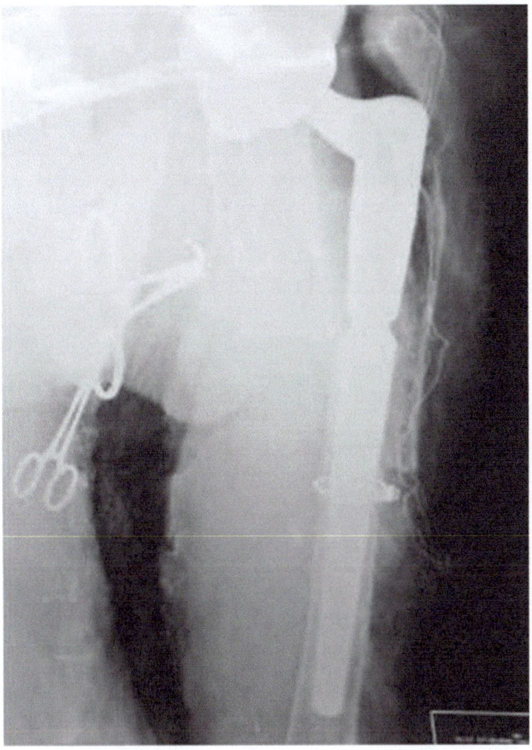

Fig. 2.22 The intraoperative X-ray showed that the isthmus was insufficient to stabilize the stem

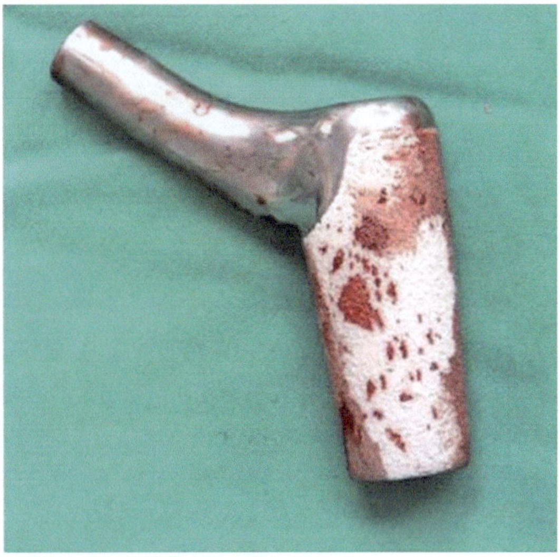

Fig. 2.23 The proximal part of the modular stem had to be abandoned

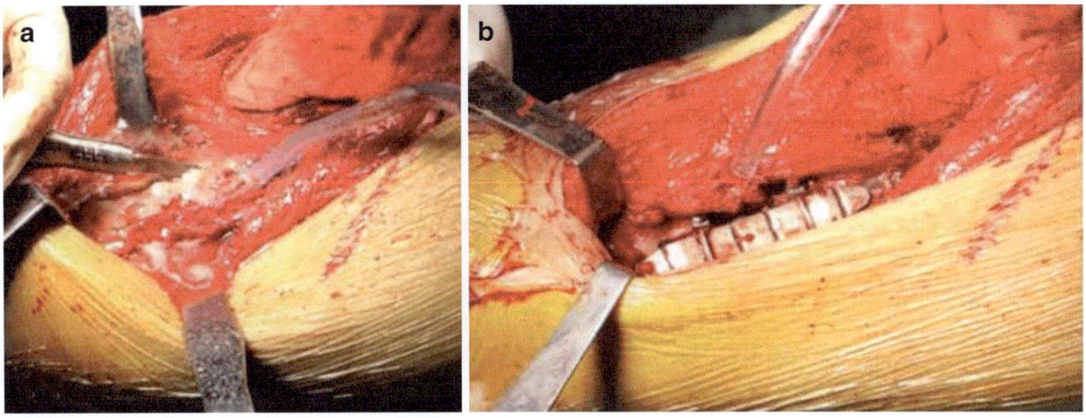

Fig. 2.24 Intraoperative findings. (**a**) Ultrasonic U osteotomy. (**b**) Binding of isthmusplasty plates

Intraoperative replacement of isthmusplasty led to ideal initial stability obtained, as shown in Fig. 2.24.

Postoperative radiographic examination is shown in Fig. 2.25 (AP view of the hip and distal femur).

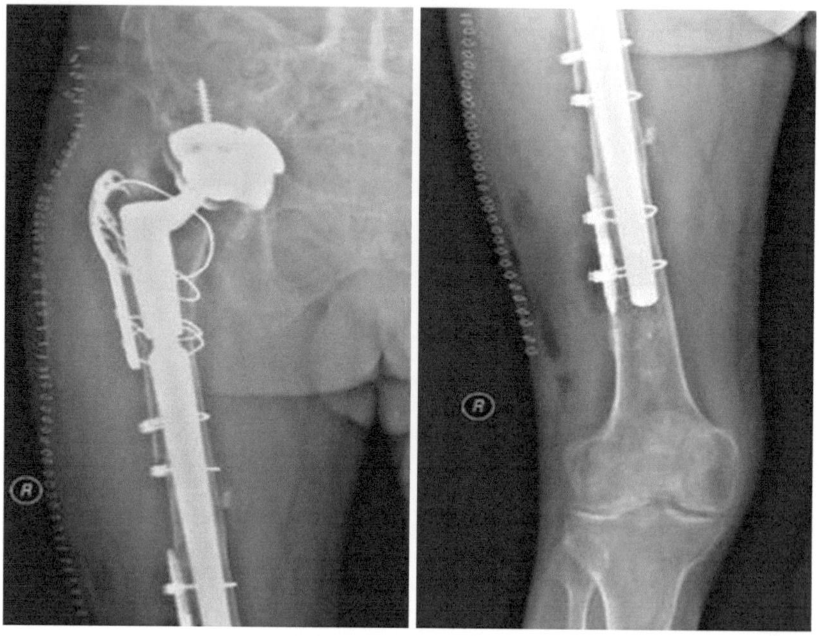

Fig. 2.25 Radiographs of the hip and distal femur in AP view

2.5 Case 4

Wang Deng and Shengjie Guo

2.5.1 Case Summary

Medical History Female, 76-year-old, admitted to the hospital with "right hip pain with limited mobility for half a year, 13 years after right hip replacement." The patient underwent open reduction and internal fixation (ORIF) for a right proximal femur fracture at a local hospital 14 years ago. The fracture end did not heal 1 year after the operation, and the patient underwent right hip replacement, with good recovery. Six months ago, the patient developed right hip pain, accompanied by limited mobility. The symptoms gradually progressed and seriously affected walking and daily activities. The outpatient considered aseptic loosening after THA (right). Past history was negative.

Physical Examination Entered the ward in a wheelchair; no tilting pelvis; two cicatrices of previous surgical incisions were seen in the right proximal femur and posterolateral hip; no obvious deformity of the right hip joint; no joint swelling; tenderness (+) in the groin area, hip area, greater trochanter area, and proximal thigh of the right hip joint, axial percussion pain (+), and severely limited mobility; Patrick's sign on the right (+); Thomas sign on the right (+); and 1.0 cm right lower limb discrepancy than the left. No significant reduction in right hip myodynamia. No edema or hypoesthesia in both lower limbs; the pulse of the bilateral dorsal artery of the foot was palpable.

Laboratory Examination No abnormality was detected in a routine blood test, ESR, and CRP.

Radiographic Data Preoperative X-rays are shown in Fig. 2.26. Preoperative digital tomosynthesis is shown in Fig. 2.27.

2.5.2 Case Analysis

1. Infection was basically ruled out according to the preoperative examination.
2. Plain radiography and digital tomosynthesis.
   (a) Acetabular side: This is a cement-reconstructed acetabulum, which is now considered to be loose from its position.

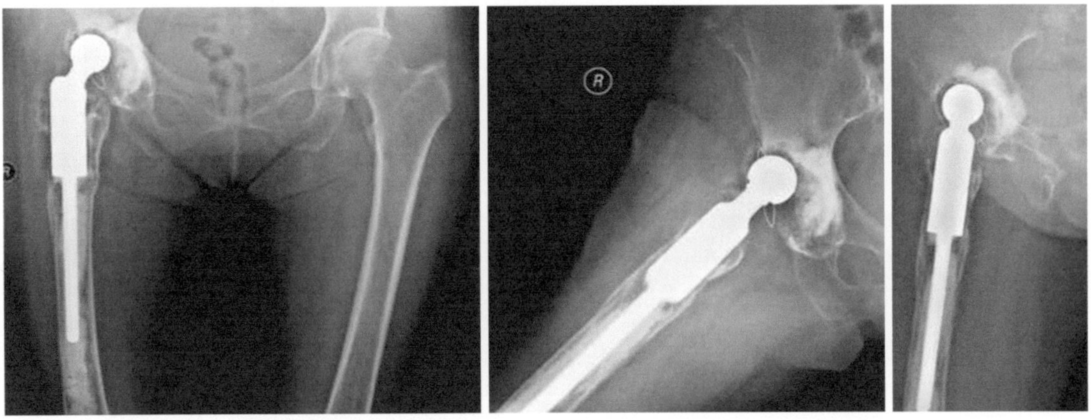

Fig. 2.26 Preoperative radiograph

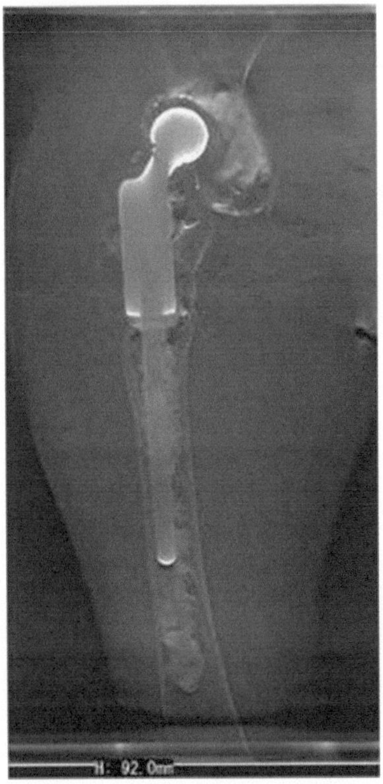

Fig. 2.27 Preoperative digital tomosynthesis

Eccentric wear was observed on the acetabular side.

(b) Femoral side: The femoral stem was reconstructed with cement, with no obvious sign of loosening despite the poor technique of the original cement. The bone condition was poor in the greater trochanter.

(c) Lateral migration of the acetabular cup was observed, and a certain degree of bone defect was above the acetabulum. There was a large amount of bone cement in the posterior column of the acetabulum; thus, a major bone defect was expected after intraoperative clearing. The teardrop and the pubic ramus were relatively intact, whereas bone defect was seen in the ischial ramus.

3. Diagnosis: prosthesis loosening after right hip arthroplasty.

2.5.3 Preoperative Planning

1. Acetabular reconstruction: According to the RPC theory of acetabular revision, the circle of the acetabulum was incomplete and needed to be reconstructed because of superior and inferoposterior bone defects. The bone defect above the acetabulum could extend posteriorly and involve the superoposterior weight-bearing area; thus, a buttress augment should be prepared. There was a certain degree of bone defect at the point of inferoposterior ischium ramus; thus, it was necessary to prepare lotus augment or slope augment (see Chap. 3).
2. Femoral reconstruction: According to the SMA principle of femoral reconstruction, if cement was completely removed through ETO, some of the isthmus would still remain

at the distal end. The modular stem for ordinary revision would provide basic initial stability and the long-term healing of the greater trochanter. Moreover, the bone condition of the greater trochanter is poor. After the intraoperative removal of bone cement, a cable-plate system should be prepared to restore the alignment of the greater trochanter.

2.5.4 Operation Situation

1. The previous incision was applied, exposed, and dislocated the hip joint. ETO was performed at the proximal femur. The femoral stem and cement were removed.
2. The acetabular prosthesis and lining were exposed and removed as well as the limbus cement of the acetabular margin. Severe bone defects were found in the lateral and infero-posterior acetabulum.
3. The acetabulum was filed to 58 mm with acetabulum files from small to large; blood exudation of the bone matrix was ideal. The incision was rinsed, and then a slope augment was placed in the ischial ramus. Biological porous Gription acetabular prosthesis was employed, and a buttress-shaped + disc-shaped augment was laterally placed in, fixed with several screws along with acetabular cup.
4. After size-wise reaming, the femoral marrow cavity was implanted with a 23 mm × 265 mm Wargnar-type stem. When reached ideal press fit, the distal femur was tied with a steel cable. The medullary cavity was rinsed and a 27 +30 mm proximal femoral prosthesis was implanted. The proximal bone was restored and fixed with three cables.

2.5.5 Postoperative Condition and Outcome

The patient was instructed to walk on crutches 2 weeks after the operation, partial weight bearing at 6 weeks, and complete weight bearing at 3 months.

Immediate postoperative AP view X-rays are shown in Fig. 2.28. Postoperative X-rays on 3-month re-examination are shown in Fig. 2.29.

2.5.6 Conclusion and Reflection

1. It was possible that the femoral stem was not loose, why we still considered femoral revision?

   As mentioned above, according to the principle of SMA (stability, mechanics and abductor), the length and anteversion of the lower limb could not be well controlled by simply revising the loose acetabulum and maintaining the original stable femoral stem; thus, it was not possible to achieve the ideal recovery of lower limb mechanics. Therefore, we chose to revise the femoral stem in this case.
2. Stem retrieval and type selection.

   This case was treated via our routine method. ETO was adopted mainly because of the poor bone condition of the greater trochan-

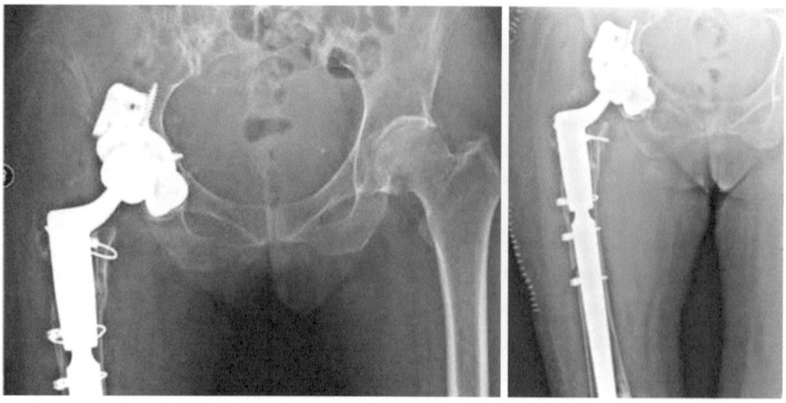

Fig. 2.28 Immediate postoperative AP view X-rays

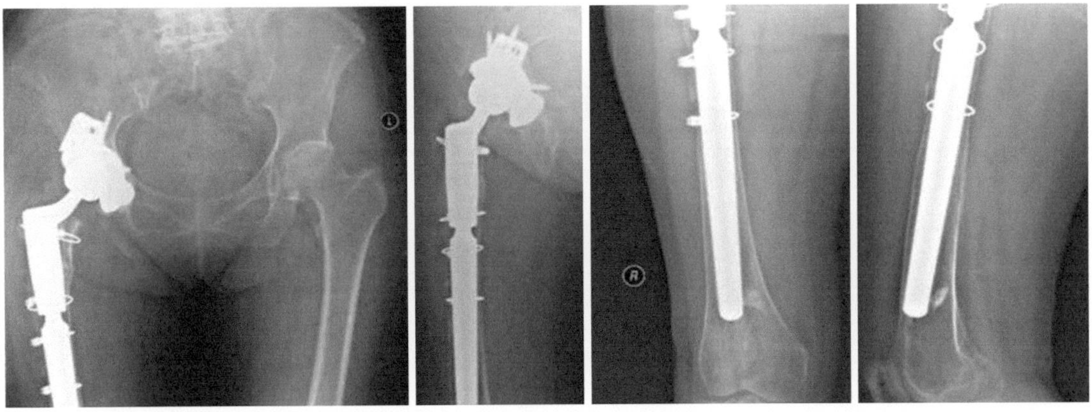

Fig. 2.29 Postoperative X-rays on 3-month re-examination

ter. ETO allowed us to avoid uncontrollable greater trochanter fracture through "controlled fracture." Meanwhile, it can be seen in the preoperative plan that ETO helped with the removal of the bone cement around the distal end of the prosthesis. The surgeons were able to clean the cement efficiently through traditional revision tools or ultrasound tools, which provided fundamental preparation for the long-term fixation of the new non-cement prosthesis. Moreover, the stem with a coated proximal body also contributed to the healing of the greater trochanter.

Recommended Reading

1. Bozic KJ, Kurtz SM, Lau E, et al. The epidemiology of revision total hip arthroplasty in the United States. J Bone Joint Surg Am. 2009;91(1):128–33.
2. Clohisy JC, Calvert G, Tull F, et al. Reasons for revision hip surgery: a retrospective review. Clin Orthop Relat Res. 2004;429:188–92.
3. Paprosky WG, Aribindi R. Hip replacement: treatment of femoral bone loss using distal bypass fixation. Instr Course Lect. 2000;49:119–30.
4. Huang Y, Shao H, Zhou Y, et al. Femoral bone remodeling in revision Total hip Arthroplasty with use of modular compared with Monoblock tapered fluted titanium stems: the role of stem length and Stiffffness. J Bone Joint Surg Am. 2019;101(6):531–8.
5. Huang Y, Zhou Y, Shao H, et al. What is the diffffer-ence between modular and nonmodular tapered fluted titanium stems in revision total hip Arthroplasty. J Arthroplast. 2017;32:3108–13.
6. Huang Y, Zhou Y, Shao H, et al. A novel Endosteal reconstruction of the femur from distal femoral remnant using 3D-printed titanium rings: a two-case report. JBJS Case Connect. 2021;11(3):1.

3 Aseptic Loosening on Acetabular Side

Shengjie Guo, Yixin Zhou, Yong Huang, and Hongyi Shao

3.1 Introduction

Shengjie Guo and Yixin Zhou

Acetabular bone defects are frequently encountered in revision total hip arthroplasty (THA). Bone defects could be quite severe, even pelvic discontinuity (PD), which is an intractable condition for many surgeons. Paprosky classification (Table 3.1) is commonly used in the clinical evaluation of acetabular bone defects. To understand the Paprosky classification, one must be familiar with the important anatomical markers on which it is based. The Paprosky classification of acetabular bone loss was based on four reference indicators: (1) the location of the hip rotation center or the dislocate distance between the hip rotation center and the superior obturator foramen line; (2) the degree of teardrop damage; (3) the degree of osteolysis of the ischial ramus; and (4) the integrity of Kohler line. Anatomical markers are shown in Fig. 3.1.

The acetabular reconstruction strategy is determined based on the severity of the bone defect and the location and quality of residual bone mass. Paprosky classification helps us understand bone defects better, while how to utilize residual bone mass is crucial for acetabular reconstruction.

Table 3.1 Paprosky classification of acetabular bone loss (See Appendix 1 for details)

I No obvious bone defect or cup migration in the acetabular rim
II Acetabular bone defect can be seen, whereas the acetabular column is intact; cup migration in the upper medial or lateral direction is less than 2 cm
(a) Upper medial
(b) Upper lateral (acetabular dome missing)
(c) Only medial defect
III Superior migration is more than 2 cm, severe ischium, and medial wall defects (with or without Pelvic discontinuity)
(a) Intact Kohler line; bone defect location: From 10 o'clock to 2 o'clock
(b) Broken Kohler line; wider bone defect: 9 o'clock to 5 o'clock
Type IIIA is also called the up-and-out type. Type IIIB is also called the up-and-in type

We usually carry out non-cement acetabular reconstruction based on the ring-point-column (RPC) theory, referred to as ring-point-column theory. For a detailed introduction of the theory, please refer to Appendix 4, which will not be elaborated here.

For pelvic discontinuity, "distraction" can be considered. For details and operation techniques, see the case discussion in this chapter.

In conclusion, in revision THA, great challenges are inevitable on both the acetabular and femoral sides. In order to achieve initial and long-term stability of the implant, hip stability, and joint mechanics, the surgeons must be capable of generating a clear train of thought and reliable methods and be in control of trauma. It is

S. Guo (✉) · Y. Zhou · Y. Huang · H. Shao
Department of Adult Joint Reconstructive Surgery, Beijing Jishuitan Hospital, Capital Medical University, Beijing, China

Y. Zhou (ed.), *Revision Total Hip Arthroplasty*, https://doi.org/10.1007/978-981-97-9804-9_3

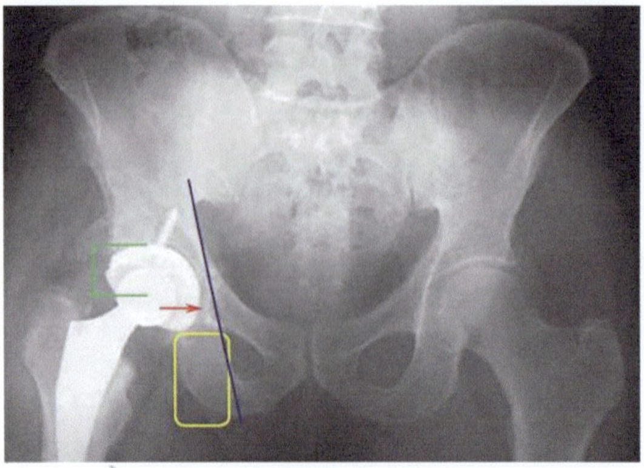

Fig. 3.1 Anatomical markers of the acetabulum. The green bracket indicates how much the center of the hip joint shifted upward, revealing whether the acetabular dome is intact. The red arrow refers to the teardrop, which reveals whether the medial wall of the acetabulum is intact. Teardrop osteolysis suggests that the medial wall of the acetabulum was missing. The blue line refers to the Kohler line, which represents whether the anterior column of the acetabulum is intact. The cup exceeding the Kohler line indicates a bone defect of the anterior column. The yellow area refers to the presence of sciatic osteolysis, which represents whether the posterior column of the acetabulum is intact

necessary to think more, practice more, and reflect more. With the progress of science and technology and the improvement of theory and practice, we believe that revision THA will bring more satisfactory results to patients.

3.2 Case 1

Yong Huang and Shengjie Guo

3.2.1 Case Summary

Medical History A 60-year-old male underwent bilateral THA at a local hospital in 2000 due to ankylosing spondylitis (AS) and stiff hips. In 2005, he had a right femur fracture caused by injury and was treated with open reduction and internal fixation (ORIF) at a local hospital. Bilateral hip pain occurred in 2012, which was intermittent, aggravated during walking activity, and slightly reduced on resting. He was instructed with oral medications and physical therapy, with no obvious symptom relief. AS was diagnosed over 30 years and he received oral drugs for symptomatic treatment. In 2014, he underwent surgical treatment for a right colon tumor in another hospital (the details are unknown).

Physical Examination Entered the ward in a wheelchair. No pelvic tilt. The right lower extremity was about 2.0 cm in discrepancy to the other; a previous operative cicatrix of 16 cm was visible in the right posterolateral hip, well healed; a previous operative cicatrix with a length of 20 cm can be seen in the front of right thigh, well healed without tenderness. Right lateral hip tenderness (+); right groin area tenderness (+); right lower extremity axial percussion pain (+); and active flexion and extension range of right hip is 0° ~ 90°, with 0° internal rotation and 35 ° external rotation. The previous cicatrix, about 16 cm in length, was seen in the left posterior hip, well healed. Left lateral hip tenderness (+); left groin area tenderness (+); and active flexion and extension range of the left hip was 0–80°, with 10° internal rotation and 30° external rotation. The abductor strength of both hips was Class V weak.

Laboratory Examination Routine blood tests, erythrocyte sedimentation rate (ESR), C-reactive protein (CRP), and so on were normal.

Radiographic Data According to preoperative Anterior posterior (AP) view of both hips and oblique X-rays of bilateral iliac crest and obturator (Fig. 3.2), lower lumbar fused; posterior pelvis tilt; and obturator foramen expanded due to posterior pelvis tilting. Severe acetabular bone defect and lesser trochanter osteolysis were also observed.

3.2.2 Case Analysis and Surgical Planning

1. Radiography Illustration.

   Bone defects can be seen in the ischium, pubis, and superior acetabular dome. AP view

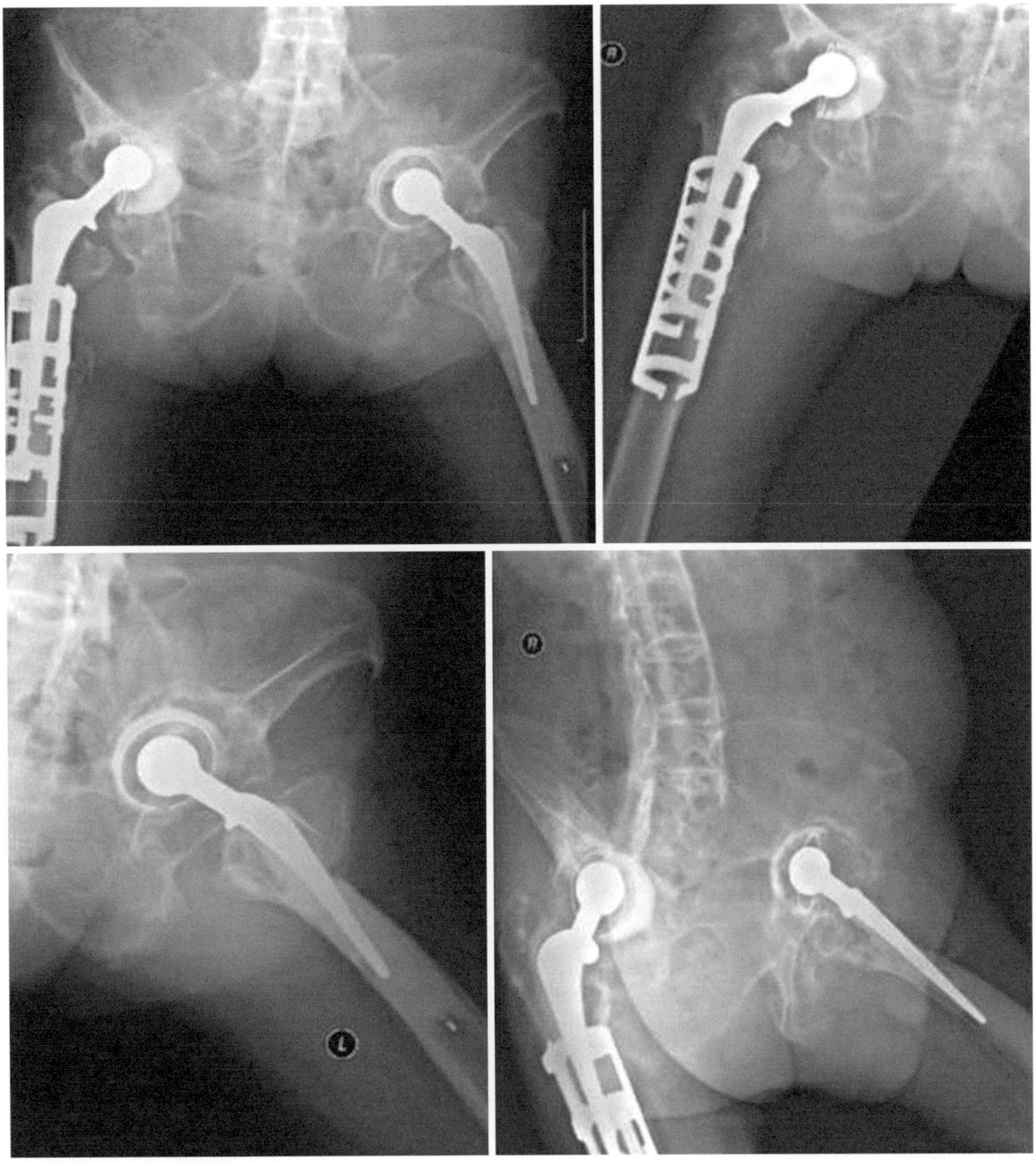

Fig. 3.2 Preoperative X-ray

of posterior pelvis tilt like these provided the perception of severe osteolysis in the ischial ramus. However, the bone defect might be overestimated. It was the bone defect in the posterior side of the acetabulum rotating to the inferior side of the acetabulum during the development of posterior pelvis tilt that gave the impression of severe bone defect in the ischial ramus. Therefore, when viewing the radiographs preoperatively, it is worth reconfirming that despite the serious inferoposterior and anteroposterior defect, the ischial bone defect is likely to be less serious than imagined.

2. Analysis of Preoperative Planning and Reconstruction Strategies.
   (a) Preoperative systemic evaluation and perioperative management: For patients with a relatively long history of ankylosing spondylitis or rheumatoid arthritis (RA), it is required to adjust their usage of disease-modifying anti-rheumatic drugs (DMARDS); whether it is complete abdominal breathing on intubation and thoracic movement must be taken into consideration for patients with ankylosing spondylitis. Observation should be made on the patient's cervical spine mobility in order to communicate with the anesthesiologist for more preparation time for intubation. Remind them that fiberoptic endoscopy might be required, and cervical fracture should be prevented in the process of transportation. Attention must be paid to the positioning when performing general anesthesia to patients with RA, in case of atlantoaxial subluxation. For patients with long-term suffering from such diseases, personality and psychological disorders are likely to be associated, which may lead to unrealistic expectations from the surgery. Thus, efficient communication is necessary to adjust the threshold of the patients' expectations.
   (b) How to prevent dislocation: Preoperative radiographs suggested the lower lumbar fusion, with a large obturator foramen and posterior pelvis tilt. The operation needed to be carefully planned to avoid postoperative dislocation, so it was very important to maintain soft tissue tension and an intact greater trochanteric. Proximal femur fracture was likely to occur if removing internal fixation was applied, which would also be time-consuming. The reconstruction of the acetabular rotation center should be treated strictly because if the rotation center is not placed in an appropriate position, it would be difficult to maintain soft tissue tension and impingement may occur. Did the femur side need to be revised? This is a question worth discussing. The surgeons hoped to be able to adjust the anteversion angle of the stem, offset, bilateral leg length, and soft tissue tension, all of which were controllable factors to maintain the stability of the hip joint. However, there were also uncontrollable factors, including the position of the spine and pelvis. We were aiming to minimize the risk of dislocation and try our best to optimize the controllable factors. Most efforts were invested in reconstructing a relatively normal rotation center and the overall offset of the hip. The intraoperative trailing should be treated strictly, ensuring that the trunk and operating table are as parallel as possible. The abduction and anteversion angle of the cup were adjusted according to the trailing result. Since anterior dislocation frequently happens to patients with posterior pelvis tilt due to impingement from the back, we slightly reduced the anteversion angle. Extra care should be taken to prevent hip dislocation for such an unusual pelvic position like this.
   (c) Stem retrieval: In a case like this, retrieving the stem was not difficult, whereas removing the bone cement was. The obturator oblique and iliac oblique radiographs needed to be assessed carefully to confirm the bone defects in the posterior, superioposterior, and inferoposterior pelvis. Since the oblique radiographs revealed no pelvic discontinuity, only point reconstruction was required while point stabilization (e.g., Professor Paprosky's distraction technique to deal with pelvic discontinuity) was not necessary to achieve three-point fixation.
   (d) Reasons for stem retrieval: ① The difficulty of this case lay on the acetabular side, but if the stem was not retrieved, acetabular side exposure would overstretch the operation; ② the calcar femorale region was separated. Calcar femorale is an important part of the stability strength of bone cement sheath and stem stability regardless of cement or

non-cement; thus, the cement in cement technique was not considered; and ③ this was a stem with a smooth surface, which was not difficult to retrieve.

(e) Since the femoral stem needed to be retrieved, were retrieving the internal fixation and performing extended trochanter osteotomy (ETO) appropriate? ETO is not necessarily suitable for every stem like this. The cost of ETO should be taken into consideration. The embracing fixator would cause great damage to the blood supply of surrounding soft tissue, and the bone strength at the fixed position would be weakened. There would be no way to make up for it. The retrieval of the embracing fixator required extensive soft tissue dissection, which would have a great impact on bone biological condition and the healing from ETO. Therefore, it was suggested to avoid ETO and only try to retrieve the stem and cement completely. As it turned out, it was not hard to retrieve the stem; thus, it should not be considered something difficult. However, if the embracing fixator was retrieved and a fracture occurred, the situation would be much harder to deal with given the weak bone mass.

3.2.3 Postoperative Condition and Outcome

The first-time postoperative immediate radiographs (right hip) are shown in Fig. 3.3. It can be seen that the reconstruction of the hip joint rotation center is ideal. Lotus-shaped 3D-printed titanium porous augment designed by the surgeons was applied to the ischial ramus bone defect to establish the inferoposterior support fixing point. The superior acetabular dome was reconstructed by slope augment and the medial wall was reconstructed by disc-shaped augment.

In the postoperative immediate radiographs of the second-time revision (left hip, 3 months later than the right hip), similar reconstruction techniques to the right side were performed. Radiographs showed that the prosthesis in the right hip was well fixed. The second-time revision postoperative immediate radiographs (left hip) are shown in Fig. 3.4.

AP and lateral views of left hip revision after 6 months and right hip revision after 9 months showed good fixation of bilateral prosthesis. AP and lateral views are shown in Fig. 3.5.

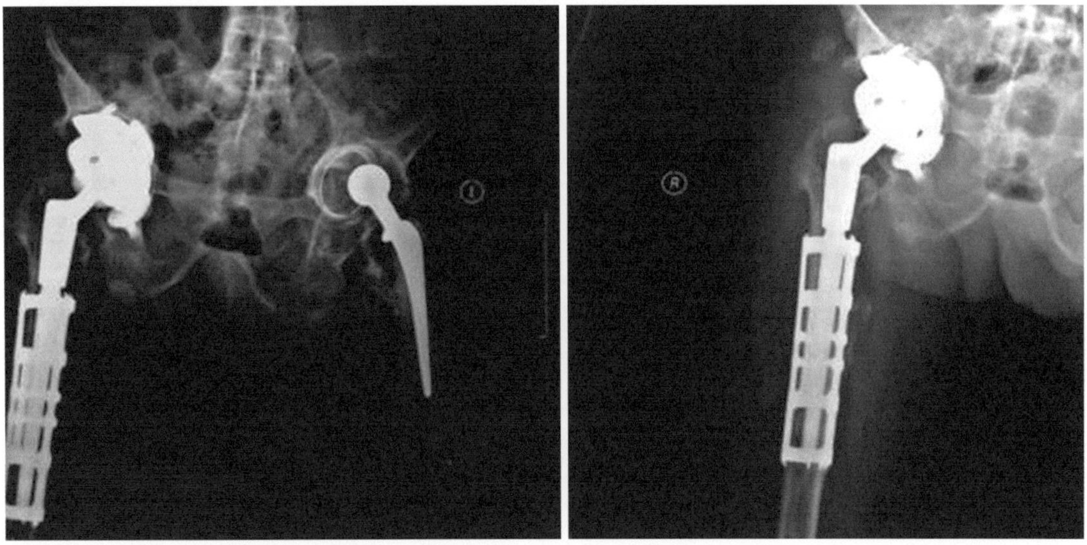

Fig. 3.3 Postoperative immediate radiographs of first-time operation (right hip)

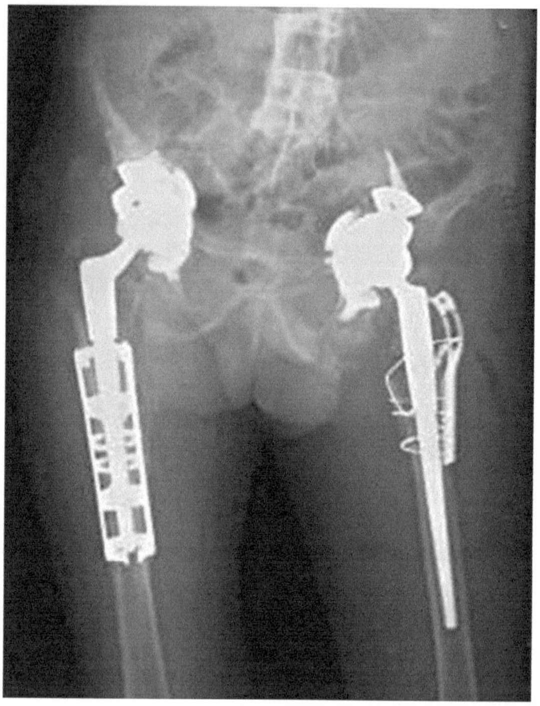

Fig. 3.4 Postoperative immediate radiographs of second-time operation (left hip)

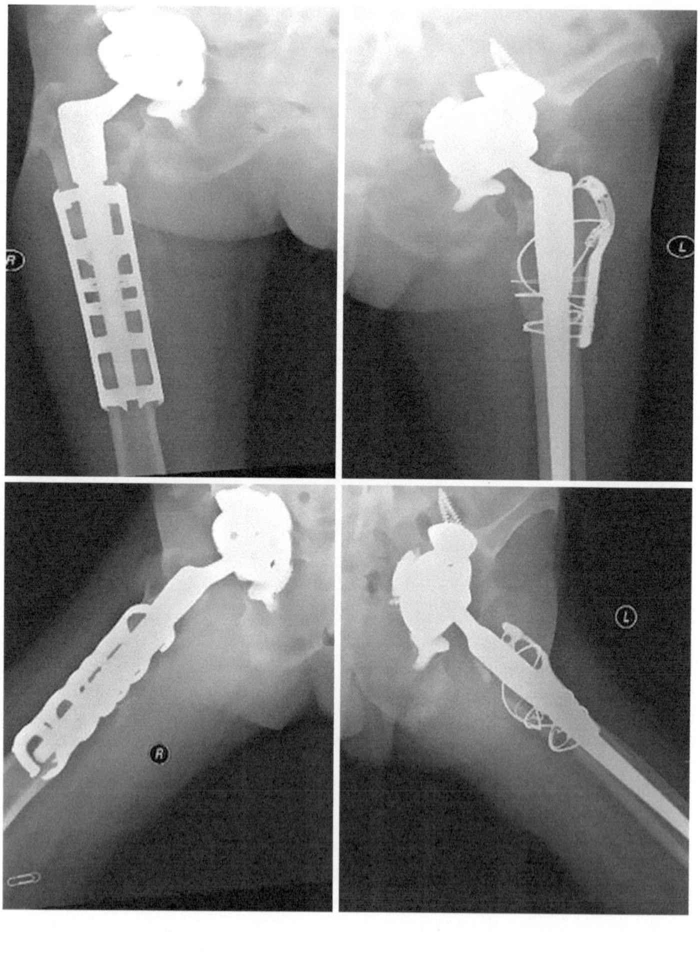

Fig. 3.5 AP and lateral views of left hip revision after 6 months and right hip revision after 9 months

3.3 Case 2

Yixin Zhou and Shengjie Guo

3.3.1 Case Summary

Medical History A 71-year-old female was admitted to the hospital due to "intermittent hip pain for one year after left hip revision." The patient underwent left THA for rheumatoid arthritis 13 years ago. One year ago, revision THA was performed in another hospital for a perifemoral fracture of the left hip caused by injury. Intermittent left hip pain occurred after revision THA, and the pain was related to movement and reduced on rest. Hip mobility was limited and the symptoms progressed gradually.

Physical Examination Claudication; posterolateral cicatrix on left hip, no swelling; left hip trochanteric tenderness (+); axial percussion pain (+); normal abductor strength in left hip; and severely limited mobility in left hip.

Laboratory Examination Routine blood test, ESR, and CRP were normal.

Radiographic Data Preoperative AP view of the hip joint and left iliac oblique view are shown in Fig. 3.6; the hip joint computed tomography (CT) plain scan is shown in Fig. 3.7.

3.3.2 Case Analysis

1. Infection was basically excluded according to the comprehensive preoperative examinations.
2. X-ray and CT scan revealed:
   (a) Kohler line was disrupted and with blurred boundaries; pelvic discontinuity (PD) was obvious.
   (b) Bone defect was obvious in the normal acetabular position, and only the bone mass around the narrow acetabulum floor was left. The projection of the anterior and posterior acetabulum margins could not be seen, suggesting an obvious defect of the posterior acetabular column.

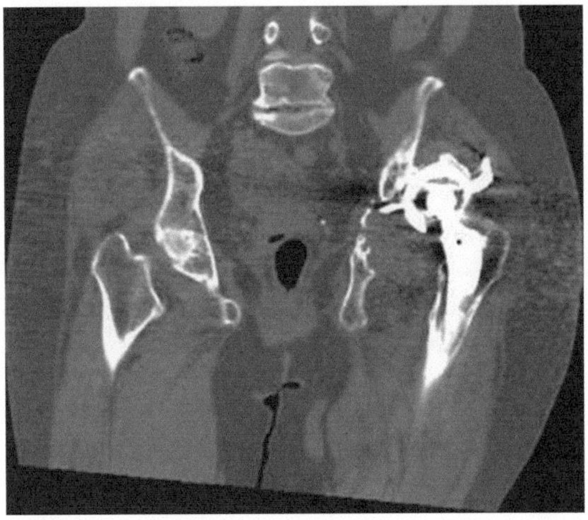

Fig. 3.7 CT pain scan of hip joint

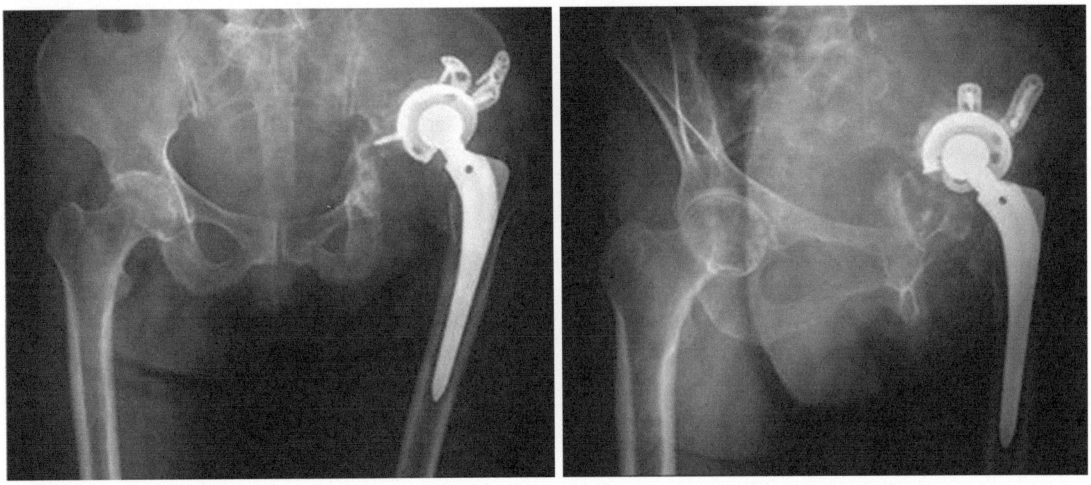

Fig. 3.6 Preoperative AP view of hip joint and left iliac oblique view

(c) Cage was superior-laterally dislocated (up and out). The bone defect was serious and extensive on the superior acetabulum, especially the weight-bearing area.
(d) Teardrop, pubic ramus, and ischial ramus were relatively intact.

Keywords: Pelvic discontinuity (PD), weight-bearing area defect, posterior acetabular column defect.

3. Diagnosis: aseptic loosening after left THA.

3.3.3 Preoperative Planning

1. According to the theory of three-point fixation, the anterosuperior point might still exist, while the bone mass in the point of the inferoposterior ischial ramus was still enough for supportiveness. Reconstruction is required in the weight-bearing area and posterior column. Therefore, buttress augments should be preoperatively prepared, which could reconstruct not only the weight-bearing area firmly but also at least half of the posterior column.
2. The distraction technique was intended to be used for pelvic discontinuity.

3.3.4 Operation Situation

1. To better expose the acetabulum for acetabular reconstruction, the femoral stem was retrieved.
2. Intraoperative results showed no bone ingrowth in the original cage. After the stem was retrieved smoothly, the pseudomembrane and cicatrix on the surface of the bone were cleaned. Soft tissue between metal cups or augments and the bone should be cleaned thoroughly since the original bone mass left was not abundant and the contact area between metal and the bone should be cherished. A large amount of cicatrix formed near the fracture line was observed intraoperatively. At this point, an electrotome should be used to gently remove the cicatrix, keeping it close to the bone surface to avoid damaging blood vessels and other important parts in the pelvis through the fracture line. The fracture line ran from up back to down front. When two curved forceps were used to push the fracture end line up and down, notable abnormal motion showed.

   Note: Removal of the cicatrix around the fracture line was meant to increase the contact between the cup and the bone surface of the acetabular floor, not to separate the fracture line perfectly. Therefore, separation and dissection should be controlled, and there was no need to increase the chance of excessive damage or bleeding. In addition, the tension of fibrous union between the two ends of the fracture line should be retained.
3. The acetabular floor was initially reamed (to 54 mm), and the position of the cup was roughly determined. The buttress augment was fixed on the posterior end of the acetabulum and the interval below the buttress augment was aligned with appropriate disc-shaped augments. Bone cement was used between the two augments for fixation.
4. Two Kirschner wires were drilled into the opposite end of the fracture line apart from the acetabulum, where the bone mass was thick (if possible, it should be as close to the perpendicular direction of the fracture line as possible to increase separation efficiency and maintain the direction). The distraction process stopped until the distraction forceps encountered intense resistance (about 4-5 mm). After the forceps locking, the acetabulum was further reamed to 60 mm. When the cup reached a relatively ideal volume and contact with the host bone, the cement was applied on the augments and a 60-mm trabecular metal (TM) cup was inserted (be careful with the drilling position). The bone cement of the screw holes was then removed and three to four screws were carefully driven into the superior side of the fracture line. Then forceps could be released and the screws were driven in the direction of ischial ramus.

   Note: When applying the distraction technique, a certain sequence of operations must be followed.
5. In order to enhance the supportiveness in the anterosuperior direction, a 20–54-mm slope augment was shaped and fastened with one

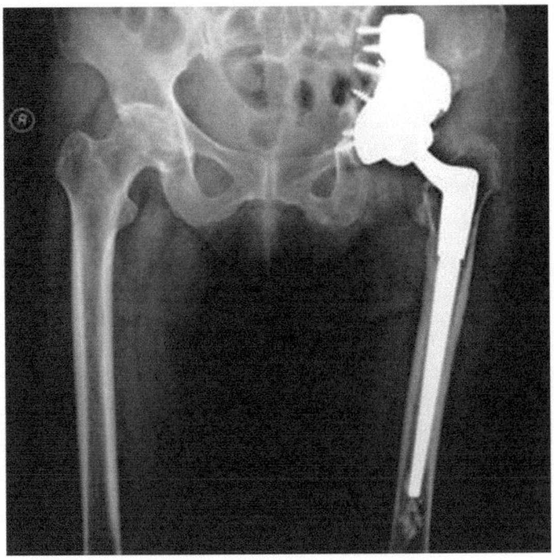

Fig. 3.8 Postoperative Immediate AP View

screw at the anterosuperior region to the cup. The slope augment, cup, and buttress augment were fixed with bone cement.

3.3.5 Postoperative Outcome

1. The patient was instructed to walk on crutches 2 weeks after the operation, partial weight-bear in 6 weeks, and full weight-bear after 3 months.
2. Clinical follow-up: The Harris score was 80; no pain; and no restriction walking up and down stairs or on plain ground. A walking cane was required for long-distance walks. There was a 1.7 cm discrepancy in the length of the lower extremities. Hip flexion and abduction exercises were gradually intensified within 3 months after the operation.

The postoperative immediate AP view is shown in Fig. 3.8.

3.3.6 Conclusion and Reflection

1. Three signs of PD on radiographs are cortical discontinuity, migration, and obturator foramen deformation.
2. The reason that internal fixation was not applied to restore and fix pelvic discontinuity in this case: the fracture in this case was already chronic discontinuity after multiple operations, with a separated fracture line and very little bone mass left; thus, the chance of healing after restoring and fixation by internal fixation fracture is slim. For a fresh or relatively fresh fracture with abundant bone mass, open reduction and internal fixation (ORIF) and cup reconstruction is an option.
3. The reason that we did not perform the revision with a cage is as follows:
   (a) It is often impossible to achieve bone ingrowth and consequently osseointegration with a cage. This patient previously received cage reconstruction, which should be a lesson learned.
   (b) The use of a cage still requires placing its hemisphere part in the host bone to reach certain endogenous stability, otherwise loosening and migration would happen easily, which should be a lesson learned.
   (c) For patients with pelvic transection fracture, if the cage cannot win the chance for fracture healing, it will come to a definite failure, which should be a lesson learned.
4. The reason that we did not apply the cup-cage system: Cup cage is a significant improvement over cage. Similar to the cage, the cup-cage system also requires endogenous stability of the hemispherical TM cup in the host bone and the cage merely provides another part of initial stability. For long-term stability, cups combined with metal augments were preferred as cups with augments are full biological fixation, whereas cup cage is partial biological fixation.

   In this case, it was difficult to reach good initial stability of the TM cup without reconstruction in the superior dome of the acetabulum, even with the distraction technique, and it was extremely difficult to perform both the distraction technique and cage as cage requires iliac wing and ischial ramus involvement.
5. As mentioned above, a cage could not lead to osseointegration, while a TM cup with a buttress augment could induce osseointegration.

The combination of the cups and augments could be considered a single complex, special-shaped non-cement cup.
6. For cases with obvious bone defects in the weight-bearing area and posterior column, buttress augment will result in unexpected success.

We diagnose only things we think about; we think only about things that we have studied.

3.4 Case 3

Shengjie Guo and Yixin Zhou

3.4.1 Case Summary

Medical History A 31-year-old female was admitted to the hospital due to "continuous pain for 2 years after right THA." The patient underwent THA 2 years ago for developmental dislocation of the right hip. Right hip pain developed when she started weight-bearing walking on crutches 3 months after the operation.

Physical Examination Walking in the ward on double crutches; flexion deformity in the right hip joint, with visible incision cicatrix; right iliac area tenderness (+); axial percussion pain (+); obviously limited motion; and right Trendelenburg's sign (+).

Laboratory Examination Routine blood test, ESR, and CRP were all normal.

Radiographic Data Preoperative AP view, lateral view, iliac/obturator oblique view, and preoperative full-length X-ray are shown in Figs. 3.9, 3.10 and 3.11, respectively.

3.4.2 Case Analysis

1. Infection was basically excluded according to the comprehensive preoperative examinations.
2. A radiographic examination of the right hip revealed the following:
   (a) The S-ROM THA system was applied in the original surgery. Superior migration of the cup was obvious and almost completely protruded. The projection of the posterior column/wall of the acetabulum is relatively intact. Subtrochanteric osteotomy was performed on the femoral side and the medial site of the osteotomy had not healed completely, whereas the lateral healing was acceptable. The stem was slightly undersize in the medullary cavity, but there were no obvious signs of loosening.
   (b) Teardrop was not seen. The ischial ramus and the posterior column were intact. Kohler line was completely disrupted and the cup was notably protruded into the pelvic cavity, presenting

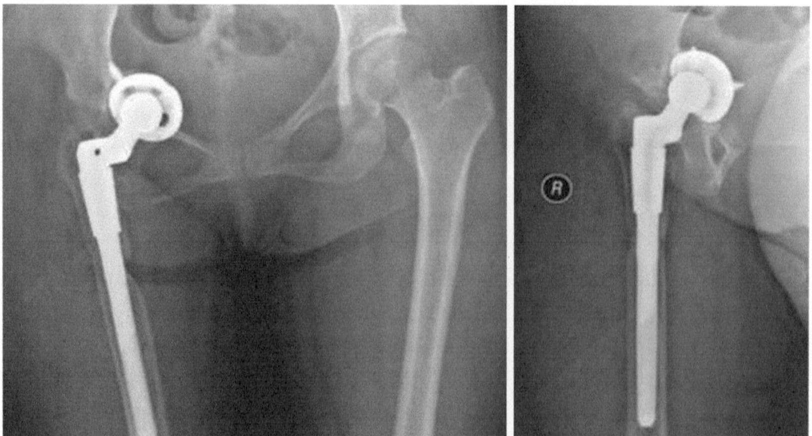

Fig. 3.9 Preoperative AP and lateral views

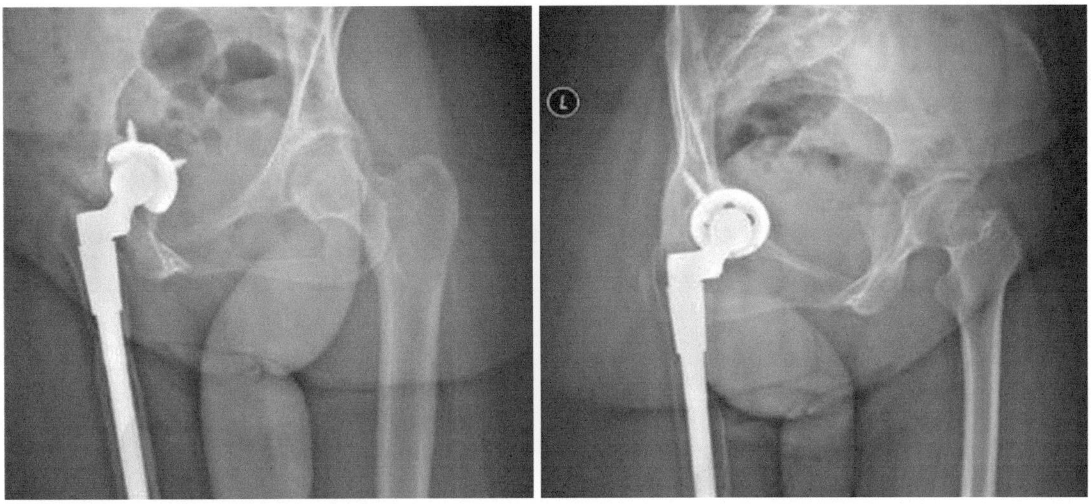

Fig. 3.10 Preoperative iliac/obturator oblique views

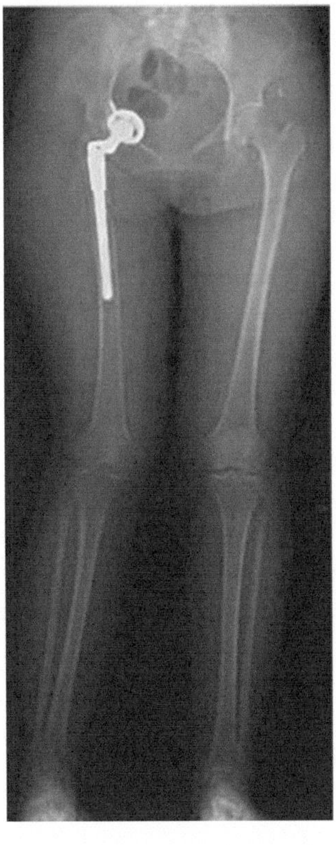

Fig. 3.11 Preoperative full-length X-ray

serious bone defect on the medial wall. Superior migration of the cup was not obvious (<2 cm).

(c) Paprosky type IIC bone defect was preoperatively concluded.

3. Diagnosis: aseptic loosening after right THA.

3.4.3 Preoperative Planning

1. It was understandable that obvious inward migration of the cup occurred in patients like this. In hips with severe developmental dysplasia, the cups are usually shallow. Thus, it is common in the initial replacement that the medial wall or even the anterior wall/column is over-reamed by accident, resulting in loss of the "embracement" to the cup and its internal migration.
2. In this case, the acetabular component was significantly displaced medially, the upper margin of which almost completely shifted to the medial acetabulum. This condition raised concerns about the relationship between the cup/screws and neurovascular as well as the important pelvic organs (bladder, uterus, etc.). Damage to these parts during cup retrieval could be devastating. What could be worse, if the screws penetrated blood vessels during first-phase THA and arteriovenous fistula formed, massive blood loss could easily occur when retrieving these screws. Computed tomography angiography (CTA) could help clarify the situation. However, the relationship between the cup and other organs is not always easy to clarify.
3. Acetabular reconstruction: Bone mass in at least three areas (posterior column/wall, posterosuperior, and anteroinferior acetabulum) was acceptable. The upper margin of the obtu-

Table 3.2 Advantages and disadvantages of keeping or retrieving femoral stem

	Retrieving stem	Reserving stem
Exposure and work space establishment	Advantaged	Disadvantaged
Periprosthetic femoral fracture	Likely to happen	Relatively easy to maintain the femur intact
Adjusting lower extremity length	Advantaged	Disadvantaged
Soft tissue release	No more release required	Femur would migrate anterosuperiorly when making more release
Damage control	Relatively larger	Smaller

rator foramen was still smooth and intact, which indicated that the anteroinferior acetabulum was relatively intact. If no further bone defect was caused during the operation, the bone left should have no problem supporting a semi-spherical porous cup. Reconstruction of the medial wall was the key. Metal augment could be considered if necessary.

4. Whether to keep or retrieve the femoral stem was not a simple decision, as both strategies had their own advantages and disadvantages (Table 3.2).

3.4.4 Operation Situation

1. The cicatrix in the posterior gluteus medius–greater trochanter complex was cut open routinely. It was unknown whether there was excessive soft tissue tension and difficulty in hip reduction in the initial replacement. However, due to the medial superior dislocation of the acetabulum, the femoral head and neck have been completely embraced by the osseous acetabulum and cicatrix. Therefore, it was impossible to dislocate the hip joint smoothly, and soft tissue release could not be performed effectively. ETO was performed to retrieve the femur stem.
2. The cup could not be smoothly retrieved after exposure of the acetabular periphery because the bony structure of the acetabulum has formed a transverse hourglass shape. Only by appropriately expanding the neck of the hourglass could the cup be retrieved.

   In the process of retrieving the outer cup, the surgeons encountered the last issue hoped for—hemorrhage. This experience remains fresh in the author's memory. Although it was less than a massive hemorrhage, there were still two to three small geyser-like gushing in the soft tissue of the acetabular floor. The fluid level in the cup rose rapidly, whereas the aspirator still had a chance to beat the speed of blood loss and reveal the soft tissue of the acetabular floor. The surgeons successfully stopped the bleeding through a combination of sutures and compression. The femoral side was treated during hemostasis by compression, saving time and improving the efficiency of the operation.
3. Acetabular reconstruction: The medial wall defect was obvious while the posterior column was intact and the remaining anterior column was weak. According to preoperative planning, a 38-mm disc augment was used, with a good fit to the surrounding host bone. The 48-mm tantalum cup was inserted, and the press fit was good.
4. Femoral reconstruction: A modular stem was applied, and the ETO part was fixed with cables.

3.4.5 Postoperative Condition and Outcome

1. The patient was instructed to walk with crutches 1 week after the operation, partial weight-bear in 6 weeks, and complete weight-bear after 3 months.
2. Functional exercises of hip flexion and abduction were gradually intensified within 3 months after the operation.
3. Postoperative radiography.

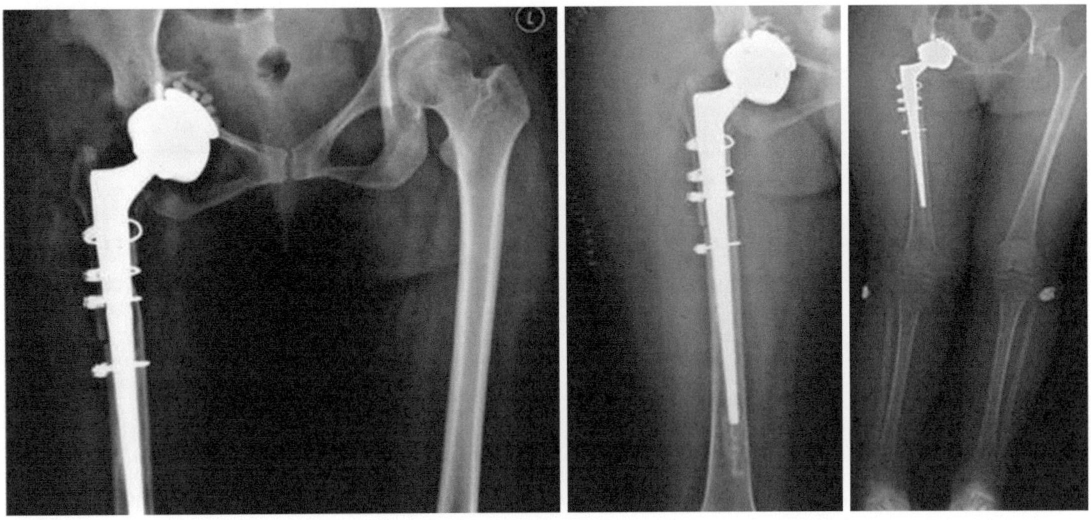

Fig. 3.12 Postoperative immediate AP view and full-length X-rays

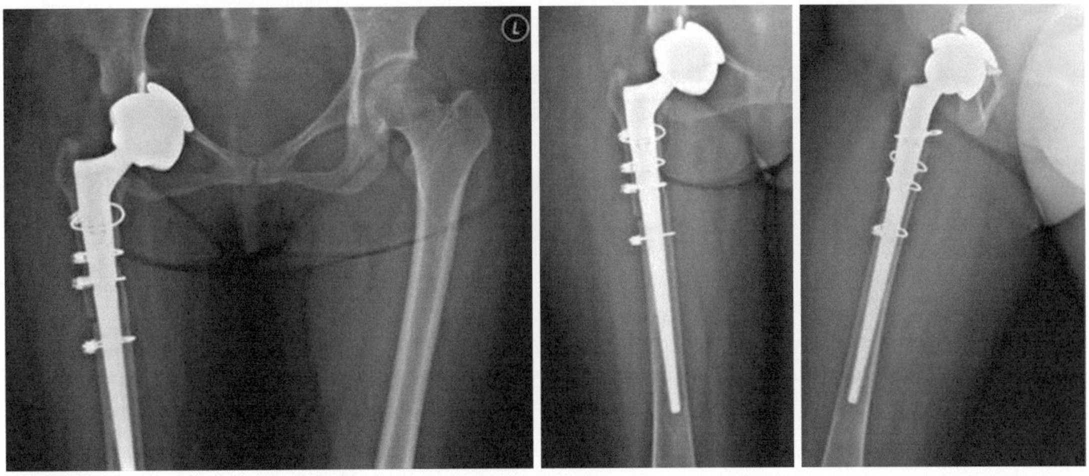

Fig. 3.13 Postoperative AP and lateral views after 3 months

Postoperative immediate radiographs, after 3 months, after 1 year, and digital tomosynthesis are shown in Figs. 3.12, 3.13, 3.14 and 3.15.

3.4.6 Conclusion and Reflection

1. There was no intraoperative hesitation on whether to retrieve the stem or not, or more precisely, it did not last for more than a few minutes, because the surgeons encountered an incident: it was impossible to dislocate the hip. The surgical process was hampered because the femur head and neck significantly protruded, which prevented the release of posterior cicatrix, and thus dislocation was unachievable.

   At this point, exposure was not the only thing in the surgeons' mind but also a large enough working space needed for the resection of the cicatrix around the hip joint and the release of soft tissue.

   ETO was a wise choice. In order to prevent comminuted fracture and future healing issues,

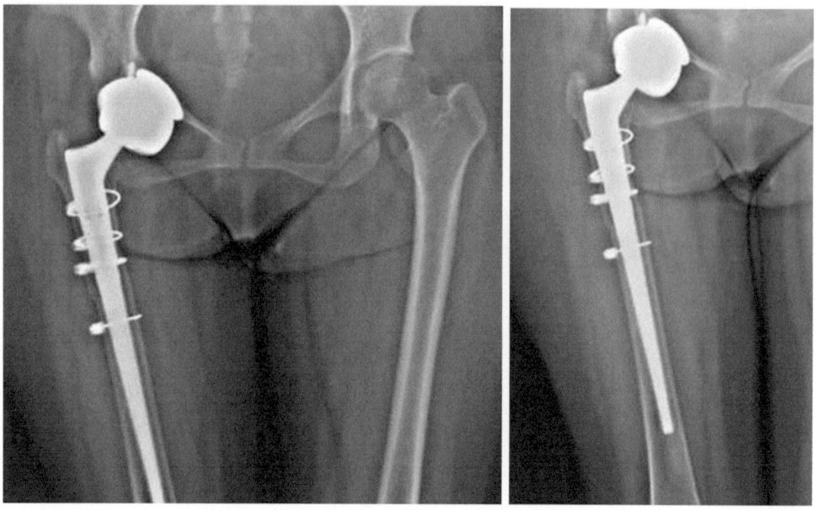

Fig. 3.14 Postoperative AP View After 1 Year

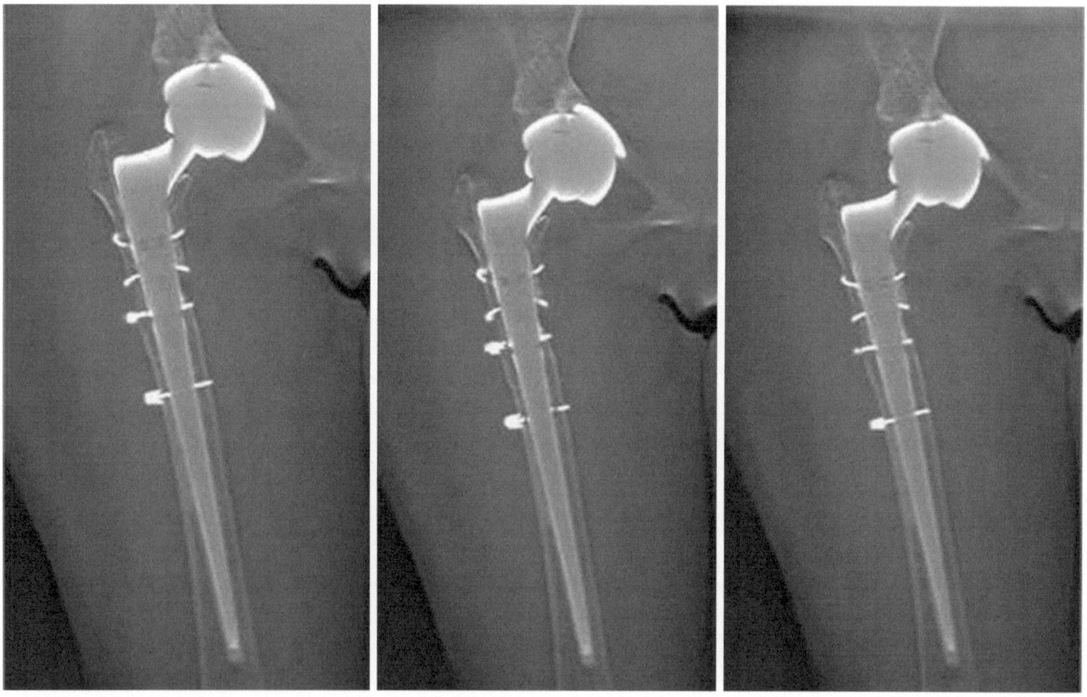

Fig. 3.15 Postoperative digital tomosynthesis after 1 year

the author extended the scope of ETO to below the osteotomy line, which can be named "step osteotomy." This way, the fracture could still be firmly fixed even if an intraoperative fracture occurred in the poorly-healed primary medial osteotomy site.

ETO itself does not naturally leave good exposure and operating space, but lifting the osteotomy block with an osteotome or Homman retractor after ETO will automatically guide the surgeon to release the cicatrix and other soft tissues.

The decisive performance of ETO is another form of damage control. In the case of poor surgical vision, the unexpected risk of surgery and extremely prolonged operation time may result from blindly extensive release, which will lead to increased surgical trauma.

In revision surgery, examination of the hip motion preoperatively or after anesthesia is an ideal guide on prediction of the complexity of exposure. If the joint has a good range of motion and the soft tissue of hip joint traction is relatively loose, intraoperative exposure will be relatively easy, and vice versa.

2. The acetabular side condition of this case was a typical "narrow opening with large chamber" one, and the following two aspects should be considered in reconstruction:
   (a) Disc or slope augment should be decided according to the size of the bone defect in the medial wall. No matter which type was applied, the augment should be able to touch the host bone at both ends or the surrounding bone, so as to function in anti-protrusion and future osseointegration.
   (b) A larger cup should be employed premised on the appropriate bone mass that was reserved around the acetabular rim. In a "narrow opening with large chamber" case like this, the opening of the acetabulum should be reamed larger (like a calabash fruit, when placing its head into the acetabulum, a larger circle in diameter needs to be reamed around its concave part), which could provide a certain amount of endogenous anti-protrusion stability.

3.5 Case 4

Yixin Zhou and Yong Huang

3.5.1 Case Summary

Medical History A 53-year-old male had a chief complaint of "pain in left THA after 25 years, gradually aggravated for 2 years." Left THA was performed in 1991 for left osteonecrosis of the femoral head, and left hip pain occurred 2 years ago, which was related to motion and could be relieved by rest. No nocturnal pain, nor limited mobility. The preliminary diagnosis was "prosthesis loosening after left THA." The patient underwent right THA in 1991 and right revision THA in 2012.

Physical Examination The patient walked in with a limp. Lateral left hip incision cicatrix was seen and no swelling around the cicatrix. Tenderness in the left groin and greater trochanteric area (+); vertical percussion pain (+); and notable limited mobility. Hip flexion, extension, and abductor strength were basically normal.

Laboratory Examination Routine blood test, ESR, and CRP were normal.

Radiographic Data Preoperative AP and lateral views and full-length X-rays are shown in Fig. 3.16. Preoperative digital tomosynthesis is shown in Fig. 3.17.

3.5.2 Case Analysis

1. Infection was primarily excluded.
2. A radiographic examination of the left hip revealed the following:
   (a) Eccentric wear was found in the liner; the cup had no obvious migration, with two large low-density areas with a larger range in the superior zone of the acetabulum (in continuous digital tomosynthesis, the cup was like an island surrounded by a large low-density area with only a few trabecular structures connected to it, suggesting severe osteolysis). There was a relatively high density of bone connection between the cup and the two low-density areas. Severe osteolysis was seen around the ischial ramus opening and cortical bone break in multiple places. The femoral stem position was low and the distal medullary of the stem revealed osteosclerosis, which indicated subsidence after loosening. Obvious osteolysis

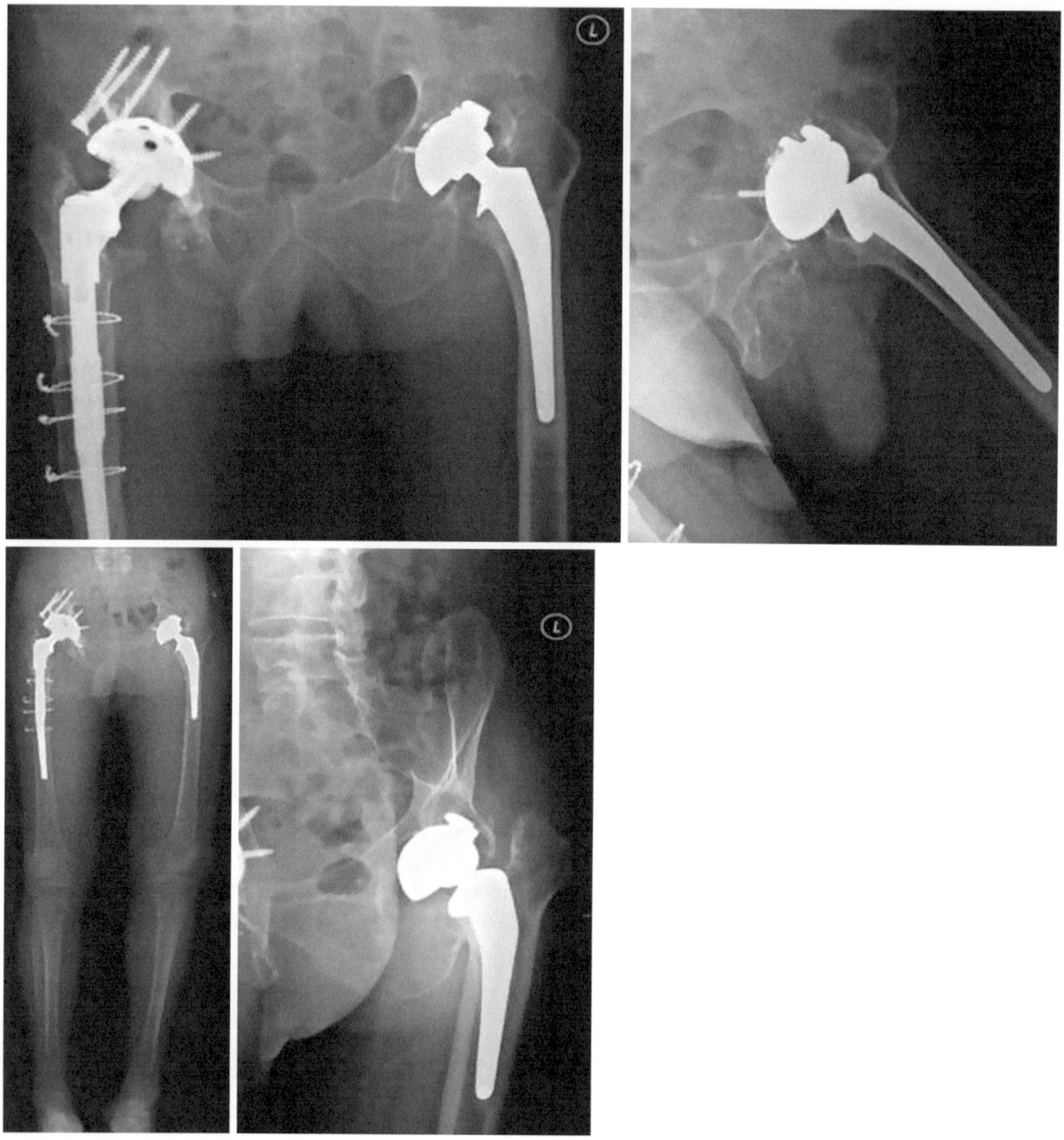

Fig. 3.16 Preoperative AP and lateral views and full-length X-rays

was observed in the medial greater trochanter of the proximal femur.

(b) The teardrop was basically intact. Severe osteolysis was seen at the ischial ramus opening with blurred bone structure. Kohler line was intact and no obvious cup migration occurred.

(c) Although the cup revealed no obvious migration, there was severe osteolysis in the upper and lower area; thus, the Paprosky classification cannot be applied simply based on the teardrop and Kohler line mentioned above. It should be referred to the intraoperative conditions.

3. Diagnosis: aseptic loosening after left THA.

3.5.3 Preoperative Planning

1. ETO: Due to the sunken femoral stem, it was difficult to fully expose the working space. In addition, it is worth emphasizing that main-

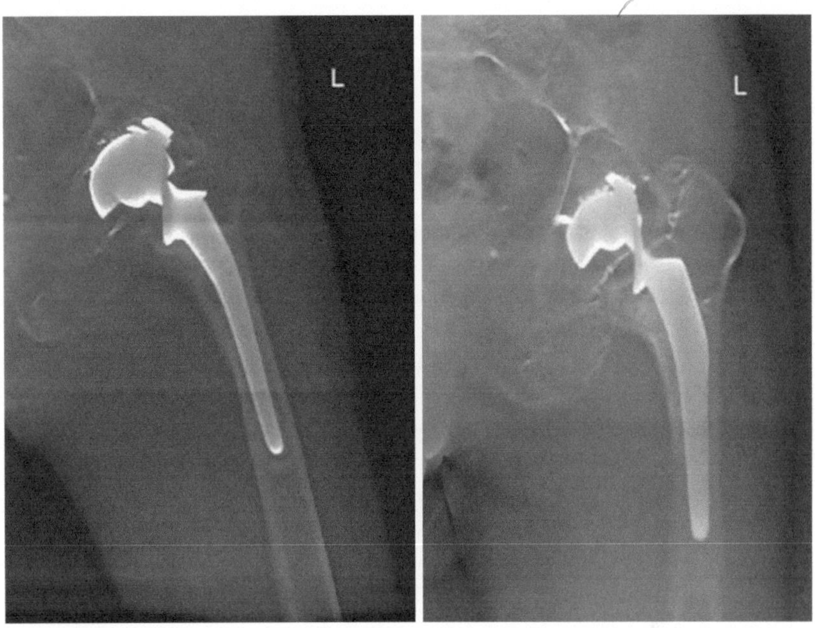

Fig. 3.17 Preoperative digital tomosynthesis

taining the continuity/intactness of both the abductor and greater trochanter is the most important task in any hip surgery, especially revision. In this case, for example, the bone mass of the greater trochanter was thin due to severe osteolysis; comminuted fracture might occur on mild tension, with the expectation of a tight fit between the residual bone mass of the greater trochanter and the stem, so that osseointegration would lead to long-term biological fixation. ETO was performed in this case, and the osteotomy site healed well in a 3-month follow-up examination.

2. The teardrop and Kohler line were relatively intact, suggesting that the anterior wall/column of the acetabulum might be intact.
3. Severe osteolysis in the ischial ramus and the discontinuity of the cortical bone suggested that the inferoposterior area might be a shaking point. There were two solutions: ① Distraction: Kirschner wires were driven into the two ends of the transection, and then forceps were used to distract to high resistance. The acetabulum was subsequently treated. Note that a certain operation order was required in performance. (2) Reaming reversely or forward and feeling the surrounding clamping force. This also applies to cases that are not suitable for Kirschner wire,
4. The osteolysis range above the cup was large (over 2 cm), for which buttress augment was preferred. Augment often leads to remarkable results when dealing with bone defects in the superior area, especially the weight-bearing area. It not only fixes the stable point but also reconstructs a relatively large part of the anterior or posterior column. In the reconstruction of the superior area, the advantage of buttress augment over slope augment is that it does not require a fit with a strong host bone matrix above the acetabulum. If the superior residual host bone is weak and cannot be firmly fixed by slope augment, buttress augment can be suspended from the ala of the ilium and the fixation between the buttress augment and the ala of the ilium is commonly easy and stable.
5. Severe osteolysis was found in both ischial ramus and superior area, and the posterior column/wall was poor.

3.5.4 Operation Situation

1. Exposure and retrieval: ETO was performed, and the loose femoral stem and cup were retrieved. There was significant osteolysis in both the acetabulum and femur, which requires not only a clear vision but also a

small stress maintained at the tips of each retractor and pry when exposing the hip joint. Otherwise, the therapeutic effect and the process of surgery would be seriously affected once a fracture occurred in the anterior column of the acetabulum or greater trochanter.
2. Acetabular reconstruction: The polyethylene liner of the acetabular side was worn through, and the metal head was articulated with the outer cup. Severe defects in the anterior and posterior iliac bones appeared to be cave-like, while the residual cortical bone was extremely thin and its strength had decreased significantly.

In pubic ramus, there was an osteolysis cavity of 1.5–2 cm deep, with only a circle of cortical bone in the anteroinferior iliac. The posterior column of the acetabulum was completely dissolved, with only a periosteum-like soft tissue remaining. The ischial ramus of the inferoposterior acetabulum also had only a ring of cortical bone, in which the cavity defect was deep and wide.

Strategy of acetabular reconstruction: As previously described, the following three questions should be answered to reconstruct the acetabulum with non-cement cup (Table 3.3).

To summarize the acetabular reconstruction strategy in this case:

1. Establishing the initial stability
   (a) The posterosuperior buttress augment and the anteroinferior slope augment formed a pinch fixation against the hemispherical cup.
   (b) A large slope augment was fixed in the inferoposterior part close to the ischial ramus cortex. The placement of the hemispherical cup had a press fit on this point. Although this point had some elasticity, the retraction force of the ischial ramus gave an augment close fit with the cup.
2. Biological fixation
   (a) The direction of the augment was controlled so that the cup was closely aligned with the anterior column bone and the acetabular floor bone.
   (b) Bone cement was applied to connect the augment with the hemispherical cup to create a non-cement acetabular complex with a large surface area. After the osseointegration with the augment, which could also be considered as osseointegration with the

Table 3.3 Strategies for acetabular reconstruction with non-cement cup

The problem	The answer	Reason	Reconstruction strategy
Was the outer rim of the acetabulum intact?	No	Extensive defect	Rim fixation excluded
Were there three points for fixation?	No	Anterosuperior and inferoposterior bone defect; severe inferoposterior bone defect; anteroinferior bone defect	Various porous TM augments could be applied for reconstruction
Were the points stable after reconstruction (are they movable)?	Yes/no	Posterosuperior and anteroinferior points were stable; inferoposterior point could be pushed	Buttress augment could be used to reconstruct both the posterosuperior point and part of the posterior column; slope augment could be applied for the anteroinferior point. Due to the excellent continuity of the anterior column, the stability of the anteroinferior point was not at risk. The inferoposterior area suffered a severe defect, but there was still a circle of cortical bone. However, the posterior column was defective and a stress fracture was revealed in the ischial ramus; thus, the inferoposterior point was unstable. Buttress augment should be used to form pinch fixation with an anteroinferior point. Meanwhile, the hemispherical acetabulum should be closely fitted to the anterior column and the medial wall bone

whole non-cement acetabular component, biological fixation was achieved.

3. The femur reconstruction was relatively simple. A modular stem was employed, while the ETO area was fixed with a greater trochanteric locking plate.

However, two points should be noted: (1) For stiff hips, the release of the posterior-medial cicatrix should be taken care of. Otherwise, a proximal femur fracture is likely to happen when the affected limb in mobile. This is generally resolved by binding cable on the distal ETO area. (2) The proximal body of modular stem with a suitable diameter should be employed. The ETO block requires shaping to maximize the adhesion with the proximal body. This is beneficial for future osseointegration.

3.5.5 Postoperative Condition and Outcome

1. The patient walked with crutches 1 week after the operation, partial weight-bear after 6 weeks, and complete partial weight-bear after a 3-month follow-up.
2. Functional exercises of hip flexor and abduction were gradually intensified within 3 months after the operation. No pain; the patient would walk on the plain ground; and 2 cm length difference between both lower extremities. Harris Hip Score was 66.
3. Postoperative examination data: Immediate, 3-month, and 2-year postoperative X-rays are shown in Figs. 3.18, 3.19 and 3.20, respectively.

3.5.6 Conclusion and Reflection

1. The concept of effective migration: Why is cup migration an important indicator of bone defect? Because wherever the cup migrates to, the bone destruction will reach there. It is certainly worth discussing whether osteolysis occurs first, and the cup migrates toward where the bone is weak, or the migration of the cup is the process and factor of bone destruction itself. From the author's point of view, both happen together. After all, the migration direction and magnitude of the cup indicate the location and extent of bone destruction. However, as it was shown in this case, although the metal cup did not physically displace, the scope of osteolysis had developed to a certain extent. The site and

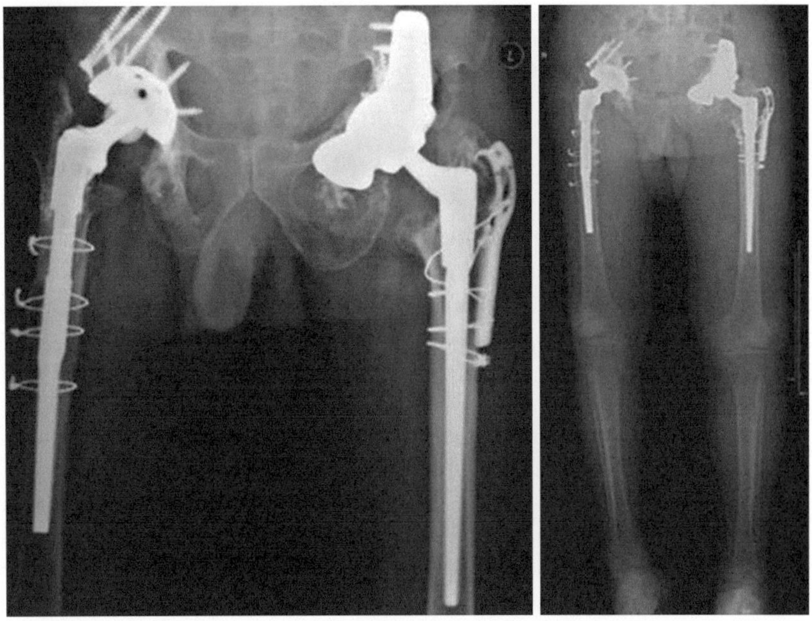

Fig. 3.18 Postoperative immediate AP view of the bilateral hip and the full-length X-rays

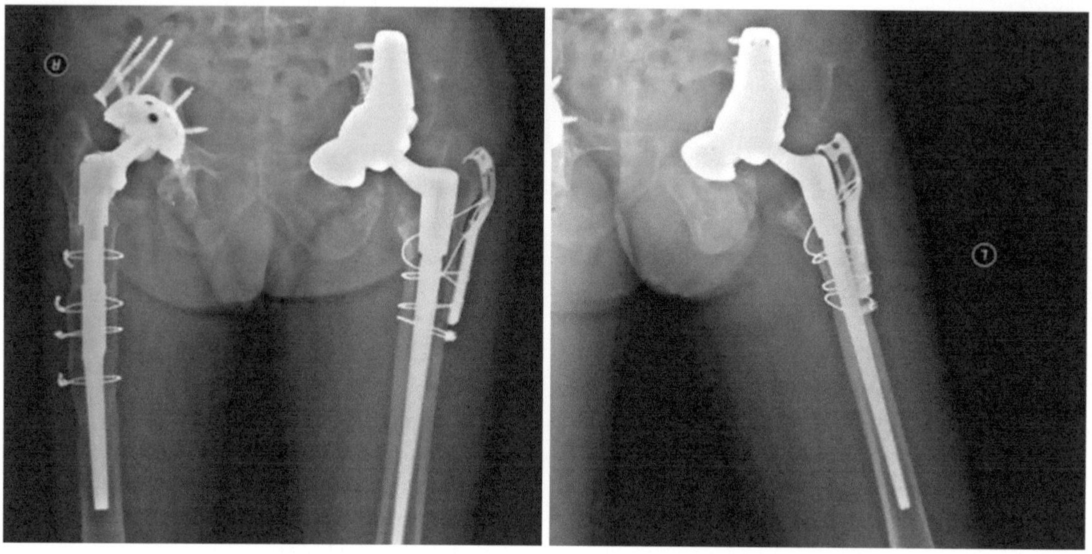

Fig. 3.19 Postoperative X-rays after 3 months

Fig. 3.20 Postoperative X-rays after 2 years

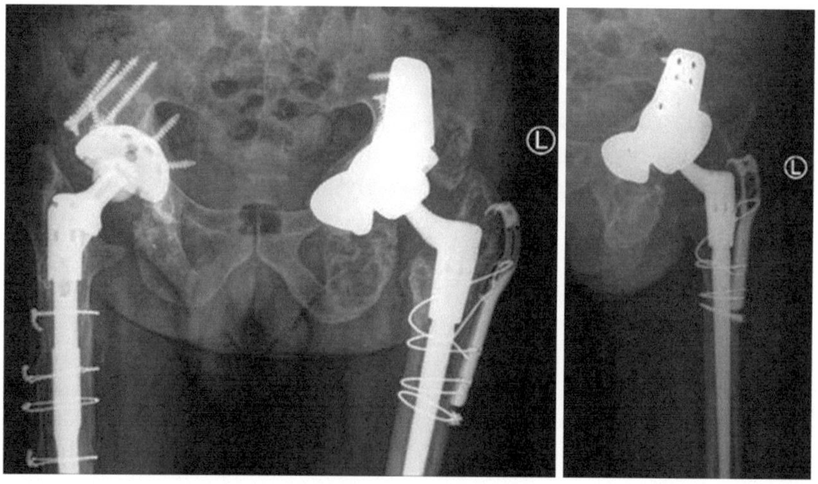

scope of bone destruction equaled the bone defect caused by cup migration. In the evaluation and classification of this type of bone defect, it should be considered equivalent to cup migration, i.e., "effective migration." The effective migration of this patient equaled the effective migration of the cup toward both up and in, as well as up and out. Therefore, the scale of the bone defect in the superior area of the acetabulum is extensive and diffuse.

2. Osteolysis was easy to be underestimated and pelvic transection fracture was easy to be ignored: This was a deceptive case, as the intraoperative findings were significantly different from preoperative plans. Therefore, preoperative radiographic data had to be reviewed afterward. At first glance of the radiographs, there was no obvious migration of the cup. The Kohler line was not disrupted, and the teardrop was clearly visible. However, taking a step back to view the radiography more systematically and comprehensively, the first impression was the femoral stem migration, with significant changes around both the acetabulum and the femoral stem. Ignoring A

(alignment) and C (cartilage, referring to the articular surface of the cup in this case), we focus on B (bone, bone around prosthesis).

(a) Although no obvious cup migration was revealed, two large expansive low-density shadows could be seen in the superior cup. Between the two shadows, a relatively high-density bone connection with the superior column structure of the cup could be seen. The interior structure of the lateral shadow was blurred, whereas, in the medial superior shadow, it could be characterized that there was a significant density reduction and blurred intraosseous structure despite some trabecular shadows. Therefore, the low-density area above the cup was periprosthetic osteolysis.
(b) Kohler line. The Kohler line of this hip was intact, which may be related to the relatively large amount of bone retained in the medial wall during the initial replacement. Nevertheless, mild hyperplasia of the medial Kohler line could be seen, and metal particles on the surface of the cup were shed and migrated toward the acetabular floor. Accordingly, the acetabular floor had a certain degree of bone defect, while some of the bone mass was still retained.
(c) Ischial ramus. The ischial ramus was severely invaded. Its cortex was thin and rough. The bone structure was completely absent in the medial superior ischial ramus. Higher-density shadows alternating with lower ones could be seen in its middle and lower parts. Frequent interruptions of cortical bone were visible in multiple locations. All these signs indicated severe osteolysis and a large bone defect in the ischial ramus. The inferoposterior point was already a shaking one.
(d) Teardrop and pubic ramus. Relatively intact

After analyzing the indicators of bone structure and cup migration, readers can get a rough idea about the periprosthetic bone defect, and more importantly, the general appearance of the residual bone.

Wait, there were also invisible signs! X-ray reviewing requires attention to the visible signs, whereas the problems that cannot be shown on the X-ray should also be aware of!

Due to the overlapping of prosthesis and being two-dimensional, part of the structures is often invisible on plain radiographs. In general, the continuity in the anterior and posterior column or the bone mass cannot be judged with only the anterior and posterior radiographs of the hip joint. Experienced observers can certainly infer the condition of the anterior and posterior acetabular column through some indirect signs. For example, up-and-in migration of the cup often indicates anterior column involvement, while up-and-out migration often suggests posterior column involvement. Iliac oblique, obturator oblique, or CT scan are often required to confirm the degree of involvement of the anterior and posterior acetabular structures.

Nevertheless, in this case, the condition of the anterior and posterior columns cannot be determined according to the migration of the cup even though neither up and in nor up and out migration occurred. However, it would be reckless to ignore the possibility of bone defects in the anterior and posterior columns. In the case of a severe bone defect in the superior and inferoposterior areas, what are the odds of an intact posterior column of the acetabulum? Of course, it is possible, but with a very slim chance. Moreover, the posterosuperior and inferoposterior areas had already revealed a serious defect. The ischial ramus opening that was not blocked by the cup was extremely thin and weak and involved shaking points. In this case, the continuity and bone mass of the posterior column of the acetabulum were questionable.

According to the Paprosky classification, the following indicators were mainly observed (Table 3.4).

The interior structure of the lateral shadow was blurred, whereas, in the medial superior shadow, it could be characterized that there was a significant density reduction and blurred intraosseous structure despite some trabecular shadows. Therefore, the low-density area above the cup was periprosthetic osteolysis.

As a rule, bone defects in reality after intraoperative retrieval are generally more serious than

Table 3.4 Indicators of Paprosky classification

To observe	A sign	Annotation
Teardrop	Relatively good clarity	Note that the outer edge of the teardrop was not smooth
Migration of the hip rotation center or cup	No obvious migration	Although the cup exhibited no obvious migration itself, two large expansive low-density shadows could be seen in the superior cup. Between the two shadows, a relatively high-density bone connection with the superior column structure of the PCA-imitation cup could be seen.

what can be seen in preoperative imaging, especially bone defects in X-rays. Experienced surgeons can keep the differences in degree and positions between preoperative and intraoperative bone defect assessment in an acceptable range. This requires considerable knowledge of imageology and rich experience in clinical practice. Surgeons should not only rely on intraoperative observation but also use fingers to feel the residual bone mass and strength. If necessary, a periosteal stripper can be employed to check for any fracture or significant decrease in bone strength with a push.

In this case, resistance of only soft tissue strength was received when the posterior wall of the posterior column was pushed with a periosteal stripper, and only thinned and lightened cortical bone was felt to be connected with soft tissue when the posterior column was held with thumbs. Therefore, it could be confirmed that both the posterior acetabular wall and column were missing, forming a transection, and no mechanical support was provided.

3.6 Case 5

Shengjie Guo and Yong Huang

3.6.1 Case Summary

Medical History A 56-year-old male had a chief complaint of "pain for 5 months after right hip arthroplasty and limited mobility for 4 months." The patient was locally diagnosed with tuberculosis infection of bilateral hips due to bilateral hip pain and bilateral hip debridement was performed in 1987. He underwent left THA in 1990 due to hip pain and limited mobility. Right THA was received in 1991. Five months ago, the patient developed right hip pain without obvious inducement, which was related to motion, and could be relieved by rest. No nocturnal pain; limited mobility. The symptoms gradually progressed. Four months ago, the pain aggravated. The patient visited the outpatient department of our hospital and was admitted to the ward with "prosthesis loosening after right THA." He had a 20-year AS history. The patient underwent cervical fracture surgery 4 years ago.

Physical Examination Patient entered with a crutch; previous incision cicatrix was seen on the lateral right hip joint; tenderness in inguinal area (+); axial percussion pain (+); right hip motion with obvious limitation; and hip abductor strength was normal.

Preoperative position photographs are shown in Fig. 3.21.

Laboratory Examination Routine blood test was normal; ESR and CRP were in the upper limit of normal range.

Radiographic Examination Preoperative X-rays are shown in Fig. 3.22. A preoperative hip joint plain CT scan is shown in Fig. 3.23.

3.6.2 Case Analysis

1. Infection was basically excluded according to comprehensive preoperative examination.
2. Reviewing radiographic examination of the right hip:

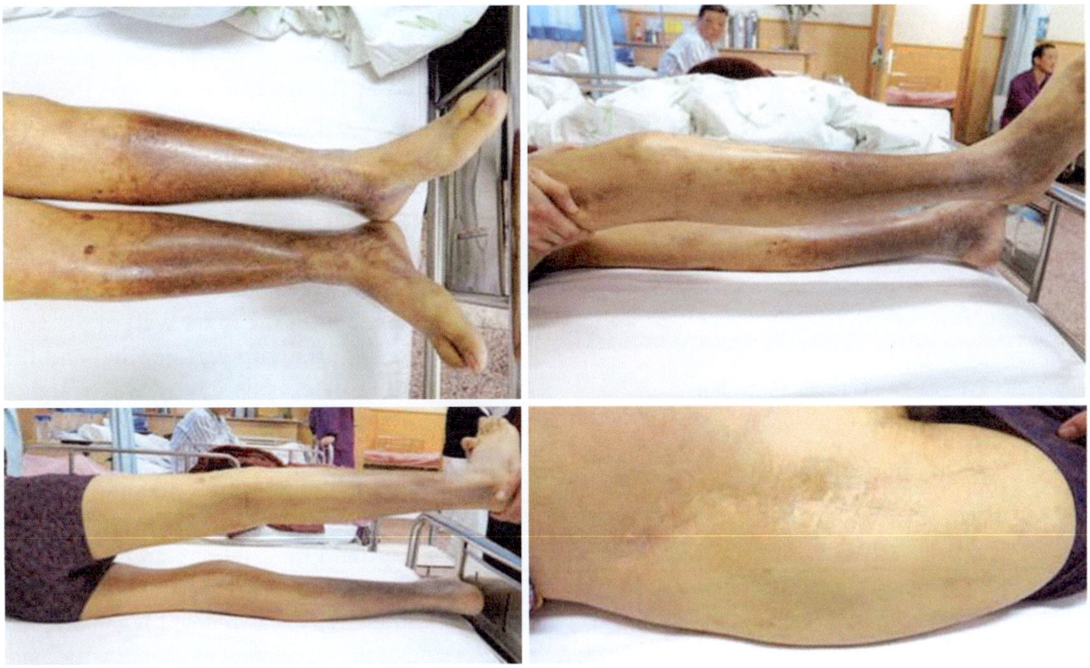

Fig. 3.21 Preoperative Position Photographs

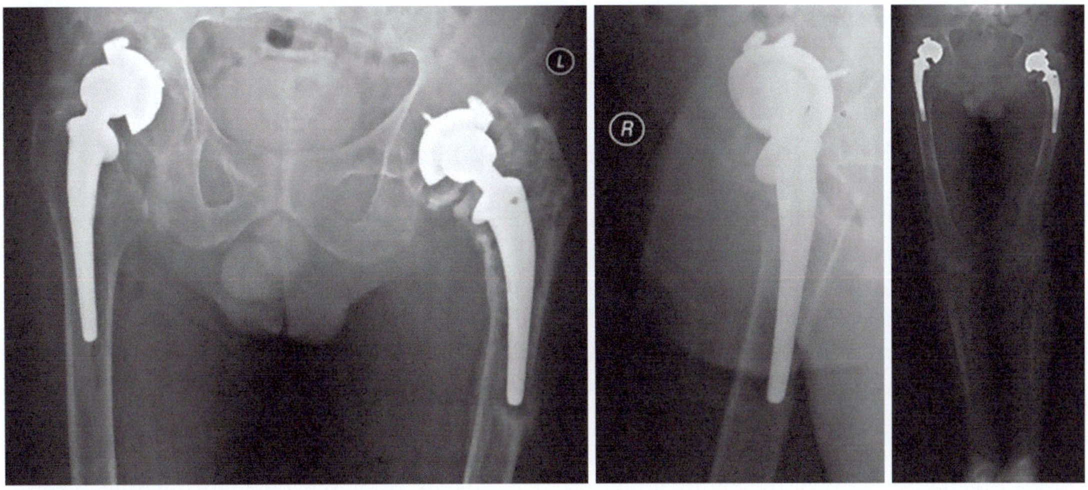

Fig. 3.22 Preoperative Radiographs

(a) The acetabular cup was loose and migrated upward; the range of periprosthetic osteolysis was large; and the superior osteolysis exceeded the distance of acetabular cup migration. The stem did not appear to be loose, but there was some space between the stem and the femur cortex.

(b) The teardrop was basically intact; the ischial ramus showed mild osteolysis at its opening but was relatively intact. The Kohler line was intact and protruded slightly into the pelvic cavity, and the bone of the acetabular floor was weak. The acetabular cup significantly migrated upward, and the extent of

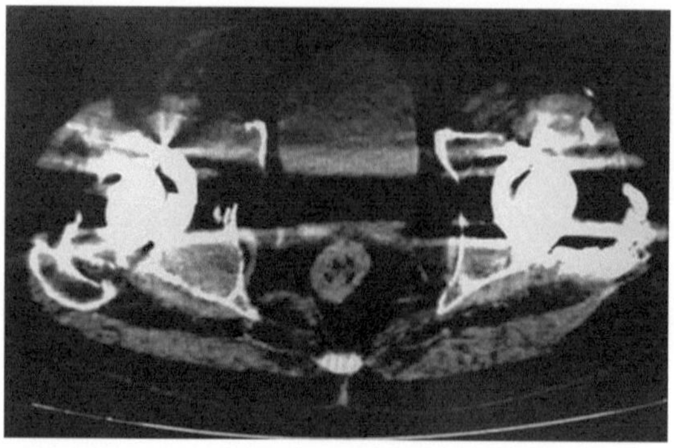

Fig. 3.23 Preoperative CT scan of the hip

superior osteolysis exceeded the distance of the prosthesis migration.

(c) Paprosky IIIA was considered, whereas severe and extensive acetabular osteolysis was observed.

(d) Diagnosis: prosthesis loosening after right hip arthroplasty.

3.6.3 Preoperative Planning

1. Residual bone island was seen in the medial acetabular cup, with obvious osteolysis both up and down. Generally speaking, the rim and medial walls of the acetabulum could be considered intact. To avoid too much migration of the rotation center, the bone island probably needed to be reamed off. Supportive points could be reconstructed with augment.
2. Our experience indicated that intraoperative finding about osteolysis tends to be worse than preoperative estimation.
3. Hip joint mobility was poor. For better exposure and optimization of the hip rotation center, ETO should be prepared for stem retrieval.

3.6.4 Operation Situation

1. ETO was performed to achieve better vision. The femoral component (monoblock femur stem with integrated head and neck) was removed smoothly.

   The acetabular cup was loose with severe osteolysis. A V-shaped bone crest remained at the central bottom of the acetabulum. A tripod of three dramatic-sized osteolysis cavities was seen in the anteriosuperior, anteroinferior (pubic ramus), and inferoposterior (ischial ramus) acetabulum around the bony crest. The soft tissue inside was thoroughly cleaned. The bone crest was removed until the inner wall of the acetabulum. The trial cup was applied and the surrounding osteolysis cavity was roughly crescent-shaped. The three bone defects were reamed with appropriate reamers. Three augments (50 mm × 15 mm, 50 mm × 10 mm, and 50 mm × 10 mm) were inserted around the trial cup and fixed with screws.
2. The central cavity was reamed reversely; the cup side of the augment was coated with bone cement, and the 56-mm porous TM acetabular cup was impacted. The initial stability was good, with approximately 25–30% area of the cup in direct contact with the bone matrix of the acetabular floor. Three screws were inserted for supplementary fixation with the caution of avoiding the augments.
3. RM modular stem was applied on the femur side, and the ETO block was fixed with a trochanteric claw plate.

   See Fig. 3.24 for intraoperative photos.

3.6.5 Postoperative Condition and Outcome

1. The patient was instructed to walk on crutches 1 week after the operation, partial weight-bearing at 6 weeks, and complete weight-bearing at 3 months.
2. Functional exercises of hip flexor and abduction were gradually intensified within 3 months after the operation.
3. Clinical follow-up: no pain; the patient could walk on the plain ground normally. Due to the presence of AS, hip flexion and abduction were still restricted. The Harris score was 66.

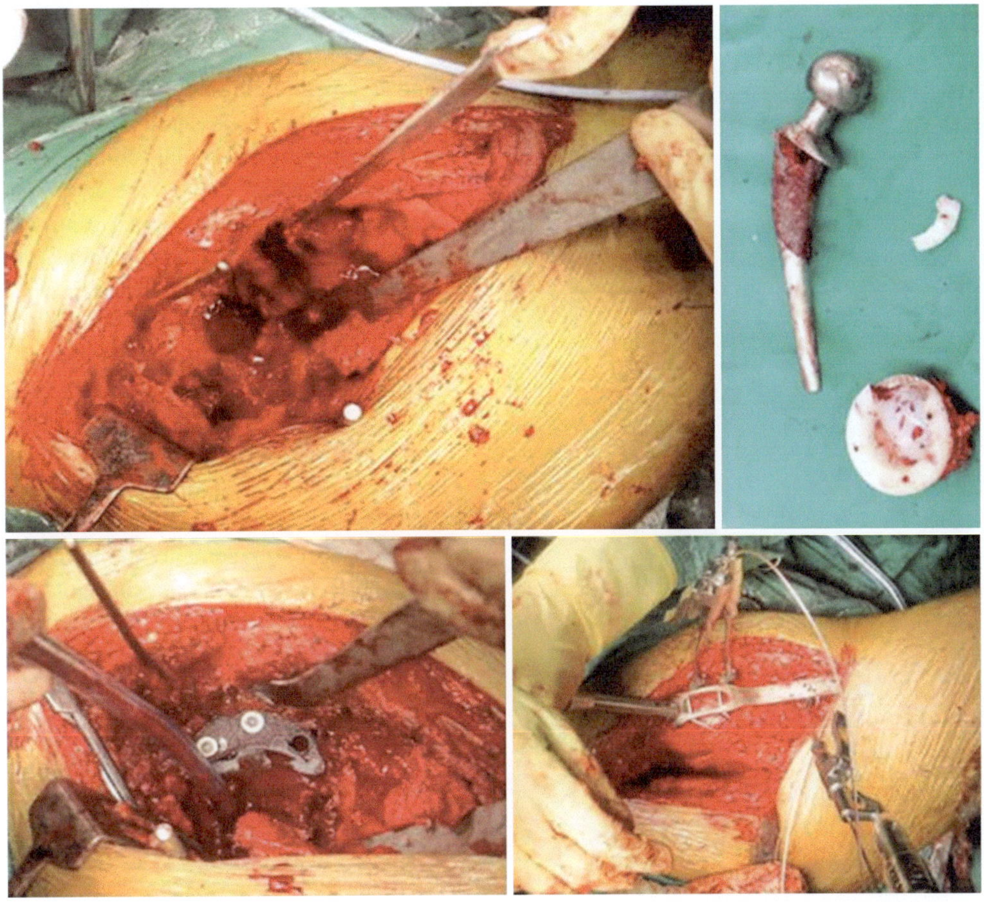

Fig. 3.24 Intraoperative images

Immediate postoperative radiographs and radiographs 2 months and 1 year and 8 months after the operation are shown in Figs. 3.25, 3.26 and 3.27.

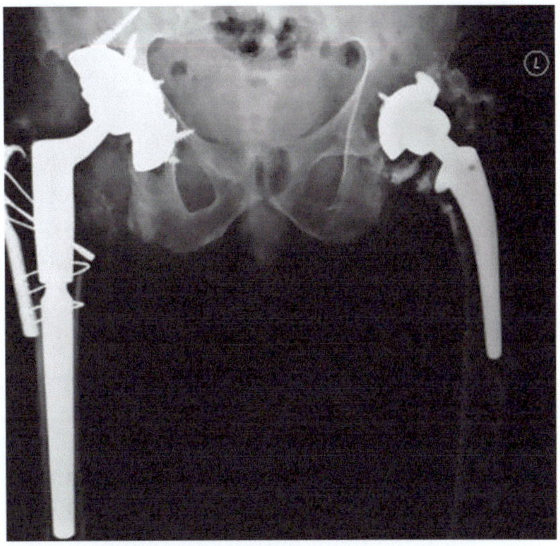

Fig. 3.25 Immediate postoperative radiograph

3.6.6 Conclusion and Reflection

1. The reasons for performing ETO were as follows:
   (a) Hip stiffness with poor mobility.
   (b) The original stem was a monoblock, which was a disadvantage in balancing between the optimization of the rotation center and the tension in the hip joint.
   (c) The surface of the original stem was coarsely coated and was not loose.
   (d) Favored acetabular side exposure.

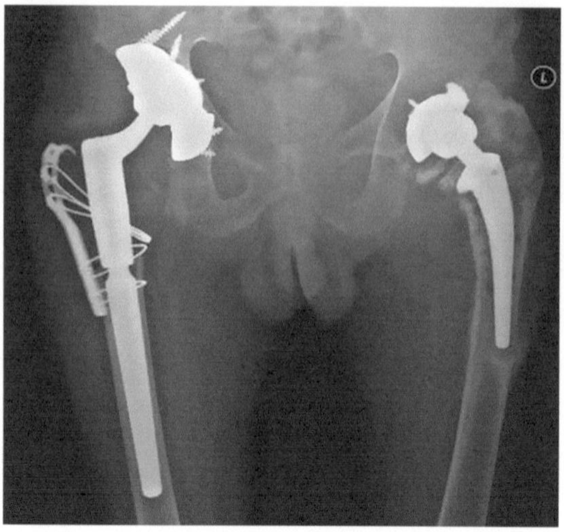

Fig. 3.26 Postoperative radiographs after 2 months

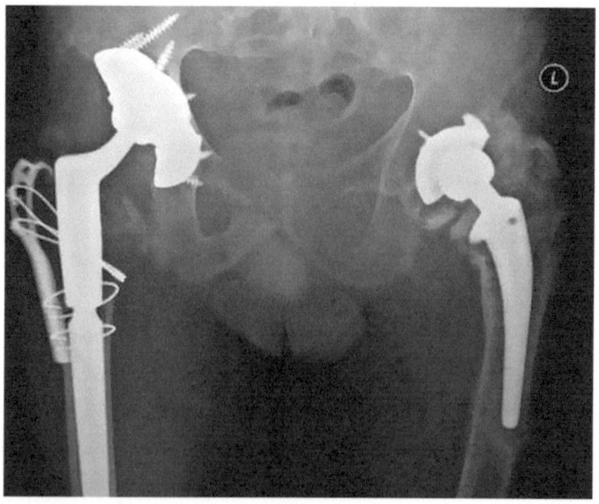

Fig. 3.27 Postoperative radiographs after 1 year and 8 months

2. Objectives of biological acetabular reconstruction were as follows:
   (a) Creating a close and stable contact between the host bone and the special-shaped acetabular cup consisting of the augment and the hemispherical acetabular cup.
   (b) Good initial stability.
   (c) Restoring the biomechanics of the hip by optimizing the rotation center. In this case, the main purpose of intraoperative removal of the central bone crest, instead of placing the prosthesis over the bone defect, was to optimize the rotation center.
3. The hemispherical acetabular cup and augment could be considered as an integrated special-shaped acetabular component, with the hemispherical cup as the main body. It should have as much contact with the host bone as possible, and the augment could be regarded as an extended part for fixation.

   Therefore, the general procedure of the operation was to ream the acetabular side at an appropriate rotation center, insert the trial cup (created as much contact with the host bone as possible), evaluate the shape and severity of the surrounding bone defect, clean the defect site, insert the augment(s), test the cup size, applying cement, and finally impact the hemispherical cup (careful with the position of the screw holes).
4. For better understanding, stabilization assisted by augment could be divided into internal fixation and external fixation.

3.7 Case 6

Yong Huang and Shengjie Guo

3.7.1 Case Summary

Medical History A 40-year-old female had a chief complaint of "right hip pain occurred after right THA 27 years ago, and gradually aggravated for 1 year." The patient underwent right THA in another hospital 27 years ago because of secondary osteoarthritis of developmental dysplasia of the right hip and underwent revision of the right hip in another hospital 7 years ago. One year ago, right hip pain was developed without obvious cause, which was related to motion and could be relieved by rest. No nocturnal pain. Symptoms progressed gradually with limited mobility. The patient was admitted by the outpatient department with "implant wear after right THA."

Physical Examination Claudication; lateral right hip incision cicatrix, no swelling; normal

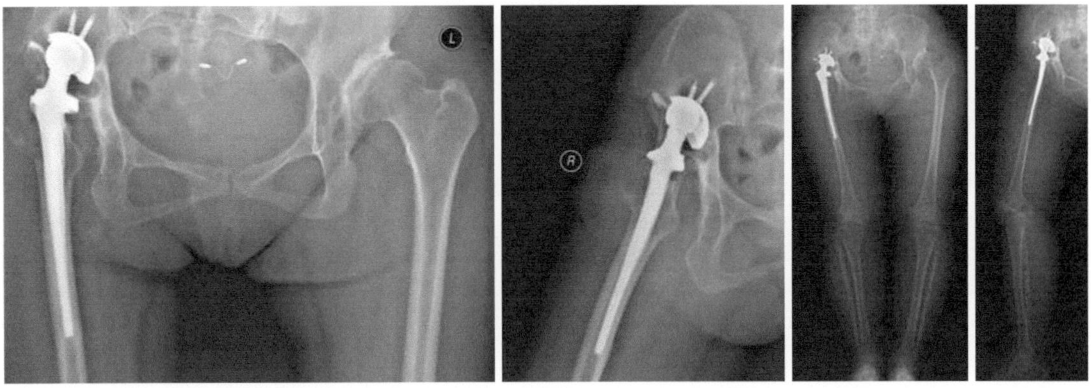

Fig. 3.28 Anterior and lateral X-rays and full-length radiographs

skin temperature; hip flexion, extension, and abductor strength were basically normal; and obviously limited mobility.

Laboratory Examination No abnormality detected in a routine blood test, ESR, and CRP.

Radiographic Examination Anterior and lateral X-rays and full-length radiographs are shown in Fig. 3.28.

3.7.2 Case Analysis

1. Infection was basically ruled out according to a comprehensive preoperative examination.
2. Although the patient was only 40 years old, she had undergone several surgeries and was admitted with hip pain, short limbs, hip stiffness, and claudication.
3. Radiographic examination review.
   (a) The acetabular rotation center significantly migrated upward (despite the acceptable angles of the cup). The severe bone defect around the cup had affected the iliac bone near the sacroiliac joint. The estimated diameter of the femoral head was 22 mm with increased neck length, with severe eccentric wear. It was close to the metal shell, which possibly suggested that the femoral head had worn through the polyethylene and even involved the metal shell.
   (b) The femoral stem was well fitted and filled for the medullary cavity proximal femur. There was no radiolucent line around the stem and the calcar femorale was atrophied, so stem loosening was not considered. However, extensive osteolysis could be seen in the greater trochanter and its lateral inferior cortex. Most bone in the greater trochanter was missing, leaving only the shadow of the cortical shell.
   (c) Bone status of the true acetabulum site: The teardrop was intact without obvious bone defect in the ischial ramus and pubic ramus; the Kohler line was intact. These were likely the result of no true acetabulum involvement in previous operations. If Paprosky classification was required, it should be classified as type IIIA.
4. Diagnosis: prosthesis wear after right THA.

3.7.3 Preoperative Planning

1. Acetabular reconstruction: It was a complicated case with severe acetabular defects. Thus, how much bone could be used to support initial stability and bone ingrowth was the key point to be calmly examined. The acetabular rim on the medial ilium had severe bone loss and could not provide fixation. Fortunately, the previous acetabular reconstruction sites were high. The true acetabulum was not involved. In addition,

the Kohler line was relatively intact. Thus, pelvic discontinuity could be considered negative.

Meanwhile, dysplasia of the true acetabulum led to its extremely small size, the posterior and anterior walls of which were scarce. However, it could still be considered that the posterior and anterior of the true acetabulum, namely, the inferoposterior and anteroinferior of the future acetabulum, could provide two points for fixation. The bone of the superior true acetabulum was scarce and flat; hence, it could not provide the superior point.

In conclusion, the key point of acetabular reconstruction was to make good use of the bone mass of the true acetabulum to provide anteroinferior and inferoposterior points. The superior point could be reconstructed with a buttress augment. The posterosuperior acetabulum could be reconstructed in the meantime so that the posterior acetabulum would be supported during hip flexion.

2. Femoral reconstruction: Since the revolutionary reconstruction of the acetabular side would result in inferior migration of the rotation center to a large extent, the femoral head could not be reduced and the length of the lower extremity could not be fine-tuned without exchanging the original femoral stem. Moreover, the original stem had a large neck-shaft angle and small offset, which could not optimize the mechanical properties of the hip without femoral stem retrieval and exchange. The third important reason for replacing the femoral stem was that severe osteolysis had already occurred in the greater trochanter. To fix the residual greater trochanter, the following was required: ① stem shoulder with proper diameter and geometry and ② a suitable surface coating to provide adequate contact area and the possibility of osseointegration.
3. Choice of liner: As the patient was young, had an active lifestyle, and had undergone multiple surgeries, there was a high risk of failure for revision. To avoid polyethylene wearing and related problems, the surgeons decided to employ a ceramic-on-ceramic joint surface, which required accurate placement of the rotation center of the hip and the angles of the cup. Otherwise, complications such as dislocation and joint squeaking could occur.

3.7.4 Operation Situation

1. To avoid fracture of the greater trochanter and remove the stem smoothly, ETO was performed. Severe osteolysis was observed in greater trochanter and only thin cortical bone remained. The original femoral stem was well fixed and the stem was removed successfully after separating the stem-bone interface with a wire saw.
2. The soft tissue was extensively stained black. The polyethylene liner had been worn through by the metal femoral head, which had direct contact with the metal shell. The acetabular cup was loose, and the cavity-like bone defect was found after cup removal. Part of the ilium was completely penetrated, and the pelvic muscle could have been touched.
3. Exposure was expanded downwards to the upper margin of the obturator foramen after the cup was removed, which was approximately the imagological level of the teardrop, and could also be considered the lowest point of the true acetabulum. Another important anatomical marker in this true acetabulum was the transverse acetabular ligament, the lower margin of which was at the same level as the superior margin of the obturator foramen and the teardrop on imaging.
4. Another important marker for acetabulum dissection is the fat on the acetabular floor. Generally, reaching the acetabular floor fat can be considered equivalent to reaching the fossa ovale of a normal acetabulum.

It should be noted that for the exposure of the acetabular side, in addition to determining the level of the lower acetabular margin, exposure of the anterior and posterior margin of the acetabulum was also required. After gaining clear vision, we could use our fingertips to feel the bone mass of the anterior and posterior walls of the acetabulum. In general, in cases with severe developmental dysplasia, the posterior column usually maintains rich bone mass, thus completely revealing that the posterior column and the adjacent part of the ischial ramus are helpful to precisely determine the rotation center and create enough pinch fixation and contact area for the acetabular cup. Surgeons should have a three-dimensional vision to identify the position of the cup, taking into account the superior–inferior and anterior–posterior parts and the depth of the acetabulum. Usually, part of the posterior column needs to be reamed off to accommodate the cup and provide pinch fixation. It should be emphasized that it is not enough to expose the true acetabulum with good clarity only, but also part of the pseudo-acetabulum, especially the transition between the pseudo-acetabulum and the true acetabulum.

For this kind of surgery, not only good clarity of vision is needed, but a good application of fingertip feeling is also required to understand the shape and amount of bone. More importantly, the eyes of "thoughts" should be practiced to see things that cannot be seen with eyesight alone or by ordinary people.

5. After exposure, the true acetabulum was found not well developed with a thin anterior column and a comparatively thick posterior column. Between the true acetabulum and the false acetabulum, the common "calabash waist" of the general hip dislocation was not seen. The acetabulum was very flat from top to bottom, which made it relatively easy to apply the augment.
6. Some of the bone mass in the posterior wall was chiseled away with an osteotome to move the rotation center posteriorly and prevent excessive reaming of the front margin of the acetabulum. The acetabulum was reamed with a small reamer, which was gradually expanded to 46 mm. During the reaming process, the bottom edge of the reamer should always be leveled with the transverse ligament. The support from the anteroinferior and inferoposterior acetabulum could be felt after reaming and placing the trial cup. However, about 50% of the superior acetabulum was not covered, and the acetabulum with posterosuperior bone defect could not provide pinch fixation for the acetabular cup in the anterior-posterior direction. Therefore, a buttress augment was selected to reconstruct the superior and posterosuperior parts of the acetabulum and restore part of the posterior column. The gap between the superior part of the buttress augment and the host bone was filled with 15° shim augment, and the gap between the buttress augment and shim augment was connected with bone cement. After the buttress augment placement was completed, bone cement was applied on the surface between the cup and buttress augment, and then a 46-mm porous acetabular cup was impacted. An obvious press fit could be felt when impacting the cup. The initial stability of the acetabular cup was good, which was enhanced with several screws.
7. Reconstruction of stem side: As the rotation center of the stem has been restored to the level of the true acetabulum, part of the medial femur was removed to release the whole joint and to help the hip reduction. RM modular stem was applied. The soft tissue tension, lower extremity length, and hip stability were repeatedly confirmed to be acceptable, and the greater trochanter osteotomy block was fixed with a claw plate and cable system.

3.7.5 Postoperative Condition and Outcome

1. The patient was instructed to walk on crutches 2 weeks after the operation, partial weight-bearing at 6 weeks, and complete weight-bearing at 3 months.
2. Functional exercises of hip flexor and abduction were gradually intensified within 3 months after the operation.
3. Clinical follow-up: In 1-year postoperative follow-up, the Harris score was 97, pain-free, and gait was basically normal.

Postoperative immediate anteroposterior and full-length radiographs are shown in Fig. 3.29. AP view and lateral view of X-ray at 4 months postoperatively are shown in Fig. 3.30, and radiographs at 8 months postoperatively are shown in Fig. 3.31.

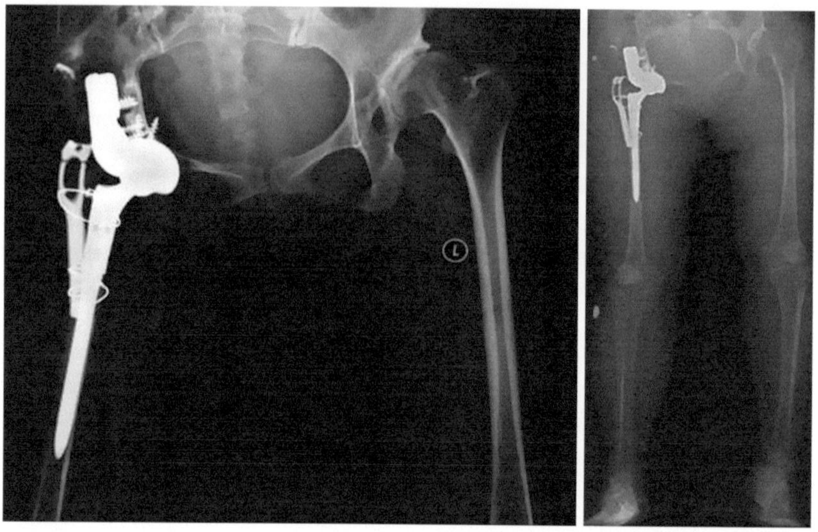

Fig. 3.29 Immediate postoperative AP view and full-length radiographs

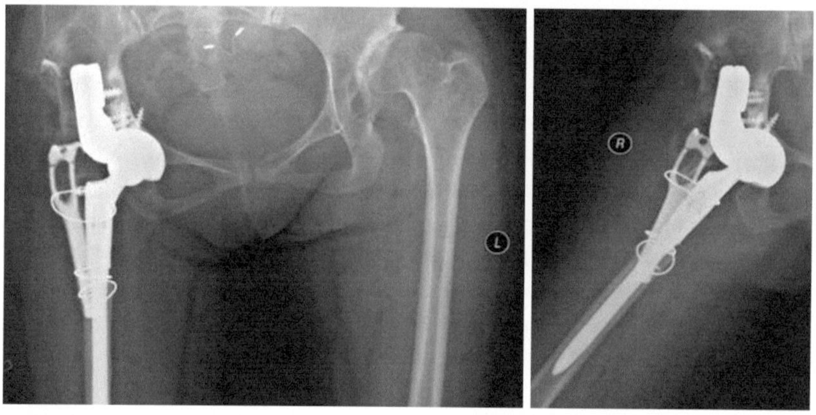

Fig. 3.30 AP view and lateral view of a 4-month postoperative follow-up

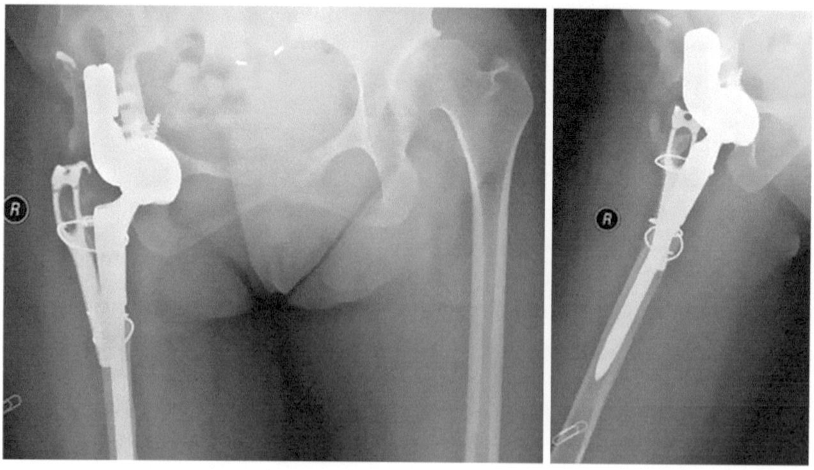

Fig. 3.31 AP view and lateral view of a 8-month postoperative follow-up

3.7.6 Conclusion and Reflection

1. Why was the osteolysis so severe?

   Osteolysis in this case was certainly related to polyethylene wear, which had been confirmed by the X-ray and intraoperative observation. However, the cause of osteolysis should not be limited to the effect of polyethylene debris, the effect of metal ions should also be taken into consideration. The metal head was made of cobalt–chromium alloy. It had friction with the titanium alloy outer cup after grinding through the polyethylene liner, which could cause massive cobalt, chromium, and titanium ion release. Osteolysis can be caused by the increase of local concentration of cobalt and chromium ions, which has been confirmed by many studies.
2. Why did serious wear and tear occur in a short term?

   (1) Patient factors: She was young and had an active lifestyle. In addition, the secondary severe arthritis due to developmental dysplasia in the contralateral hip joint caused excessive weight-bearing on the operative side for a long time. (2) Prosthesis factors: The cup shell was small, while the polyethylene liner was thin. Ordinary polyethylene has poor wear resistance. The metal femoral head and the rotation center migrated up and out significantly, the femur side offset was small, and the arm of the force of the abductor was small, resulting in the surge of the joint reaction force (JRF).

   Various mechanisms can lead to up and in migration of the femoral head within the polyethylene liner. After the operation, early-stage up-and-in migration of the cup is usually caused by the creepage of the polyethylene liner under femoral head stress. The medial-term up-and-in migration is mainly caused by polyethylene wear. However, there are different types of polyethylene wear. Sheer articular friction often produces tiny particles that are more biologically active and more likely to cause osteolysis. The polyethylene destruction caused by edge loading is more significant, which often leads to cleft and delamination. However, the fragments it produces are relatively large (the coagulated, wax-like, translucent patches often seen intraoperatively in the red tissues in the surgical field are exfoliated polyethylene). These patch-like polyethylene detritus caused by high edge loading or impingement have low biological activity and hardly cause osteolysis. The removed prosthesis also revealed that the polyethylene liner of the hip was worn through from up and in, but there was no polyethylene edge damage on the outer upper edge due to edge loading. This was also consistent with the mechanical condition of this hip. The surge of internal joint stress led to severe scraping and wear between the femoral head and the inner and upper part of polyethylene. As the overall anteversion and abduction angle of the cup were ideal, there was no significant edge damage to the polyethylene liner caused by edge loading.
3. Analyzing the causes of hip failure and looking at hip arthroplasty from a broader perspective is the main motivation for surgeons to perform revision surgery.

3.8 Case 7

Yong Huang and Shengjie Guo

3.8.1 Case Summary

Medical History A 66-year-old female had a chief complaint "developed pain and limited mobility for more than half a year in the right hip after THA 16 years ago."

Physical Examination There was a 3-cm shortening discrepancy in the right hip; incision cicatrix could be seen, no swelling and sinus tract; skin temperature was not high; iliac area tenderness (+); axial percussion pain (+); and severe limited motion.

Patrick's sign on the right (+); Thomas's sign on the right (+); Trendelenburg's sign on the right (+); Allis's sign (+); Ober's sign on the left (−); no edema in both lower extremities; no hypoesthesia; and the pulse of the bilateral dorsal artery of foot was palpable.

Laboratory Examination No abnormality was detected in a routine blood test, ESR, and CRP.

Radiographic Data Preoperative X-ray (Fig. 3.32) showed severe expanded osteolysis in soap-bubble appearance in the iliac crest and the ischium of the patient.

3.8.2 Case Analysis

There was no migration of the acetabular cup, probably because the bone had healed in one or two sites and the screws provided mechanical fixation. However, there were also severe osteolysis and possible pelvic discontinuity around the acetabular cup. The two facts were not inconsistent though. No acetabular cup migration did not necessarily mean that the osteolysis was not serious. Whether the acetabular cup migrated was not very important to the evaluation of whether it was a Paprosky III bone defect. The superior transparent area was not linear, but inflated, balloon-like. The

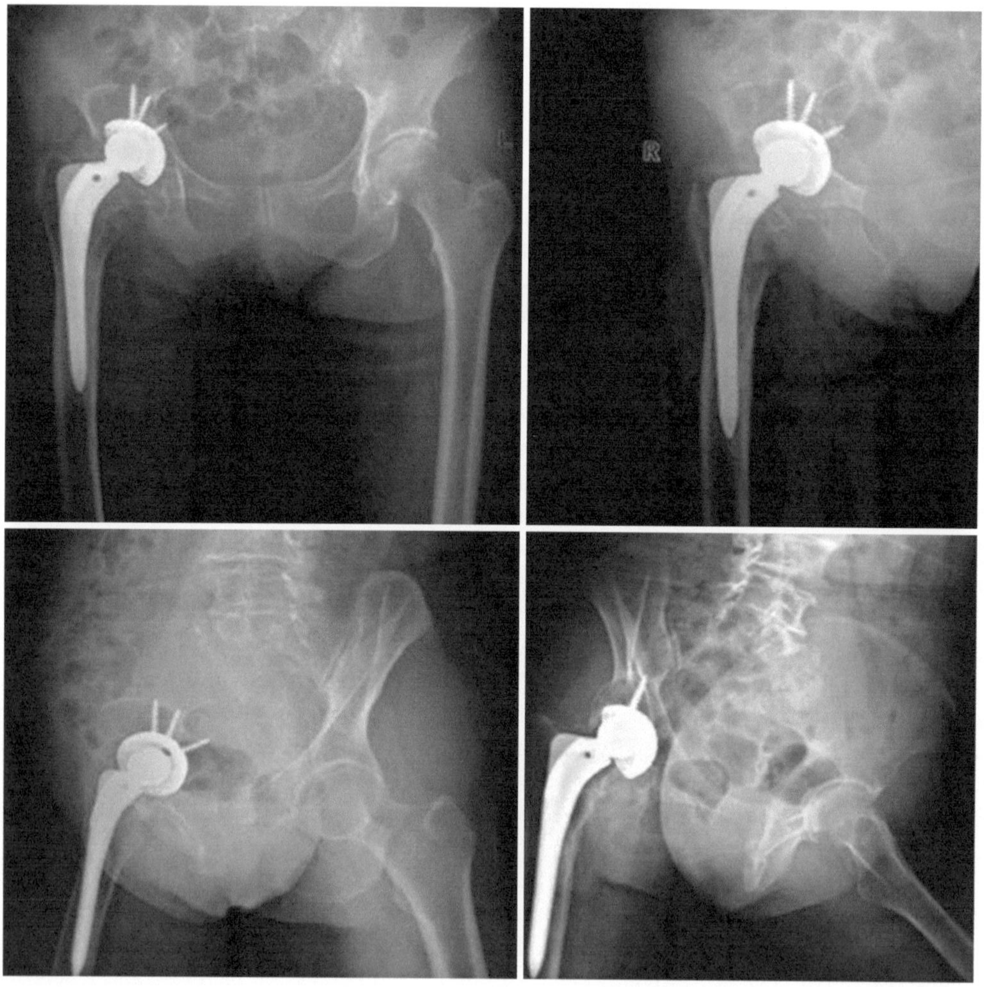

Fig. 3.32 Preoperative X-ray

osteolysis had exceeded 2.5 or even 3 cm of the upper margin of the acetabular cup within the ilium, reaching the junction of the true and false pelvis. Although the acetabular cup revealed no obvious migration, the osteolysis range was massive in its superior area. Therefore, it was considered a Paprosky IIIB bone defect. There was large-scale osteolysis in the posteriosuperior area around the cup and inferior ischial ramus. Thus, it should not be casually speculated that bone mass in the posterior area was not affected. It must be taken into consideration that the continuity of the posterior column could be broken.

According to the oblique radiographs, we had already lost the posterior column. The iliopectineal line and ilioischial line appeared to be a thin layer of cortex. Although complete, deformed, and tortuous dense shadows could be seen, it was in fact a layer of soft and thin residual cortical bone, with poor condition and mass. It could provide neither biological bone ingrowth nor mechanical stability (non-supportive).

3.8.3 Preoperative Planning

In cases like this, we should not be deceived by the dense shadow of the bone cortex. It could be considered that the posterior column had lost its mechanics. The superoposterior part was not supported; thus, a supporting point was required. A buttress augment could not only build a superior supporting point but also rebuild part of the posterior column due to its shape. Therefore, the reconstruction of the superoposterior area with buttress augment required an ilium that was high enough, biologically active, and provided mechanical support. This was actually a type of extended fixation. If it was not enough for bone reconstruction to merely add a disc-shaped augment to the deep layer of the buttress augment, we placed a slope augment in the deep layer of the buttress augment. The shape detail of disc-shaped augment and slope augment did not matter much. In addition, the patient used an acetabular cup along with non-crosslinked polyethylene (non-XLPE) and this hip system was not good for hip mechanics. After years of clinical utilization of this type of prosthesis, periprosthetic osteolysis had been found in many patients.

Why was stem retrieval and exchange not considered? Spot welding was found around the stem; osseointegration occurred; no windshield-wiper loosening; no coronal migration or subsidence; and no stem loosening. From the perspective of historical follow-up examination, the fixation of this stem was good. Of course, removing the stem also had advantages, such as easy to expose the acetabulum and adjust the biological parameters of the hip, leg length, stem anteversion, and offset of extremity. If stem removal was planned, it should be performed rapidly. If it cannot be completed in 10 min, ETO should be performed right away.

For small osteolysis around the acetabular cup, it has also been reported that a window can be directly opened around the acetabular cup to clean up the osteolysis area to perform bone grafting or augment placement without removing the acetabular cup when it is well fixed. In this case, osteolysis was severe, and acetabular cup revision was necessary.

3.8.4 Surgical Procedure and Intraoperative Observation

The porous tantalum augment (shim augment) was trimmed during the operation to make it fit the bone defect in the ischial ramus. It was subsequently impacted to establish inferoposterior supporting and fixation points. The buttress augment was applied in the superior area to reconstruct the supporting and fixation points. Meanwhile, three slope augments were placed in the deep part of the buttress augment, and a disc augment was applied to reconstruct the medial wall.

The abduction angle of the acetabular cup was small. When the polyethylene liner was implanted, it caused minor migration of the shim augment. However, the disc medial wall augment was connected to the acetabular cup by bone cement.

Postoperative immediate radiograph of the right side (Fig. 3.33) showed that the rotation center of the hip joint was well reconstructed.

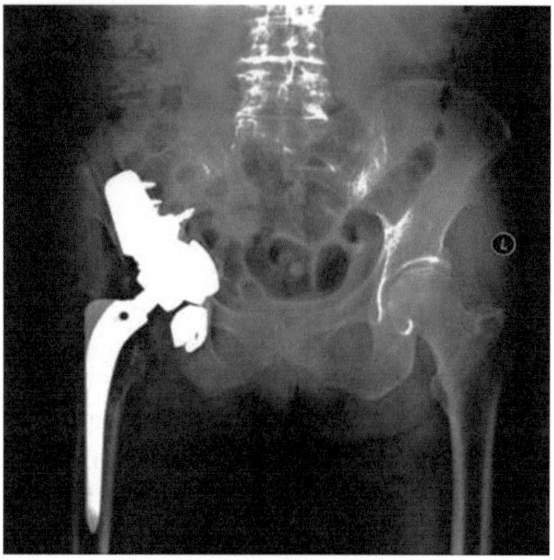

Fig. 3.33 Immediate postoperative radiograph

3.8.5 Postoperative Outcome

During the 2.6-year follow-up after the operation, the patient developed no pain and was very satisfied. Tomosynthesis suggested very good bone ingrowth.

Postoperative X-rays after 3 months (Fig. 3.34) suggested that the right prosthesis was well fixed, and a small portion of the shim augment was knocked off in the lateral view to provide a better fit to the ischiatic defect. At first glance, the shim augment seemed to have no contact with the acetabular cup. In fact, it was connected and fixed with the acetabular cup via bone cement for support and fixation.

Postoperative tomosynthesis of the right hip joint at 8 months (Fig. 3.35) showed radial trabeculae (white arrows) connected to a porous metal surface around the superior buttress augment and the inferior shim augment. This was a typical sign of bone ingrowth (spot welds), which indicated that the prosthesis had achieved long-term biological fixation.

Both prostheses were seen well fixed 2.6 years after revision. Postoperative X-rays 2.6 years after revision are shown in Fig. 3.36.

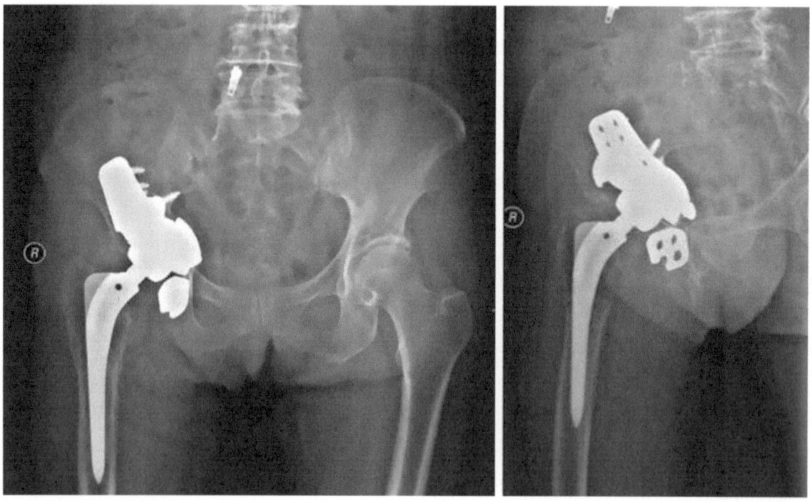

Fig. 3.34 Postoperative X-rays after 3 months

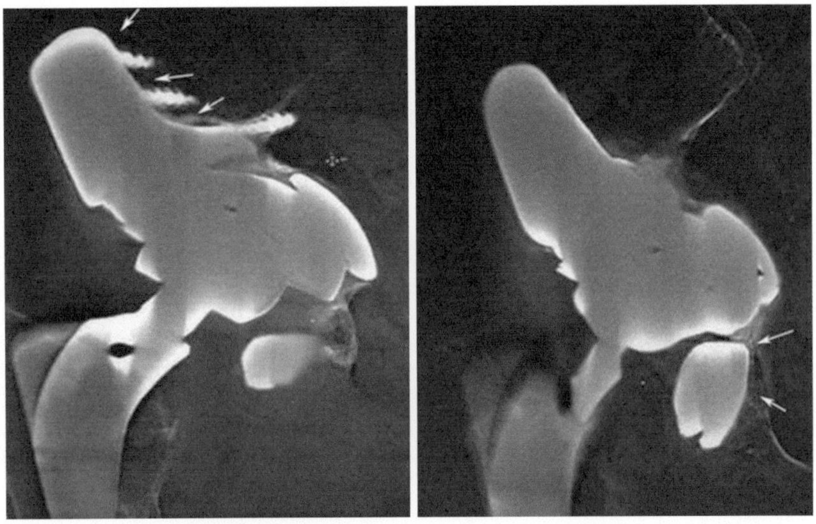

Fig. 3.35 Postoperative tomosynthesis 8 months after revision

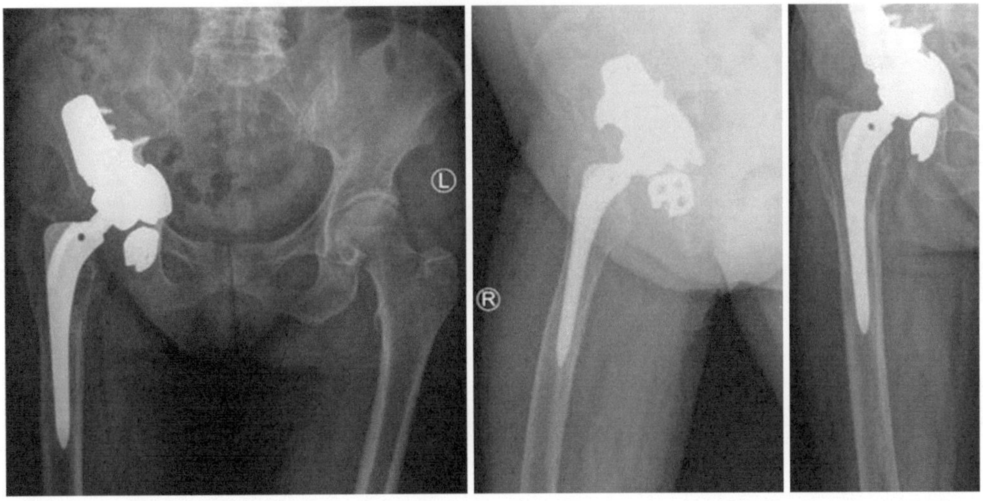

Fig. 3.36 Postoperative X-rays 2.6 years after revision

3.9 Case 8

Yong Huang and Hongyi Shao

3.9.1 Case Summary

Medical History A 56-year-old male presented with pain for 2 years after left THA 25 years ago. No special medical history.

Physical Examination The patient entered the ward with claudication; no pelvic tilt; left hip joint revealed discrepancy and flexion deformity; incision cicatrix could be seen; no joint inflammation or swelling; left groin area tenderness (+); axial percussion pain (+); obviously limited mobility; left Patrick's sign (+); left Thomas's sign (+); left Trendelenburg's sign (+); and Allis's sign (+).

Laboratory Examination No abnormality was detected in a routine blood test, ESR, or CRP.

Radiographic Data Preoperative X-rays and CT are shown in Figs. 3.37 and 3.38.

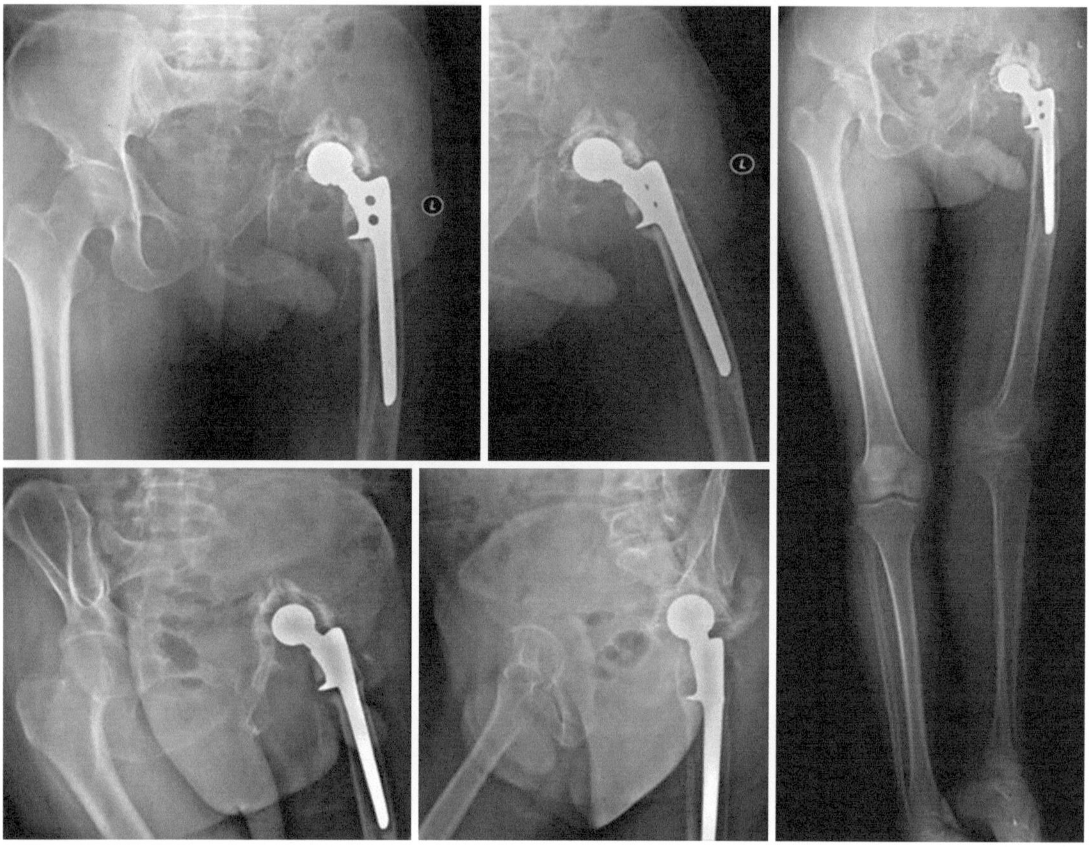

Fig. 3.37 Preoperative X-rays

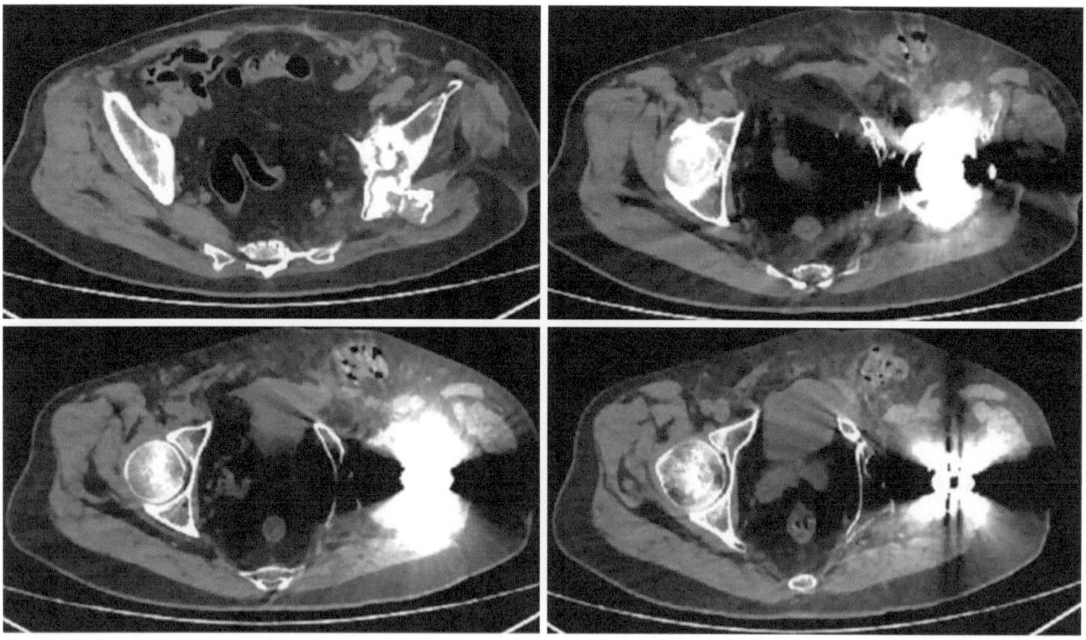

Fig. 3.38 Preoperative plain CT scan

3.9.2 Case Analysis and Preoperative Planning

1. Radiography Illustration.
   (a) According to anteroposterior and oblique views of the X-ray, there was a transverse fracture and a fracture line on the acetabulum side. The upper and lower segments were discontinuous, and the lower segments revealed counterrotation. The obturator foramens were asymmetric on both sides. The defect in the ischial ramus was large, and the continuity of the ilioischial line was lost. Therefore, it was estimated that the prosthesis had touched the medial wall. The oblique view showed discontinuity in the anterior and posterior columns. In consequence, the patient had pelvic discontinuity. According to the RPC theory, it was likely that the anterior column and the posterior column of the patient were in poor condition. Pelvic discontinuity and how to improve the initial stability of the acetabular side should be thoroughly considered in the reconstruction. The femoral greater trochanter was missing, suggesting that the gluteus medius might be damaged.
   (b) According to the full-length lower extremity film, the affected knee joint significantly migrated upward compared with the opposite side, indicating a discrepancy in the affected lower extremity, which was relatively severe. In addition, the lower extremity was in a fixed external rotation position, and joints were notably stiff. It was presumed that the patient had a significant problem with both greater and lesser trochanter. In addition, the patient should be further evaluated in the coronal view for any deformity, and how to expose the joint should be considered due to the poor cortical condition.
2. The reconstruction strategy
   (a) Through preoperative AP and lateral views of X-rays, it could be inferred that the patient had more than one surgery. As this revision was going to be difficult, the residents were suggested to ask about the patient's medical history and treatment experience in detail first. Based on the imaging findings, such severe bone destruction should not have occurred within only 2 years. Second, the general condition of the patient should be evaluated; any historical conditions should be considered to determine whether he is suitable for revision in his current physical condition. From the perspective of physical examination, combined with the possibility of greater trochanter dissolution and gluteal muscle injury evaluated from imaging, the patient should be asked to perform hip flexion, extension, and other actions, even if abduction could not be done, so that the situation of myodynamia and any muscle contraction and joint motion problem could be determined.
   (b) If a comprehensive evaluation and physical examination of the patient suggested that he was suitable for revision surgery, the condition of the acetabular side and femur side should be analyzed specifically.
      - Due to the evident pelvic discontinuity on the acetabular side, it should be considered whether it would affect the operation. If it was difficult to predict the 3D shape of the acetabular side, the pelvic model could be 3D-printed so that it could be used to design the reconstruction method combined with the RPC theory. In particular, if the condition of the pelvic and acetabular side was not clear, the surgery should not be rushed to the surgery. The intraoperative situation was likely to be more complex than imagined. ETO should be considered.
      - There was obvious stem loosening on the femur side, and the bone morphology of local X-ray and full-length film should be specifically studied. Proximal osteotomy should be considered if the deformity was observed in coronal view. The greater trochanter of the patient was

missing; thus, the abductor force should be strengthened even if the gluteus medius had contraction. The prosthesis could be affected if the abductor strength was not sufficient in the long term.

3.9.3 Surgical Procedure and Intraoperative Observation

1. The left hip was dissected layer by layer through a modified Gibson approach to expose the hip. There were no obvious signs of infection such as pus or necrosis, the acetabular component was loose, as well as the femur component.
2. The acetabulum and femur prosthesis were successfully retrieved. Severe bone defect could be observed on the acetabular side with pelvic transection fracture. Structural bone defect presented in lateral, superoposterior, and inferoposterior areas. The cicatrix tissue of the acetabulum was resected. The fossa ovalis was cleared and the acetabulum was reamed to 66 mm.
3. Buttress augment was applied to the superolateral acetabulum and slope augment was applied to the inferoposterior area. A 66-mm non-cement cup was impacted with bone cement connecting the cup and the augments. The abduction angle was 40°; the anteversion angle was 20°; and the prosthesis was fixed with three screws.
4. The femur was rasped in a sequential fashion and a Wagner-type stem (16/225 mm) was applied in the distal end and a 19 + 30 mm body in the proximal end. A 36 mm + 5 ceramic femoral head was fixed. After restoring the alignment, the range of motion was satisfied. It was rinsed and sutured layer by layer.

3.9.4 Postoperative Condition and Outcome

1. Postoperative rehabilitation: Based on the principle of "mobilization in early stage and weight-bearing in later stage," we instructed the patient to mobilize the hip and walk on crutches as early as possible to prevent complications and regain confidence. The patient could be instructed to prepare a weight scale. Stepping on a scale with toes would help understand how 10 and 20 kg felt like. In general, patients are usually instructed to support their toes with heels dangling and try to maintain 10–15 kg weight in the first month. In the second month, patients can be asked to put their entire feet flat and try to maintain a weight of 20–25 kg. Although such rehabilitation instructions are relatively sketchy, the effect is always better than directly putting the patients on crutches.
2. Postoperative radiography: It could be seen more clearly from the radiographs that the pelvis had obvious transection, therefore augments and screws were applied on the superior and inferior acetabulum, and the femur side was also dissected. The external rotation of the patient's lower extremity could be caused by long-term posture. In terms of gait, there was no anatomical abnormality, but a certain degree of gluteal gait could be seen. Therefore, gluteus medius was not specially treated during the operation. If the soft tissue between the gluteus medius and lateral femoral muscles was in good continuity, there was no need for intraoperative special treatment. The shallow and deep hip sleeves were sufficient to provide reliable tension.

Postoperative X-rays after 3 days are shown in Fig. 3.39. Postoperative follow-up X-rays after 1 year are shown in Fig. 3.40, and postoperative tomosynthesis after 1 year is shown in Fig. 3.41.

The tomosynthesis indicates that the revision had good results. If curved osteotome was used, attention should be paid to the osseointegration around the screw holes. Postoperative tomosynthesis suggests that screws were the reliable choice for better fixation results.

3.9.5 Conclusion and Reflection

The first impression of the patient's preoperative radiographic data was a "very tricky case." However, a qualified orthopedic surgeon should

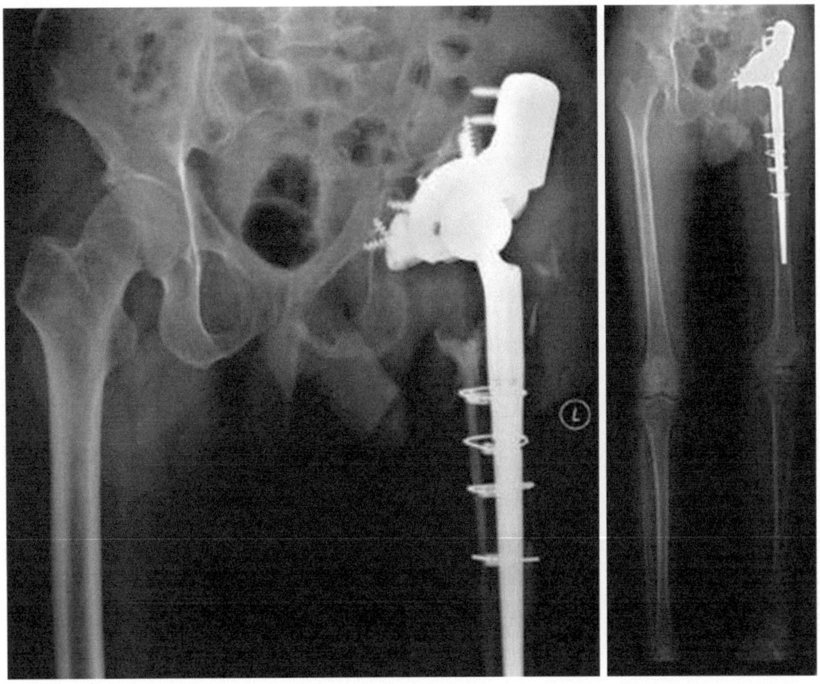

Fig. 3.39 Postoperative X-rays after 3 days

Fig. 3.40 Postoperative follow-up X-rays after 1 year

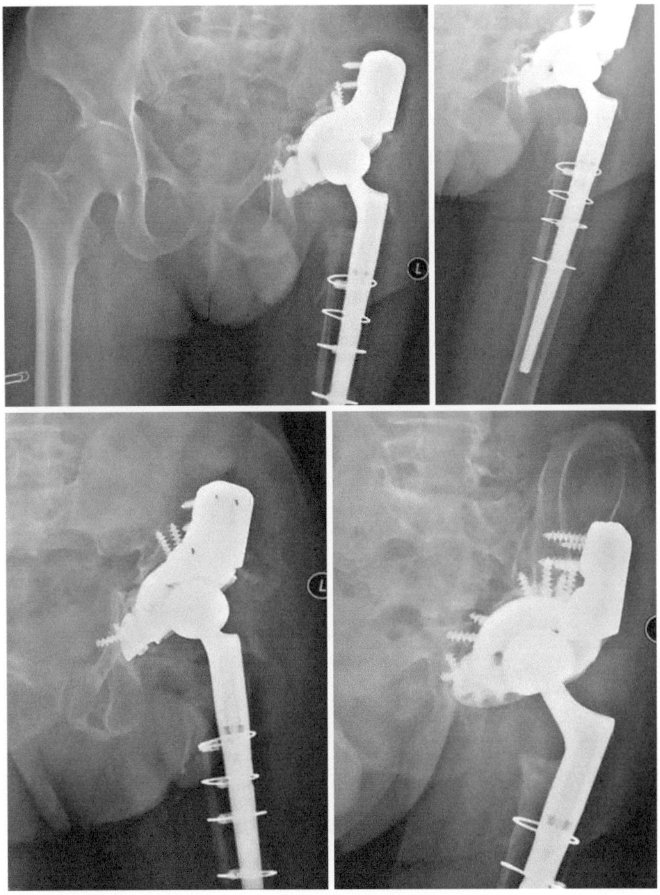

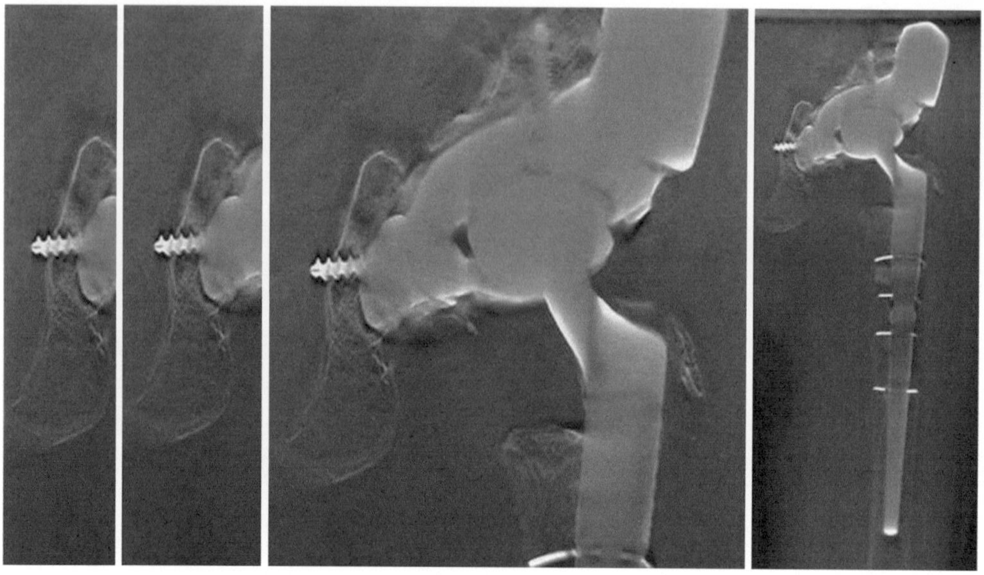

Fig. 3.41 Postoperative tomosynthesis after 1 year

not flinch from such cases. Despite the pelvic transection fracture and missing greater trochanter in this patient, it was not impossible to revise. Admittedly, various risks and uncertainties would occur intraoperatively. In the face of these surgical risks, the surgeon team should discuss in detail with the patients and their families: Is there a better strategy provided by any other medical team or institution? Is there a following solution for these risks? Does the patient understand and accept all these risks?

Recommended Reading

1. Paprosky W G, Perona P G, Lawrence J M. Acetabular defect classification and surgical reconstruction in revision arthroplasty. A 6-year follow-up evaluation.J Arthroplas, 1994;9(1):33-44.
2. Zhou Y. Cementless acetabular reconstruction based on the ring-point-column theory. J Clin Orthop Res. 2019;4(1):1–2.
3. Deng W, Wu T, Wang Z, Shao H, Yang D, Zhou Y. Medial wall reconstruction using metal disc augments in revision total hip arthroplasty. Int Orthop. 2023;47(5):1203–12.

4 Periprosthetic Femoral Fracture

Hanlong Zheng, Shengjie Guo, Yixin Zhou, and Yong Huang

4.1 Introduction

Hanlong Zheng and Shengjie Guo

Periprosthetic femoral fracture (PFF) is one of the most serious and common postoperative complications after THA. With the increasing application of biological total hip arthroplasty (THA) and patient life expectancy, the number of PFF cases has been rising in recent years.

4.1.1 Epidemiology

Most PFFs occur on the femur side. PFFs on the acetabular side are less frequent. Meek et al. [1] reported the largest retrospective cohort study to date. Out of 52,136 patients who underwent primary THA, the PFF rate within 10 years was 1.7%; among 8726 patients with revision THA, the PFF rate was 6.2%. There was a linear correlation between postoperative PFF rate and time in first-time THA patients, whereas the PFF risk in patients with revision THA was higher within 2 years and between 5 and 10 years. PFF is also one of the common causes of revision THA.

H. Zheng (✉) · S. Guo · Y. Zhou · Y. Huang
Department of Adult Joint Reconstructive Surgery, Beijing Jishuitan Hospital, Capital Medical University, Beijing, China

4.1.2 Risk Factors

Female, advanced age, revision THAs, obesity, and bone metabolic disorders are the most mentioned risk factors for PFF. Patients preoperatively diagnosed with arthritis before primary THA are more likely to suffer from PFF. Another risk factor is undergoing primary THA because of a femoral neck fracture. Patients may also suffer osteoporosis or multiple complications and have a higher risk of fall. Thus, preoperative diagnosis of osteoarthritis is a protective factor of postoperative PFF.

In terms of stem selection, the overall postoperative PFF rate in cases with non-cement femoral stem is higher. Risk factors associated with post-THA PFF include aseptic loosening of the femoral stem, osteolysis due to polythene detritus-induced bio-inflammatory responses, and femoral morphology. Patients who had received hip revision are at a much higher risk of developing PFF than first-time THA patients.

4.1.3 Diagnosis and Evaluation

AP and lateral radiograph is a key examination for PFF diagnosis. It plays a significant role in judging fracture site, classification, stem stability, bone condition around the femoral stem, and whether the acetabular component is loose or not. However, about 20–47% of stem loosening is not visible on the radiograph. Compared

Y. Zhou (ed.), *Revision Total Hip Arthroplasty*, https://doi.org/10.1007/978-981-97-9804-9_4

with X-ray, CT is relatively more reliable in judging the stability of the stem, but it can be affected by the artifacts of metal implants. In recent years, tomosynthesis has been gradually applied in artificial articular implantation. It is the most effective radiological examination to determine stem loosening, which can be employed to detect the degree of osseointegration of the biological coating of non-cement stem. It is also suitable for PFF, especially for cases in which the stability of the stem is difficult to judge by preoperative X-ray. On the other hand, the medical history of patients should be inquired in detail. If hip pain occurs before the fracture, it indicates that loosening is likely to have occurred.

4.1.4 Classification

In the early years, PFF was usually categorized by Johansson and AAOS classification, which were of little significance for clinical treatment. In 1996, Duncan et al. proposed the Vancouver classification, the most widely applied classification clinically to date. Other ones are rarely mentioned nowadays.

Vancouver A fracture occurs in the proximal femur trochanter area and is divided into fracture of the greater trochanter (Vancouver AG) and fracture of the lesser trochanter (Vancouver AL). Vancouver B fracture occurs in periprosthetic or slightly below the distal stem, which is the most common type clinically. According to the degree of stem stability and bone mass, it can be further divided into Type B1 (the stem is well fixed), Type B2 (stem is loose with good bone mass), and Type B3 (loose stem with severe bone loss). Vancouver C fracture occurs in the distal femoral stem, in which the stem is usually stable without significant bone loss. Subsequently, the author of this classification proposed a unified classified system (UCS classification) in 2014, which was almost exactly consistent with the principle of Vancouver classification, while Type D was added as a fracture between the hip and knee prosthesis. See Appendix B for details.

4.1.5 Treatment Principles

1. Type A
   (a) AG (A1): It is generally accepted that if the fracture migration is less than 2 cm, non-surgical treatment should be considered. A better result can be achieved by walking with weight-bearing protection or wearing abduction support for 6–8 weeks. Migrated AG fracture usually requires surgical treatment with the option of wire binding, cable, screw, or greater trochanteric claw plate fixation.
   (b) AL (A2): A typical AL-type fracture is relatively rare; an avulsion fracture is the most common type. In fact, fractures in lesser trochanter that do not involve the stem are very rare. Most of the fractures occurring in the lesser trochanter clinically usually invade the stem, which are in fact Vancouver B fracture. Conservative treatment or tying alone may cause potential instability. If stem loosening occurs at the same time, it usually needs to be revised.
2. Type B: It is the most common type clinically, accounting for more than 70%. Conservative treatment is usually inconclusive, which only applies to patients not suitable for surgery in most cases. Most Type B fracture cases require surgical treatment.
   (a) B1: The basic principle of the treatment of B1 fracture is to perform open reduction and internal fixation (ORIF) under accurate evaluation of femoral stem stability. Options include a cable-plate system, locking compression plate (LCP), intramedullary nail, regular dynamic compression plate, memory alloy embracing fixator, and wiring, in which the first two are the most common ones. At the distal site of the plate, a length of more than twice the femoral diameter should be reserved. It is the key to healing; otherwise, fracture may reoccur in the stress-concentrating area. Excessive soft tissue stripping and destruction of blood flow at the fracture end will also affect the healing. If screws are used for internal fixa-

tion, at least eight layers of cortex should be fixed on the distal side of the plate and at least four layers on the proximal side. The indwelling of three or four screw holes in the fracture end can increase the working length of the plate effectively.

The postoperative failure rate in Type B1 fracture is higher than that in other types, the most significant reason for which is the application of a single fixation method and inaccurate evaluation of stem stability. Lindhal et al. analyzed 1049 patients with PFF, finding that preoperative diagnosis of Type B1 fracture is a highly significant risk factor leading to failure. It is also recommended that surgeons should assume all Type B PFF include stem loosening unless its stability can be demonstrated.

The authors believe that for some Type B1 fractures, although the stem is stable, internal fixation alone may lead to fixation failure, in which long-stem revision may be a better choice, especially for transverse or short oblique fractures at the tip of the stem. However, these perspectives are still controversial.

(b) B2 and B3: Type B2 and B3 fractures are accompanied by femoral stem loosening. Although some surgeons believe that open reduction and internal fixation can be performed in some cases, most patients require revision with a long stem. Meanwhile, attention should be paid to whether the acetabular component is loose. During revision, operation time should be monitored, and damage control needs to be applied as much as possible. Extended Trochanter Osteotomy (ETO) can be performed along the fracture line if the stem is difficult to retrieve. The outcome uncemented revision with long stem as PFF treatment is usually more ideal than cement stem; the latter is only suitable for elderly, weaker patients with shorter life expectancy. There are several options, ranging from non-cement, full-coated cylindrical long stem with a fixed distal end, non-modular, conical, ridged titanium stem, and modular stem. Among them, modular stem comes with various distal and proximal components in different sizes, which achieves good results in the revision of PFF.

The principle of Type B3 fracture treatment is basically the same as that of Type B2 fracture, but due to the large bone defect, sometimes it is necessary to restore bone mass. Compression bone grafting, allogeneic cortical bone plate, artificial bone, allograft prosthesis composite (APC), or proximal femur replacement can be applied in bone mass restoration. However, infection is an unavoidable problem in bone grafting. After performing more than 100 cases of revision of PFF, we believe that for most of the B2 and B3 fractures, modular stem revision is enough to restore bone stock without bone grafting.

3. Type C: It is relatively rare. This type usually involves a stable stem; thus, it can be fixed by plate, wiring, or retrograde intramedullary nail according to the principle of ordinary distal femoral fracture treatment. Screw-plate system or cable-plate system is most used clinically.
4. UCS Type D: The treatment of this type is complicated, especially in cases with knee prosthesis with extending rods or THA stem loosening. If the knee prosthesis is attached with an extending rod, and both hip and knee prostheses are stable, a long locking plate is recommended for internal fixation. If a fracture occurs between the hip and the knee prosthesis with an extending rod, along with stem loosening or poor bone condition, treatment is difficult. Sometimes a custom-made tumor prosthesis or a connection rod of an extension stem is required.

Because of frequent multiple complications in PFF patients and complicated surgical methods, the overall mortality and reoperation rates are high. Nevertheless, most deaths are not caused by the surgery itself. The high reoperation rate was mainly due to aseptic loosening, refracture, dislocation, non-union, infection, or a combination of multiple factors, most of which occur within 2 years after the operation. The healing rate of fracture is often between 75% and 100%, but most of these cases cannot fully restore hip function before fracture. In conclusion, as the most serious and increasingly common failure after THA, periprosthetic fracture remains a major challenge today.

4.2 Case 1

Shengjie Guo and Hanlong Zheng

4.2.1 Case Summary

Medical History A 57-year-old female complained of "post-traumatic hip pain (right) with limited mobility for 3 days." The patient underwent right THA due to avascular necrosis of the femoral head 4 years ago and recovered well. She developed right hip pain with limited mobility after a fall while riding a bicycle 3 days ago. The patient was admitted to the hospital with a "periprosthetic fracture following THA" (right).

Physical Examination The patient was led into the ward on a gurney; right hip deformity with discrepancy and external rotation; angulation deformity in the middle of the thigh; local tenderness (+); vertical percussion pain in the right lower extremity (+); and loss of mobility in the right lower extremity.

P84

Laboratory Examination Routine blood test and CRP were high, and ESR was normal.

Radiographic Data See Fig. 4.1 for the preoperative X-ray.

4.2.2 Case Analysis

1. Radiographic examination of the right hip:
   (a) The original prosthesis was ABG II, and no obvious migration of the non-cement acetabular or femoral prosthesis was observed. The position was good.
   (b) Short oblique fracture in distal femoral stem.
   (c) Vancouver B1 was considered for this PFF.
2. Diagnosis: PFF following right THA.

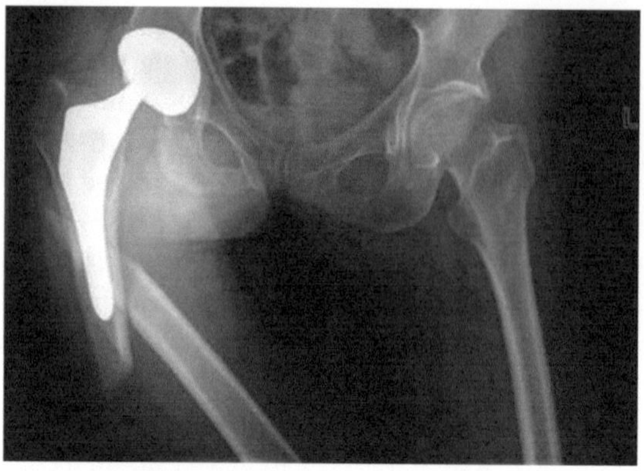

Fig. 4.1 Preoperative X-ray

4.2.3 Preoperative Planning

1. According to radiography, the femoral stem had no obvious migration; thus, it should be classified as a Type B1 fracture. Only internal fixation was required if intraoperative examination confirmed the stability.
2. It should be borne in mind that sometimes fractures around the proximal coating are not easy to find. If this was the case, it should be treated as a Type B2 fracture and a revision stem should be prepared.

4.2.4 Operation Situation

1. Intraoperative examination indicated a short oblique fracture in the distal end, with an intact metaphysis cortex. The stem was stable.
2. After the alignment of the fracture end was restored, a locking compression plate (LCP) was applied for fixation. A screw was inserted into the proximal greater trochanter, combined with cable binding. Monocortical and bicortical screws were applied alternately for distal fixation.

4.2.5 Postoperative Condition and Outcome

1. The patient was instructed to walk with crutches within 3 months after operation.
2. Hip flexion and abduction exercises were gradually intensified within 3 months after the operation.
3. Postoperative reexamination data
   (a) Postoperative X-rays after 3 months are shown in Fig. 4.2.
   (b) In postoperative outpatient reexamination asfter 2 years, the Harris score was 98. X-rays (Fig. 4.3) indicated that the fracture was healed and the stem was stable.

PPP

4.2.6 Conclusion and Reflection

1. Type B1 and B2: One major factor in determining how to treat PFF is the stability of the femoral stem. Therefore, it is necessary to be cautious in determining B1 fracture. The outcome of single internal fixation in many cases

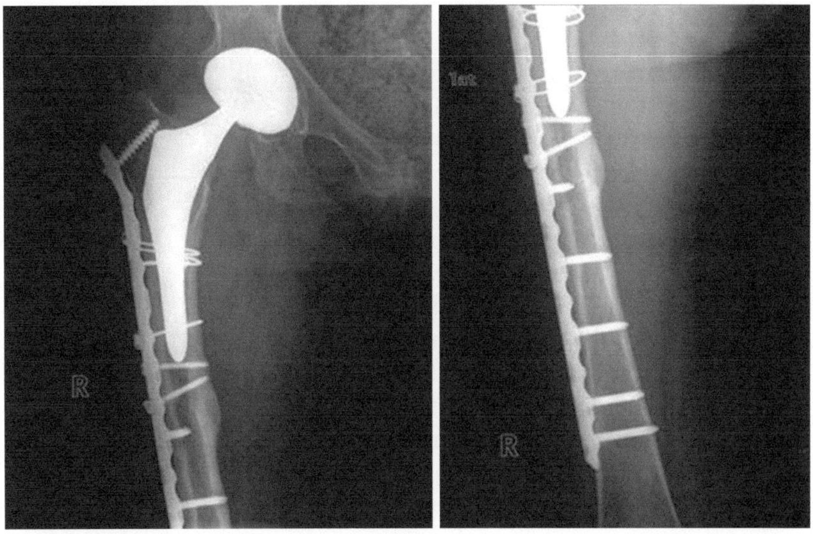

Fig. 4.2 Postoperative X-rays after 2 years

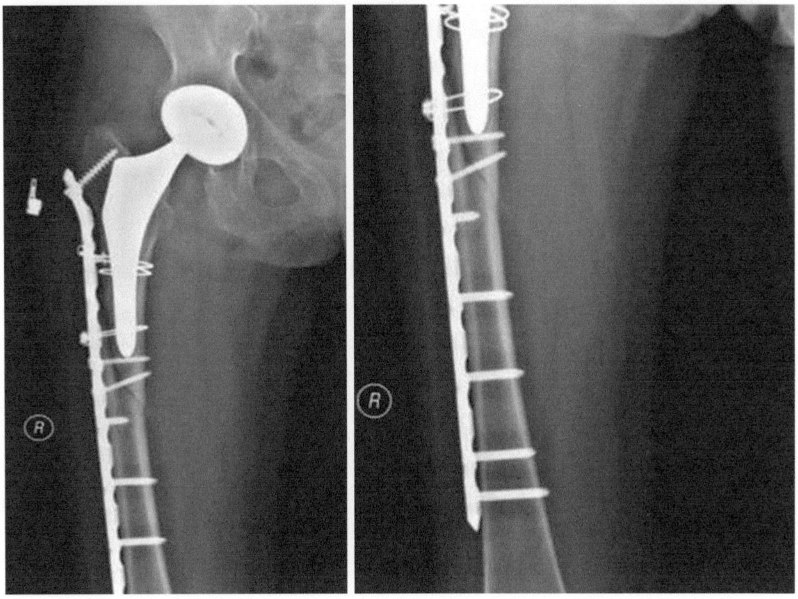

Fig. 4.3 Postoperative X-rays after 3 months

of so-called Type B1 fracture is not ideal (requiring revision), one of the crucial reasons for which is the misidentification of Type B2 as B1. In other words, many cases treated as Type B1 fracture that failed in fact should have been B2 fracture. In consequence, evaluation solely based on preoperative X-rays is not completely reliable. Intraoperative judgment of whether a periprosthetic fracture occurred, especially around the coating that affects stability, should be made to accurately evaluate the stability.

In addition, on some specific occasions, even though preoperative and intraoperative evaluation is sufficient to identify it as a Type B1 fracture, we should still treat it as B2, with the application of revision stem. Generally, the following factors need to be comprehensively considered to make decisions: (1) The age and physical condition of the patient; (2) whether the osseointegration (coating) area of the original stem has been significantly affected; (3) whether the intactness of the cement sheath of cement stem has been obviously affected; (4) what the morphology of fracture is (short oblique, transverse or long oblique, long spiral fracture), and whether it can be restored and secured (in some comminuted fractures, it is difficult to obtain good alignment and solid reconstruction in the future, which is likely to form stress concentration in distal stem); and (5) whether the acetabular side requires treatment in the meanwhile.

2. Internal fixation of Type B1 fracture: The internal fixation of Type B1 fracture requires detailed attention. The following bullet points are worth mentioning.
   (a) The application of a plate in the lateral femur requires longer material. Minimally invasive plate osteosynthesis technique (MIPO) can be employed, in which the screws can be inserted based on the "far far, near near" principle (both close ends of the fracture and both distal ends of the fracture).
   (b) Cable cannot be used alone for short oblique or transverse fractures because of its poor rotation resistance. Application of bicortical or monocortical screws can greatly improve the stability of fixation.
   (c) The two-plane fixation is more reliable. Usually, the plate is placed in the lateral femur, and an allogeneic bone plate is placed in the front of or medial femur. Local bone grafting is good for fracture healing.

4.3 Case 2

Shengjie Guo and Hanlong Zheng

4.3.1 Case Summary

Medical History A 28-year-old male complained of "5 years after right THA, post-traumatic pain with limited mobility for 10 days." The patient underwent bilateral THAs due to both hip involvement of ankylosing spondylosis 5 years ago. Postoperative recovery was ideal. He developed right hip pain with limited mobility after a fall 10 days ago. The outpatient department admitted him with a "periprosthetic fracture (right) after THA."

Physical Examination The patient entered the ward on a gurney; the right hip showed discrepancy and external rotation deformity; angulation deformity was seen in the middle of the thigh with local tenderness (+); difficulty in motion of right lower extremity; and the motion of each toe of the right foot was normal.

Laboratory Examination White Blood Cell (WBC) was high in routine blood tests, and CRP was high.

Radiographic Data Preoperative X-ray is shown in Fig. 4.4.

4.3.2 Case Analysis

1. Radiographic examination of the right hip:
   (a) The acetabular side was non-cement, with a good position and no signs of loosening. The femoral side was cement-type, bound with cable.
   (b) Almost a traverse fracture occurred on the distal cement stem, and the cement sheath was not intact.

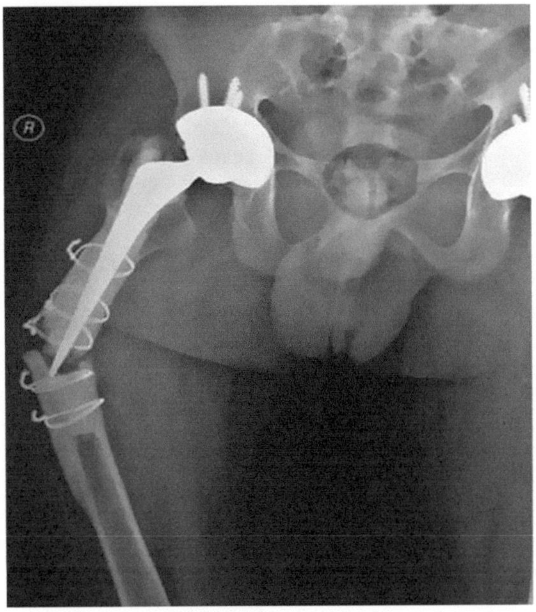

Fig. 4.4 Preoperative X-ray

(c) According to the Vancouver classification, if the bone cement was considered stable, it could be classified as a Type B1 fracture. However, if the stem and the cement sheath were regarded as one piece, in which the incomplete cement sheath was considered loosening, it could be classified as a Type B2 fracture.

2. Diagnosis: PFF following right THA.

4.3.3 Preoperative Planning

1. The acetabular component had no sign of loosening and required no special treatment.
2. Regardless of whether the case should be classified as a Type B1 or B2 fracture, the authors planned to treat it as a Type B2 fracture, and femoral stem revision was planned.

4.3.4 Operation Situation

1. The fracture end was exposed. The original binding wire was removed, and ETO was performed to the fracture end based on preoperative planning. The bone cement in the medullary cavity of the proximal femur was carefully cleaned to retrieve the femoral stem. Due to the difficulty of bone cement retrieval, along with the pre-existing severe osteoporosis-induced bone defect, the area below the lateral greater trochanter of the femoral bone had a fracture.
2. Intramedullary bone cement of the distal fracture end was carefully cleaned. Restoration Modular (RM) modular femoral stem was implanted, and a greater trochanter claw plate was applied combined with cortical bone allograft to secure the greater trochanter and the fracture end. Demineralized bone matrix (DBM) was injected locally to restore bone stock and for better healing.

Intraoperative observation is shown in Fig. 4.5. P88

4.3.5 Postoperative Condition and Outcome

1. Partial weight-bearing was instructed within 3 months with the aid of crutches.
2. Hip flexion and abduction exercises were gradually intensified from the second week to 3 months after the operation.
3. Postoperative reexamination data
   (a) Postoperative X-rays are shown in Fig. 4.6.
   (b) Re-examination at 6 months after operation revealed good healing. The Harris score was 76. Reexamination X-rays at 6 months after operation are shown in Fig. 4.7.

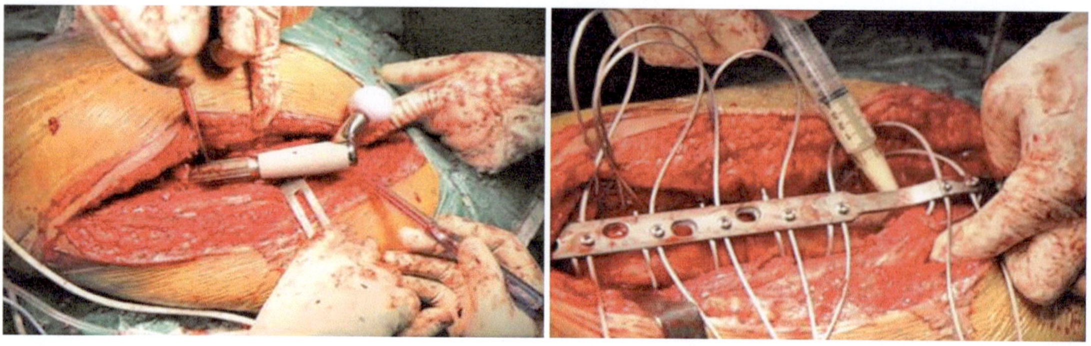

Fig. 4.5 Intraoperative observation

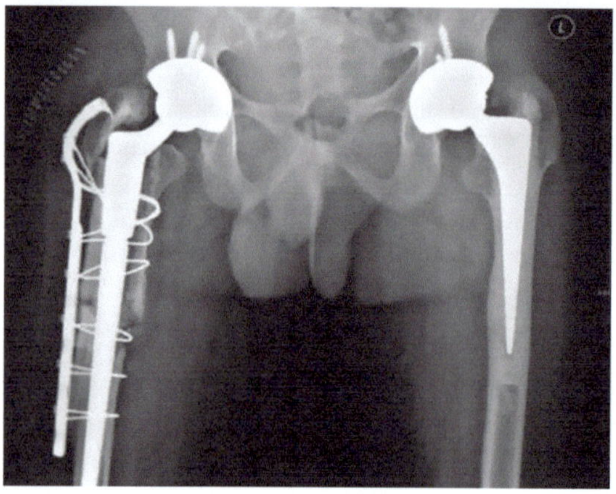

Fig. 4.6 Postoperative immediate X-ray

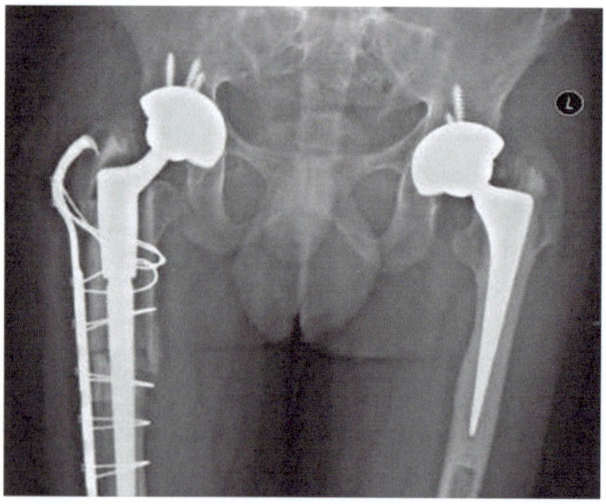

Fig. 4.7 Postoperative re-examination X-ray at 6 months

(c) In postoperative re-examination at 2 years, the Harris score was 93. The fracture was completely healed without pain. The patient could perform physical labor of moderate to high intensity. The components were stable with no subsidence or loosening. Peripheral bone condition was good. Postoperative X-rays at 2 years are shown in Fig. 4.8.

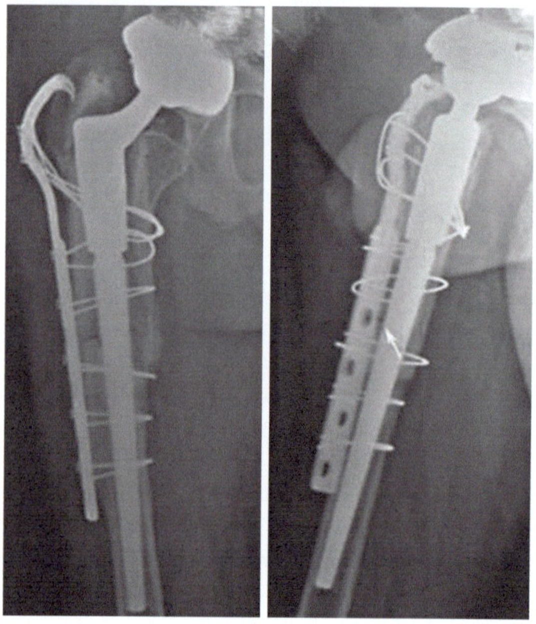

Fig. 4.8 Postoperative X-rays at 2 years

4.3.6 Conclusion and Reflections

1. The decision between revision stem and simple internal fixation: In terms of the preoperative decision between the two strategies, regardless of the classification, we listed the pros and cons of them.

   Single internal fixation was less traumatic and would cause no additional bone defect, but the main issue was whether it could be securely fixed and whether the stem could achieve effective long-term survival. Obviously, this was a transverse fracture of the distal cement stem. If internal fixation was applied, the best way was to combine the long plate and allograft bone plate with double-plane fixation. The transverse fracture had poor rotation resistance; thus, the proximal end could not be fixed solely with cable. Inserting screws (either monocortical or bicortical) would be hard to achieve with significant osteoporosis and was highly likely to damage the cement sheath, which was already damaged in the distal end. The long-term survival of the stem, a key issue to be considered for a young patient, was a serious concern. In addition, the medullary cavity in the fracture area was filled with bone cement, which seriously affected the blood flow within the medullary cavity. How much impact it had on fracture healing in the future? It could not be predicted! In short, if internal fixation was applied, there would be great uncertainty in terms of the fixation, bone healing in the future, and the long-term survival of the stem. These were exactly the most critical objectives for the success of the operation.

Revision stem strategy would undoubtedly lead to a relatively large surgical trauma and inevitably iatrogenic bone defect, but damage control could be achieved to a great extent. More importantly, a long revision stem, especially the distal fluted femoral stem, could function as central scaffolding. It could realize good control on the rotational stability of short oblique or transverse fractures like this. Combined with plate and allogeneic bone plate, it could reach a firm fixation. In addition, the excellent coating on the stem provided a good expectation for osseointegration.

In conclusion, after weighing the pros and cons, revision strategy was selected. Intraoperative application of an allogeneic bone plate and artificial bone could restore bone mass, and the postoperative follow-up examinations also proved that the decision was appropriate.

2. Scaffold technique: For Type B2 and B3 PFF, the authors increasingly lean toward the distal-fluted modular tapered stem. It can control the rotational stability of the fracture end well. This type of intramedullary fixation is like an architectural scaffold. For the fixation of the fracture, especially short oblique or transverse fractures, it can provide excellent fixation with the cable-plate system or allogeneic bone plate if necessary. The size and length of the proximal parts of the modular stem can be adapted with multiple options according to the specific situation of the host bone, leading to good osseointegration in the later stage.

4.4 Case 3

Yixin Zhou and Hanlong Zheng

4.4.1 Case Summary

Medical History An 81-year-old male complained of "left hip pain accompanied by limited mobility for 6 months after revision 4 years ago." The patient underwent left THA for a femoral neck fracture 8 years ago. The recovery was good. The patient developed left hip pain without obvious inducement 4 years ago, which was related to motion. Left hip revision was performed in another hospital (the details were unknown). He developed left hip pain 6 months ago, which gradually aggravated with limited mobility. He was admitted by the outpatient department with "PFF (left) following THA."

Physical Examination The patient was wheeled into the ward on a gurney; left lower extremity discrepancy and deformity; incision cicatrix of the posterolateral left hip was observed without redness and swelling; middle left thigh tenderness (+); axial percussion pain (+); and severe limited mobility.

Laboratory Examination Routine blood test was normal; CRP and ESR were normal.

Radiographic Data The preoperative X-rays are shown in Fig. 4.9.

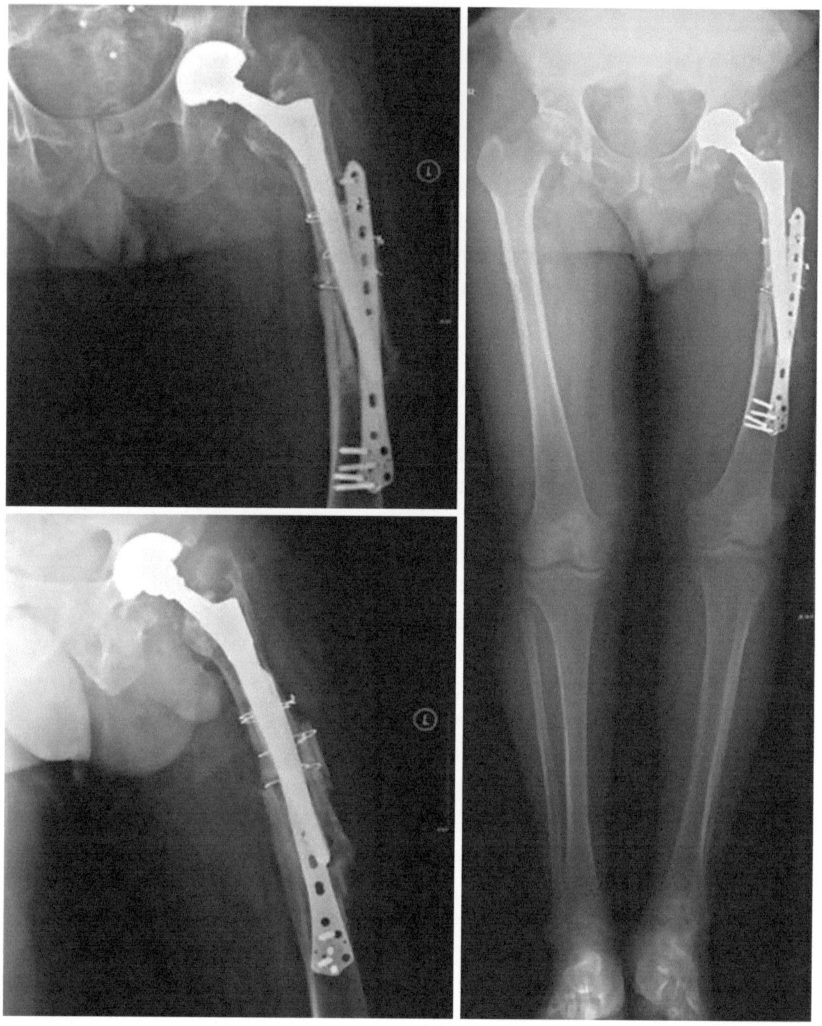

Fig. 4.9 Preoperative X-rays

4.4.2 Case Analysis

1. Infection was ruled out first.
2. Left hip radiographic data review:
   (a) The cup showed no obvious loosening or eccentric wear.
   (b) On the femoral side, the stem revealed significant subsidence and varus; varus deformity in the proximal femur. A fracture line was visible on the upper-middle segment of the medial femur and distal lateral stem. A plate was fixed in the lateral femur with cable and screws. Signs of loosening were shown on the proximal wire and screws.
   (c) Vancouver B3 was considered.
3. Diagnosis: PFF (left) following THA.

4.4.3 Preoperative Planning

1. The acetabular component showed no signs of loosening, but its positioning and angle were not ideal. Revision was considered.
2. The proximal fracture end could be split directly to retrieve the component. The fracture was closer to the distal end. It was a long oblique fracture; thus, a long revision stem should be prepared. The distal fracture

end required careful treatment so that the isthmus could be protected as much as possible.

4.4.4 Operation Situation

1. Invasion was through the original approach to fully expose the hip and fracture.
2. Lateral plates, wires, and screws were removed.
3. The proximal end was split and the distal end of the original Wagner stem was wrapped in plenty of bone cement, which was thoroughly cleaned.
4. The periacetabular area was exposed to retrieve the original acetabular component and a 60-mm trabecular metal cup and a 40-mm liner were placed.
5. The medullary cavity of the distal fracture was carefully exposed, and bone cement filling was also found around the opening. After the cement and soft tissue in the medullary cavity were thoroughly cleaned, a cable was applied for pre-cerclaging. After reaming, a medium-sized 21-mm (235-mm-long) RM taper fluted long distal stem was inserted. After testing, medium-sized 27-mm (+30-mm) proximal parts were inserted, a 40-mm dual-mobility head was installed, and the alignment was restored.
6. The fracture end and split proximal femur were fixed with a greater trochanter locking plate, with secondary cable fixation.

Intraoperative observation and postoperative immediate X-rays are shown in Figs. 4.10 and 4.11.

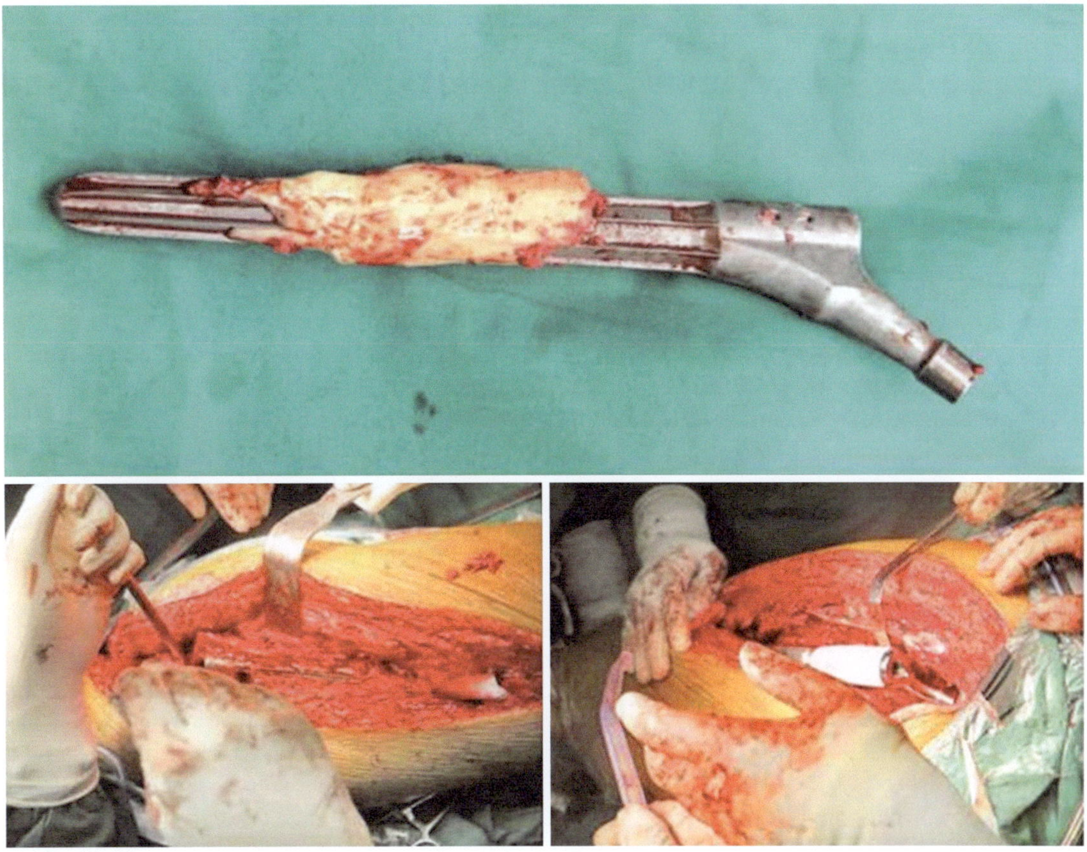

Fig. 4.10 Intraoperative view

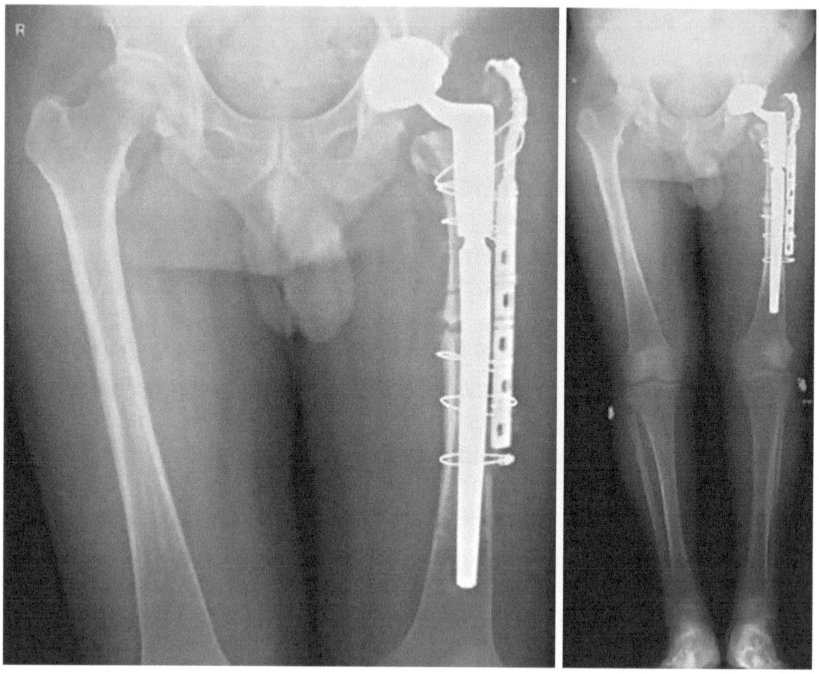

Fig. 4.11 Postoperative immediate X-rays

4.4.5 Postoperative Condition and Outcome

1. Partial weight-bearing was instructed within 3 months with the aid of crutches.
2. Hip flexion and abduction exercises were gradually intensified from the second week to 3 months after the operation.
3. Postoperative re-examination data
   (a) When the plate and titanium cable were applied for fixation, a fracture block was missed and escaped. In the early rehabilitation, the thigh was often reported with abnormal sounds, which recovered later.
   (b) In the telephone follow-up after 1.5 years, the patient could walk normally without support; his gait was normal; the patient could ride bicycles. The patient was completely free of pain; each lower extremity was equal in length; the Harris score of the hip was 89.

4.4.6 Conclusion and Reflection

1. Reflection-summary improvement: Revision is a window into another world for the surgeons. It is an opportunity to learn about a wide variety of failures and their different mechanisms. Provided with these learning opportunities, one can improve clinical practice with valuable experience.
   (a) For Type B2 and B3 fracture, to fully understand the role of scaffold technology on fracture stabilization, the basic requirement is to apply a long taper fluted stem (Wagner-type). For the non-cement type, the stem should cross the fracture end for 5 cm or more than twice the femur diameter when the placed into distal medullary cavity, and be fixed with at least 2 cm of the femoral cadre in the isthmus. Secondary fixation with cable-plate system or allogeneic bone plate can be applied according to specific situations.
   (b) Function of the longitudinal raised ridge on the long fluted tapered femoral stem: When it is buried inside the medullary cavity wall, it can control the rotational stability. As a non-cement femoral stem, osseointegration usually occurs at the root of the longitudinal raised ridge (where the main part of the femoral stem attaches to).

2. Effective isthmus: It was a long oblique fracture in this case. Isthmus in the most distal fracture end hardly remained. Nevertheless, if the bone defect around it was in fact less than one-third, it could still provide embracement on the stem. Therefore, the "effective isthmus" in this case could fix the stem with sufficient embracement. The foreign matters in the distal medullary cavity should be carefully cleaned to avoid additional bone defects. In addition, pre-cerclaging with cable in the distal fracture end was also necessary to maintain the embracement force of the medullary cavity.

4.5 Case 4

Yixin Zhou and Hanlong Zheng

4.5.1 Case Summary

Medical History An 80-year-old female complained of "post-traumatic pain accompanied by limited mobility for 12 days after revision right THA 12 years ago." The patient underwent right THA 22 years ago. She received the right revision THA 12 years ago due to loosening. After falling in the bathroom 12 days ago, she developed right hip pain with limited mobility. The patient was admitted by the outpatient department for "periprosthetic fracture (right) following THA." Previous hypertension for 10 years, controlled with oral drugs; long-term history of chronic asthma; Hashimoto's thyroiditis, with daily use of Euthyrox; and left THA was performed 9 months ago.

Physical Examination The patient was wheeled into the ward on a gurney; right hip shortening; posterolateral incision cicatrix was observed on both sides of the hip, without redness or swelling; right hip iliac area and middle thigh tenderness (+); axial percussion pain (+); and severely limited mobility.

Laboratory Examination Routine blood test : WBC 4.08 × 10^9/L, N 59.6%; CRP 42.6 mg/L; Hemoglobin (HGB) 96 g/L; total protein 59.4 g/L (ref: 60–83); albumin 36.9 g/L (ref: 34–48); T3 1.0 nmol/L (ref range: 1.2–3.1).

Radiographic Data Preoperative X-ray is shown in Fig. 4.12.

4.5.2 Case Analysis

1. Infection was excluded first.
2. Radiographic examination of the right hip:
   (a) Both the upper and lower components of the right hip were cement. There was no obvious migration of the cement cup, the position of which was normal without obvious eccentric wear.
   (b) A fracture line on the distal femoral stem was visible in good clarity, which was a short oblique spiral fracture.

   The medullary cavity of the proximal fracture area was stuffed with a cement stem. An unbroken lucent line between the cement sheath and the surrounding cortical bone could be seen, but the surface of the cement sheath was not smooth and overlapped with the bumps in the medullary cavity. Four loops of cable all seemed to have subsided into the abnormally thin cortical bone.

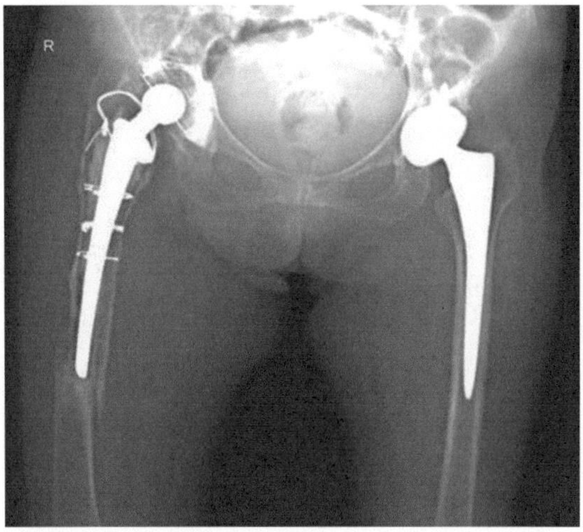

Fig. 4.12 Preoperative X-ray

There was also significant osteoporosis in the general distal fracture area, where the cortex was thin, with a small amount of bone cement in the opening.
   (c) Vancouver B3 PFF was considered.
3. Diagnosis: PFF following right THA.

4.5.3 Preoperative Planning

1. The patient was in elder age with a poor physical condition. He presented internal medical complications such as Chronic Obstructive Pulmonary Disease (COPD). Therefore, she was suggested to actively adjust her health condition and strengthen her respiratory training before the operation.
2. On the acetabular side: There was a lucent line between the bone cement and the bone matrix of the acetabular side, but it could not be determined whether the cup was loose or not, and the cup showed no obvious eccentric wear. Thus, it was planned that if the cup was found obviously loose during the operation, it should be retrieved. Otherwise, the cup was planned to be reserved. Damage control is significantly important!
3. On the femur side: Without splitting the proximal fracture section of the femur side, it was not easy to retrieve the femoral stem and bone cement and subsequently insert the revision stem after filing the medullary cavity. In consequence, the proximal fracture section was planned to be split during the operation. The isthmus remaining in the distal fracture was not abundant, where isthmus restoration could be performed to a certain extent in addition to avoiding collateral damage.

4.5.4 Operation Situation

1. Regional nerve block and low-dose general anesthesia were performed.
2. The incision was opened and extended to the proximal knee. The stem was retrieved after the proximal fracture segment was split lengthwise, and the residual intramedullary cement and soft tissue were cleaned thoroughly.
3. The fracture end was fully exposed and cleaned. The cable was pre-cerclaged at about 5 cm further from the fracture end. The distal medullary cavity was filled to 20.5 mm. A 21-mm RM cylindrical stem was inserted into the cavity, and another cable was tied 2 cm further from the fracture end. A 23-mm (+30-mm) proximal stem was implanted after the mold test.
4. The hip was moderately adjusted with abduction and internal rotation to close the proximal bone blocks, so that the femoral stem could be embraced, and the tension of gluteus medius could be maintained at an appropriate level. The greater trochanter cable-plate system was applied to fix the fracture block (as the cortex was thin, the plate could also provide strengthening and fixing to avoid the femur breaking when the cable was tightened up).

Intraoperative observation can be seen in Fig. 4.13.

4.5.5 Postoperative Condition and Outcome

1. The patient was instructed to walk with crutches 2 weeks after the operation, perform supine straight-leg raise training within 2 weeks, and partial weight-bear gradually increased to complete weight-bear within 6 months.
2. Functional exercises of hip flexor and abduction were gradually intensified within 3 months postoperation.
3. Postoperative re-examination data
   (a) Postoperative immediate X-ray is shown in Fig. 4.14.
   (b) The fracture was healed and the walking ability was normal at 5 months of re-examination. The affected extremity revealed a 2.5-mm discrepancy. The Harris score was 78.
   (c) Postoperative X-ray after 2 years is shown in Fig. 4.15.

Up to now, it has been 3.5 years with follow-up examinations. The Harris score is 82. Walking ability is normal, and the stem shows no subsidence.

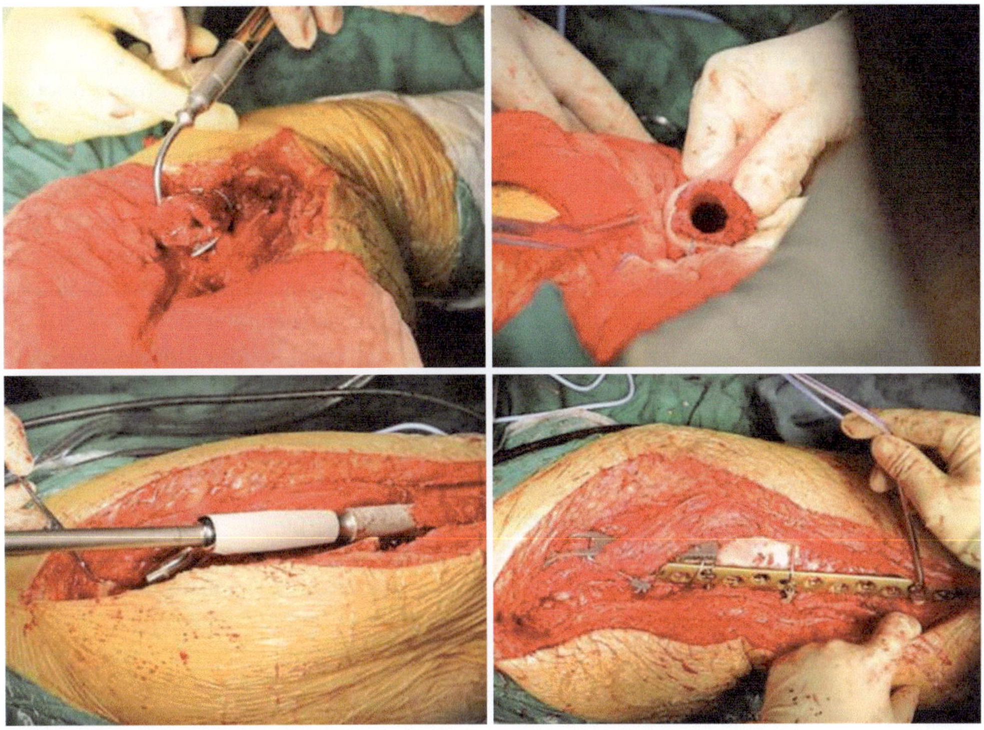

Fig. 4.13 Intraoperative observation

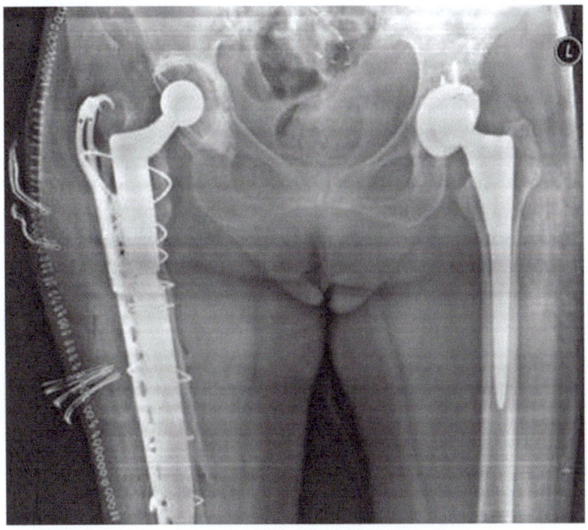

Fig. 4.14 Postoperative immediate X-ray

4.5.6 Conclusion and Reflection

1. Damage control—the basic principle of revision: Revision is always full of challenges. Minimizing the damage to the patient's general condition from the surgery (including anesthesia) requires the surgeons to develop tailored

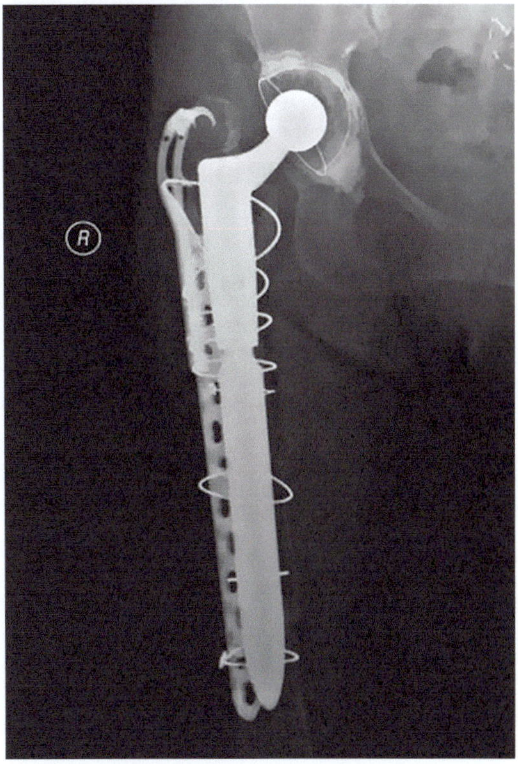

Fig. 4.15 Postoperative X-ray after 2 years

operation plans for each patient. In this case, the patient was of senior age and poor health; thus, the time of operation needed to be limited as much as possible, and hemorrhage should be controlled. Meanwhile, fracture stabilization and initial stability of the stem should be realized to an ideal extent, so that the patient could regain movement in the early stage.

The specific strategies included:

(a) Reserving the acetabulum: Although the preoperative X-ray showed a lucent line around the periprosthetic acetabulum, it was not intact and the overall width was less than 2 mm. It had been more than 10 years since the last operation. The cup showed no obvious signs of migration; combined with the patient's self-report that no pain was developed in the inguinal area before the fracture, it could be deducted preoperatively that the acetabular component had no loosening. The deduction was confirmed during the operation; thus, the decision to preserve the acetabulum was made.

    Retrieving the cup and subsequent reconstruction of the acetabulum would undoubtedly extend the surgical period and increase hemorrhage.

    However, it was also a "local war" with relatively controllable risks if the acetabular component would loosen or instability would occur in the future, and acetabular revision would be required, as communicated with the patient.

(b) Central scaffold technique application: First, press fit and initial stabilization were established in the distal fracture segment, and then the split proximal segment was wrapped around the stem for fixation. The advantages of this technique in damage control were as follows:
    - With full exposure of the distal fracture, eccentric filing and adverse stem alignment could be avoided completely.
    - The retrieval of the cup and bone cement cleaning could be simplified to the greatest extent, and the further creation of new bone defects could be avoided as much as possible.
    - It helped restore the alignment and fracture fixation, as well as position adjustment of the greater trochanter.

(c) Applying "minor general anesthesia" technique: This technique is performed by multiple regional nerve blocks (lumbar plexus, femoral nerve, iliac subfascia, etc.) combined with low-dose general anesthesia. Intraoperative monitoring of electroencephalogram (EEG) was employed to minimize the dose of general anesthesia; thus, cardiopulmonary, liver, and kidney function impairment can be reduced, as well as perioperative complications.

2. Stem selection and isthmus restoration: The femur was thin after multiple operations and the fracture line involved isthmus. For good osseointegration especially between the greater trochanter and the surface of the metal stem after the longitudinal splitting of the proximal fracture segment, RM cylindrical stem with double-sprayed coating on both distal and proximal ends was selected.

    When the distal femur was exposed, it could be seen that the first loop of pre-bound cables was far away from the fracture end (about 5 cm). The medullary cavity was filed and a thicker stem was applied. Once the stem was inserted, the femoral cortex close to the pre-bound cable could be spread, or even split, which would be predictable and controlled. After the stem was driven in, a second cable (about 3 cm apart) was tied between the first pre-bound cable and the fracture end. This partly rebuilt the isthmus.

3. Regrets
    (a) Due to the fact that there were no sufficient sizes of RM stem in China at the time of the operation, a proximal component of +30 mm was used. As a result, there was still about a 2.5 cm shortening discrepancy in the affected limb.
    (b) The distal end of the plate was too close to the distal femoral stem, which had a certain risk of stress concentration. A longer plate or stem would have been employed if it was possible.

4.6 Case 5

Hanlong Zheng and Yixin Zhou

4.6.1 Case Summary

Medical History A 45-year-old female complained of "Fracture of left hip 9 months after revision." The patient had suffered from claudication on both sides since childhood and underwent "open reduction" surgery in 1979 due to dislocation of both hips. The specific procedures were unknown. The right hip was well restored, while the left hip failed. Before 2 years, due to left hip arthritis, left proximal femur osteotomy and THA were performed in another hospital. Postoperative rehabilitation was performed. The patient had left hip PFF caused by trauma 9 months ago and underwent right THA + left revision in another hospital, in which the femoral stem was replaced and the fracture was fixed with a plate. Regular re-examination showed that the fracture had not healed. The patient had difficulty in walking. She attended our hospital for further treatment. The diagnosis in the outpatient department was postoperative loosening (left). The patient was accepted for further treatment. Previously in good health.

Physical Examination The patient entered the ward with claudication; the pelvis tilted to the left; left hip discrepancy; front and lateral incision cicatrices could be seen in both hips; no redness and swelling; tenderness in left inguinal, hip, greater trochanter, and proximal thigh area (+); axial percussion pain (+), no limitation of passive mobility; and loss of initiative flexion and abduction of the left hip. The left lower extremity had about a 2 cm discrepancy than the right one.

Laboratory Examination Routine blood test, ESR, and CRP were normal.

Radiographic Data See Fig. 4.16 for the preoperative X-ray of the initial THA. See Fig. 4.17 for

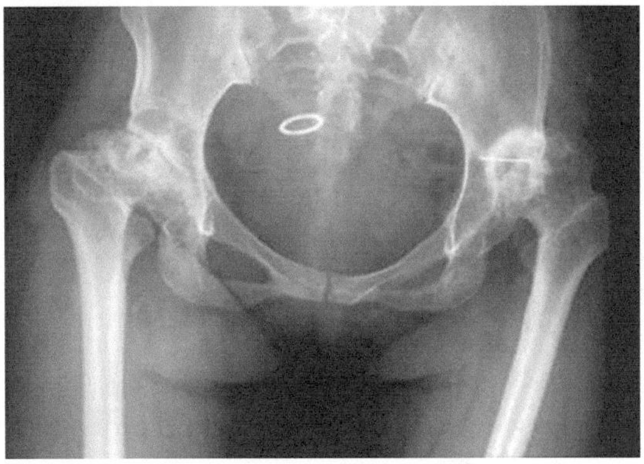

Fig. 4.16 Preoperative X-ray of the initial THA

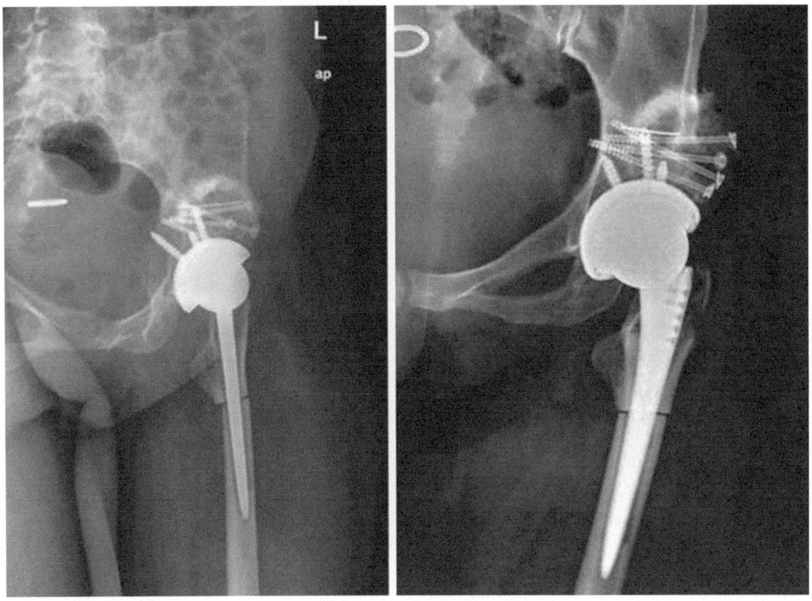

Fig. 4.17 Postoperative X-rays of the initial THA

postoperative X-rays of the initial THA. See Fig. 4.18 for the preoperative X-ray of PFF 9 months ago. Figure 4.19 shows the X-rays at 9 months after the first-time revision of PFF.

4.6.2 Case Analysis

The outpatient X-rays gave the authors a strong first impression. The first question to ask: Was the whole construction mechanically sound? Apparently not. The S-ROM stem seemed to have migrated; the stem did not show good osseointegration; the fracture restoration or fixation was not ideal. The second impression was "severe biological damage." By the looks of it, this was a busy X-ray. The cables in the cable-plate system for secondary fixation were too dense, which damaged the blood flow and affected fracture healing.

In cases like this, the surgeons need to ask themselves: What kind of problem is this? How did the problem occur? How to solve it?

On the femoral side, it could be observed that the stem did not have a good fit and fill, which showed varus inside the medullary cavity. The femoral stem appeared to be too "smooth," possibly because the medullary cavity was too narrow, and the stem could not fit into a sleeve. In contrast to the femoral side, the medullary cavity on the affected side was indeed very narrow and was likely to have been over-reamed. Looking at the acetabular side, some of the metal entered the obturator foramen and the rotation center migrated downward, which would potentially strain the soft tissue. The solution could be further releasing and subtrochanteric osteotomy. However, it could create more mismatches at the distal and proximal ends of the osteotomy.

For internal fixation, the length of the plate and the intensity of the cable binding should be considered. Obviously, the initial stability after the last revision of this case was not reliable, with proximal fracture and loss of distal press fit, in which the plate did not cross the fracture line far enough. In the proximal end, there was a loss of embracement. Without a sleeve or cone, it lacked adequate scratch fit. The conical stem plays a fracture-bridging role in the medullary cavity. Even in distal fixation, there is no mechanism to prevent the vertical femoral stem subsidence. It had no osseointegration on its surface, which would explain the stem loosening.

In conclusion, it was not difficult to tell why the fracture did not heal. Neither the restoration nor fixation of the fracture was good; there was no proper intramedullary support or coating. The

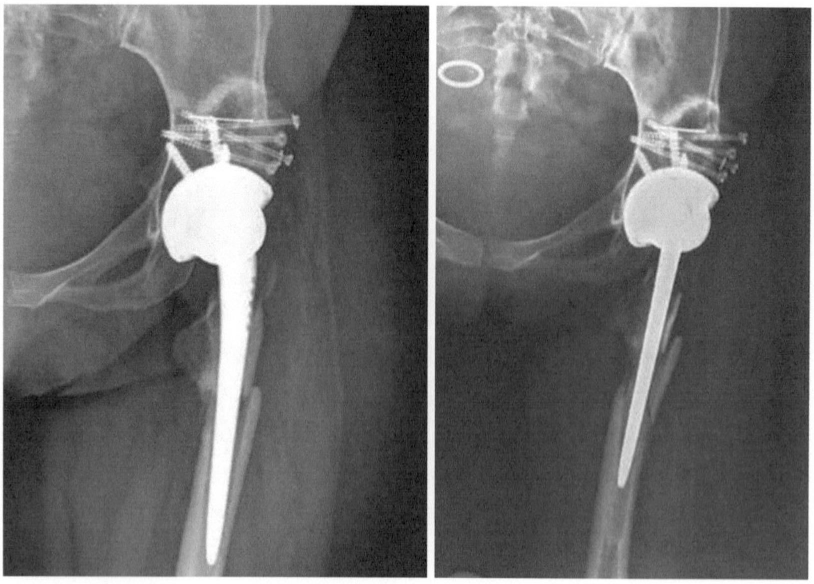

Fig. 4.18 Preoperative X-ray of PFF 9 months ago

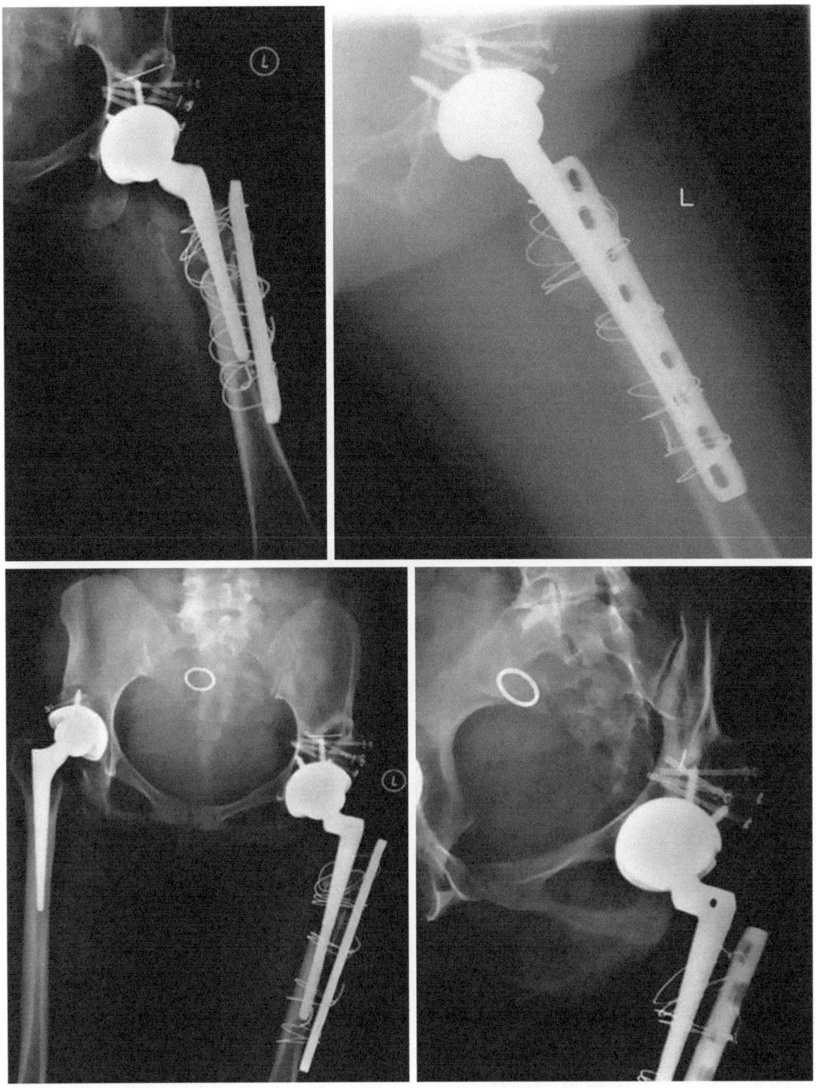

Fig. 4.19 Postoperative X-rays at 9 months after the first-time revision of PFF

plate length and method of the internal fixation were not appropriate. The fixation technology of trauma orthopedics should have been adopted according to the AO principle, and screws, locking nails, and cable-plate systems should be applied comprehensively.

Wait, have we forgotten anything that were less obvious? It was not difficult to see on the radiographs that the femoral greater trochanter was missing on the affected side, suggesting that the abductor of the patient might have been seriously damaged, and dislocation or severe gluteal gait could occur after the operation, and walking ability could be severely damaged after the revision.

We can analyze the X-rays of the patient's initial replacement along with the timeline: The distal femur was excessively filed, and an obvious cortical step could be seen near the tip of the stem, with a lucent line around it. These observations were likely to give the surgeons a false impression, but the fact was that the distal femur was likely to have a poor fixation. The femoral osteotomy line was bisected exactly the length of the stem, but the best clinical procedure was to reach two-thirds of the distal femoral stem across the osteotomy line, as the distal medullary cavity required adequate stability. Of course, the stem with a rectangular transection could not absolutely fit and fill the medullary cavity, but if there was a lucent line around the stem, it was difficult to achieve ideal initial stability. In addition, if there was a very short femoral stem inserted into the medullary cavity, and the lateral cortex was weak due to excessive filing, a stress riser would generate at the weak point, which would easily cause fracture.

Back to the preoperative X-ray of the initial THA: It was not difficult to see pseudarthrosis, subchondral osteosclerosis, and many osteophytes on the affected acetabular side. The needle indicated previous surgery, which can also be inferred that the hip mobility of the patient might be poor. The true acetabulum of this patient was not well developed; thus, the initial THA was difficult. In terms of the femoral side, how to choose the stem of the initial THA was also worth considering. Even with a modular S-ROM stem, which allows for more flexibility and more options, it was hard to achieve distal and proximal fit. In this case, excessive filing in the lateral femur might be unavoidable (although, too much filing such as in this case should be avoided). There were initial anatomical problems in this patient. If modular femoral stem was applied in the initial THA, compared with other stems such as S-ROM and Wagner cone, it would have led to greater difficulties in the surgery.

4.6.3 Surgical Planning

First, did the acetabulum require revision? The acetabular side looked well fixed, and the revision of the femur was already a big enough operation. However, the cup in this patient still worried the surgeon: The previous bone graft did not achieve good healing, which would possibly crack or break in the future. The cup continuously bore an outward lever force, which was a potential risk in the future. For surgeons, a key point to always bear in mind in terms of damage control is never to get obsessed with performing a flawless operation. In conclusion, the authors decided to skip the acetabulum revision.

The difficulty in this case lay in the femur side.

1. The lateral femoral cortex had a defect; the distal end of the stem was at the apex of the inverted cone; and the medullary cavity on the subsequent distal end was gradually widened. The shape of a Wagner stem would not establish initial stability or control the subsidence. It required a long tubular bone with a high fixation distance. Nevertheless, the femur with the inverted triangular medullary cavity and missing isthmus in this case suggested that fixation was difficult to achieve with this type of stem. The osseointegration capability of the Wagner stem was not as good as a conical stem with a scratch fit. A conical stem is a good choice for a femur with a short osseointegration area and narrow medullary cavity.
2. Apart from the fixation of the distal fracture end, a central scaffold structure should also be constructed in the proximal femur. The use of a cable-plate system depended on the intraoperative conditions.
3. As a comminuted fracture, how should we establish a good restoration and how could we realize a better biological condition? It might not be achievable with a plate either in terms of bridging the fracture block or protecting the angle of blood flow around the fracture.
4. According to previous radiographic data of the patient, the condition of the femoral greater trochanter had been poor. If the greater trochanter was missing and the gluteus medius was torn apart, how should it be rebuilt? The continuity of gluteus medius and lateral muscles could be achieved by augment and tendons. Of course, it also depended on the intraoperative situation.

4.6.4 Surgical Procedure and Intraoperative Observation

1. Access through the original modified Gibson approach on the left posterolateral hip to expose. The femoral head was retrieved, and then diaphysis was exposed along the distal of the plate. The wrapping cable and plate were removed, and the original femoral stem was retrieved reversely.

2. After the cicatrix tissue was cleaned out, the greater trochanter was missing, and the primary fracture was not healed. The proximal end was opened longitudinally and the distal medullary cavity was expanded to 11 mm with a high-speed drill after being strapped. The medullary cavity was washed and an artificial bone containing antibiotics was placed in the distal end. The proximal end was strengthened with a titanium cable. RM 11 femoral stem was implanted, the proximal end of which was connected with a 19 + 0 stem.
3. Torsion test was negative. The original bone fragments were restored, and the AP and lateral defects were observed. An allogeneic bone plate was employed to increase the coverage, and four titanium cables were bound and fixed. Demineralized bone matrix (DBM) was inserted into the gaps. A 36 mm-3 mm ceramic (powdered) femoral head was applied. The proximal end of the allogeneic bone plate was perforated, and the residual gluteus medius and gluteus maximus were fixed with non-absorbable sutures. After restoring the alignment, the incision was sutured layer by layer, and the patient was returned to the ward.

The intraoperative observation is shown in Fig. 4.20.

4.6.5 Postoperative Condition and Outcome

The postoperative immediate X-ray is shown in Fig. 4.21. Postoperative X-rays after 2 years are shown in Fig. 4.22.

In the last follow-up examination, the hip was completely free of pain. Gluteal gait was seen.

4.6.6 Conclusion and Reflection

For such PFF cases, the surgeons must be able to clearly identify the purpose of surgery, priority and preoperative expectations, decisions, and

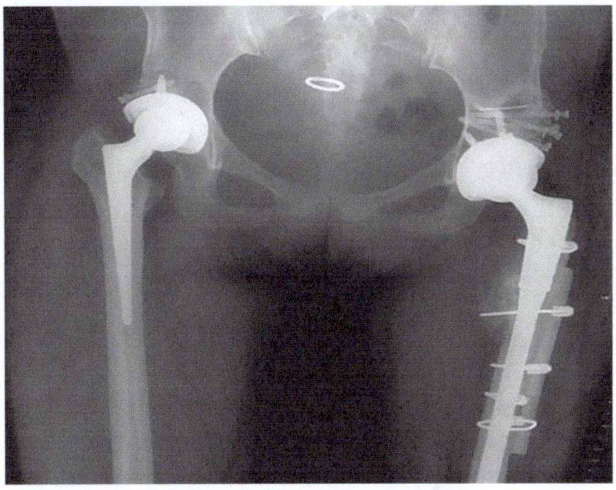

Fig. 4.21 Postoperative immediate X-ray

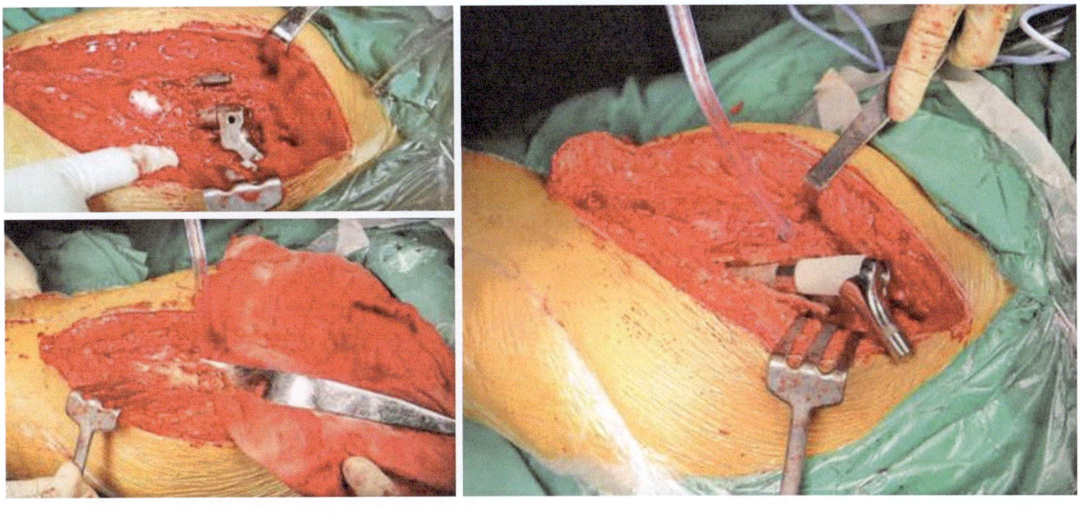

Fig. 4.20 Intraoperative observation

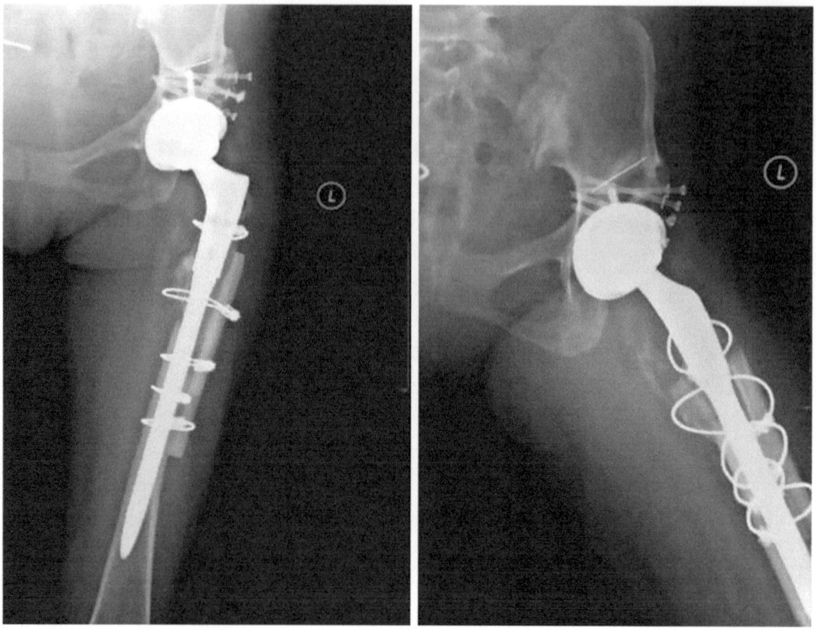

Fig. 4.22 Postoperative X-rays after 2 years

judgments. The ideal situation was osseointegration in both the distal and proximal femur, with both proximal and distal fractures healed. A less ideal situation would be osseointegration in the distal stem, with proximal osseointegration into the surface of the modular stem; distal and proximal fracture was not healed. Taking another step back, if osseointegration occurred in the distal and proximal femur, and soft tissue sleeve of the hip was in good condition, it could also provide support for the abductor. However, the surgeon had to stay to the bottom line: the distal end of the stem was well fixed in the medullary cavity; otherwise, none of the above could be achieved.

In the actual operation, We employed an RM modular stem for this case. Before reaming the medullary cavity, preventative binding of the proximal femur was applied. Allogeneic cortical bone was selected and bridged with a porous surface, and then the gluteus medius was sutured to the greater trochanter of the allogeneic bone plate via non-absorbable sutures. The lateral rotator muscle group was reconstructed without augment. The residual bone cortex of the distal femur was pressured with titanium cable and attached to the surface of the stem. For a better fit of the cortical bone, trenches were shaped in advance. In addition, DBM can effectively reconstruct bone mass, which was also applied in this case. At present, the patient had undergone follow-up examinations for nearly 3 years free of walking pain. Unfortunately, there was still gluteal gait, despite functioning normally. Follow-up radiography examination suggested that osseointegration was developed in the cortical bone. To sum up, for such cases, surgeons should not rush to come up with a solution. It is crucial to identify the problem and the underlying reasons behind it first.

4.7 Case 6

Hanlong Zheng and Yixin Zhou

4.7.1 Case Summary

Medical History A 44-year-old male patient suffered a left hip fracture due to a car accident 16 years ago and received internal fixation in another hospital. Left hip pain occurred 2 years after the surgery. After left THA in a local hospital, the recovery was good. Two years ago, the patient presented with left hip pain, left lower extremity discrepancy, claudication, and limited mobility in the left hip. Two weeks ago, the patient was injured accidentally when getting out of a car. The left thigh was swollen and developed severe pain, with limited mobility in the left lower extremity. Traction treatment of the left lower extremity was performed in another hospital. "Postoperative loosening following left THA and left femoral stem peripheral fracture" were diagnosed in the outpatient department of our hospital. Previously in good health. He had abdominal surgery from a car accident 16 years ago. No further details were provided.

Physical Examination The patient was wheeled into the ward on a gurney; two cicatrices from a previous operation were observed on the left hip; a 0.5-cm wound was found in the medial and lateral side of the left distal femur with scab and no bleeding; left femur swelling and tenderness, crepitus and abnormal mobility, and axial percussion pain (+); no hypoesthesia in both lower extremities; and both dorsal arteries of feet were palpable.

Laboratory Examination Routine blood test: WBC 8.02 × 10^9/L, HGB 125 g/L, N 65.8%; CRP 10.7 mg/L; ESR 47 mm/h.

Radiographic Data Preoperative full-length anteroposterior X-rays of both sides, iliac oblique X-rays of the left hip, and full-length X-rays of both lower extremities can be seen in Fig. 4.23. See Fig. 4.24 for preoperative CT.

P105

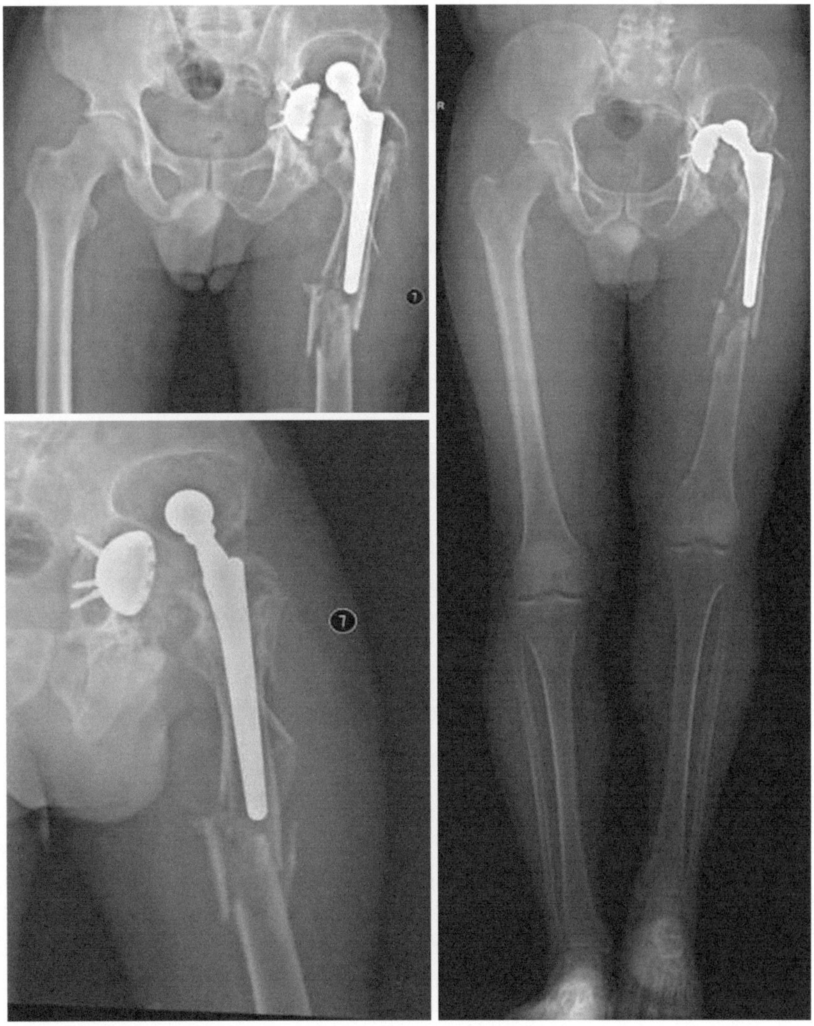

Fig. 4.23 Preoperative X-rays

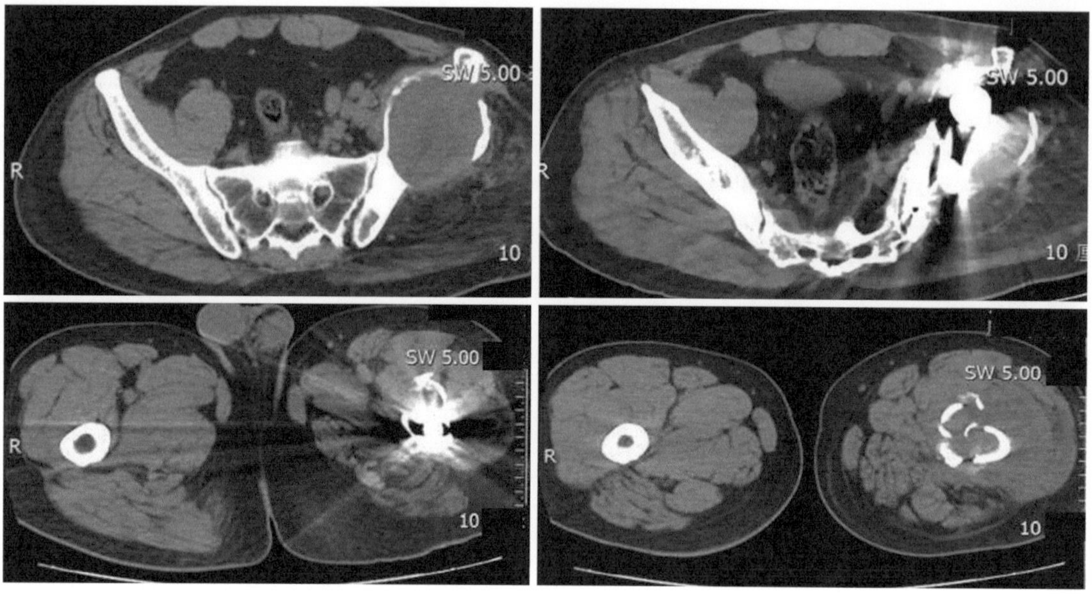

Fig. 4.24 Preoperative CT plain scan

4.7.2 Preoperative Planning

1. Radiography Illustration:
   (a) Acetabulum side: Hip dislocation with a small abduction angle. A lengthened femoral head was applied. The anterior and posterior columns had continuity, and the bone mass was poor. The teardrop existed; pubic ischial ramus was intact, and a small amount of ischium was missing. There was a large bone defect in the superior acetabulum, revealing a typical "ballooning osteolysis."
   (b) Femur side: A comminuted fracture in the periprosthetic biological femoral stem, accompanied by bone loss, femoral isthmus missing, and a medullary cavity with "small top and large bottom"; osteolysis around greater trochanter; and significant discrepancy in the lower extremity.
2. Reconstruction strategy: The major difficulty of this case was reconstruction, including initial stability and long-term biological fixation. What was more complicated was that the massive bone defect was also accompanied by fracture, involving mechanics and biology. In addition, the fragmentation of the greater trochanter increased the difficulty of reconstruction. The authors must admit that, on the first view of this patient, we were very confused and not ready to come up with a solution.

According to the X-rays, it was obvious that the massive bone defect in the acetabular side could not occur in a short period of time. The symptoms could have been around for more than 2 years, which also suggested that the patient did not take good care of his hip. Thus, poor patient compliance was expected. What caused such massive osteolysis? Extended femoral head were applied to the affected side, and the anteversion angle of the acetabulum was relatively small, both of which could be the potential cause of the osteolysis. Of course, it could not be specified whether it was caused by polyethylene wear or metal ion corrosion exactly. But there was no doubt that this was a typical osteolysis, as there were many explanations.

With such a massive bone defect, it seemed complicated at first. However, when reviewing the radiographs carefully, it was found that there was still continuity in the anterior and posterior columns of the acetabulum (despite the poor bone condition). The teardrop still existed, and the pubic ischial ramus was intact. A small amount of bone loss was found in ischium. Despite the massive bone defect in the superior acetabulum, if the "pubic-ischial segment" was intact, the continuity of pelvic was present, the missing part was only the superior point. In this way, all that needed to be done was reconstructing the upper point in this acetabular bone defect that appeared to be complicated. From the radiographs, pelvic discontinuity was not considered, but a potential pelvic discontinuity during debridement should be prevented.

More concerns lay in the femoral side, where the isthmus of the stem was damaged. The stem was loose even if no fracture occurred. Establishing initial stability was challenging.

Could we perform direct ORIF? According to preoperative radiographs, it was clear that it should not be classified as Vancouver B1 despite possible bone ingrowth. On the other hand, exposure to ORIF was difficult, and the acetabulum could not be managed.

Should tumor prosthesis be considered? Applying a tumor prosthesis would allow the patient to recover part of the motion smoothly in the short term. However, given that this patient was relatively young, and many problems could occur with a tumor prosthesis fixed with bone cement in the long run, non-cement fixation was adopted. Moreover, the femoral isthmus was missing, with a medullary cavity of "small top and large bottom." It was hard for the Wagner stem to achieve axial stability, so it was not suitable.

For a Type IV femur like this, revision was performed with a coated stem. Even without more than a double cortex for fixation, the success rate of the operation could be increased by binding fracture blocks to the stem surface, reducing motion and delaying the rehabilitation to improve osseointegration. The Wagner femoral stem has good anti-rotation performance and achieves initial stability mainly by its taper, whereas it was not suitable for an inverted, tapered medullary cavity in this case. Therefore, a modular cylindrical stem was an ideal choice. To obtain more scratch fit between the stem and the medullary cavity, appropriate over-filing and prophylactic pre-cerclaged could be applied to prevent intraoperative fracture. A columnar medullary cavity should be established to press fit as much as possible to achieve biological fixation.

Furthermore, how should infection of retrograde nailing be prevented? First, the bone traction should be retrieved as early as possible. Second, a barrier could be generated by placing artificial bone in the distal femoral to close the medullary cavity, which could slowly release antibiotics and insulate the distal stem from the nail tract. For patients with lower extremity fractures, the problem of the nail tract must be considered; otherwise, the complications induced by infection will bring great financial losses to the patients.

Based on the above, reconstruction solutions were clarified individually for both the acetabular and femoral sides. It was no doubt an expensive surgery. Frankly speaking, if the patient had financial concerns, it would have been a worse dilemma for us. Of course, for these patients, it did not mean 100% failure without hip revision. If the patient had financial problems, an illizarov frame, or even hip amputation, could be employed as an alternative. However, if it had been decided to perform a very expensive revision surgery, the lead surgeon had to explain the difficulty of the operation caused by potential complications such as abrasion, metal ion disease, and needle tract infection to the patient, as well as the possibility of requiring multiple operations. Moreover, other relevant concerns besides medical treatment had to be discussed with the patient because the cost of the surgery was too high.

The 3D printing of the patient's pelvis model needed to be prepared preoperatively to simulate the acetabular reconstruction strategy, as shown in Fig. 4.25.

4.7.3 Surgical Procedure and Intraoperative Observation

1. A posterolateral approach was taken to reveal the femoral side and fracture line, as shown in Fig. 4.26.

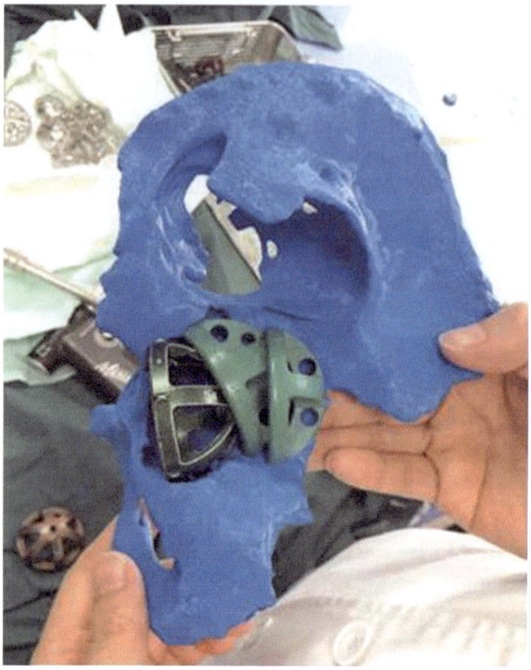

Fig. 4.25 Preoperative 3D print of pelvis model

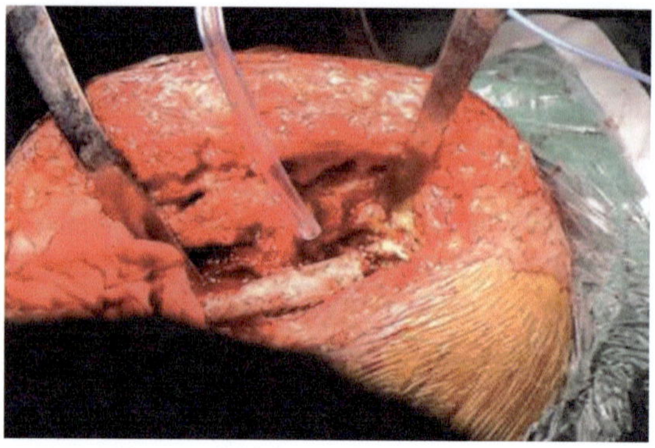

Fig. 4.26 Intraoperative exposure of femoral side and fracture line

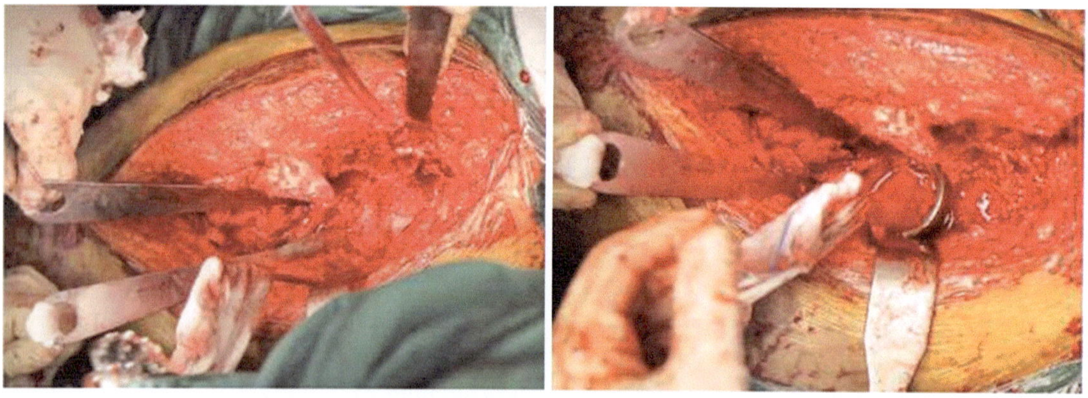

Fig. 4.27 Intraoperative original component retrieval and test mold placement

2. The acetabular side was exposed, showing a segmental bone defect on the posterior side of the acetabulum. The original component was retrieved and an acetabular test mold was placed in, as shown in Fig. 4.27.
3. Augment test mold was placed in. Finally, a 52-mm TM porous cup was implanted, and two augments were implanted above, then fixed with screws, as shown in Fig. 4.28.
4. The femoral stem was exposed through a posterolateral approach. The fracture end was cleaned, and the distal medullary cavity was sealed with artificial bone and vancomycin. It was subsequently immersed in iodophor for 10 min. A long cable-plate system was applied to fix the fracture end. A 167-20 + 2 RM stem and a 32 mm + 4 femoral head were inserted (see Fig. 4.29).

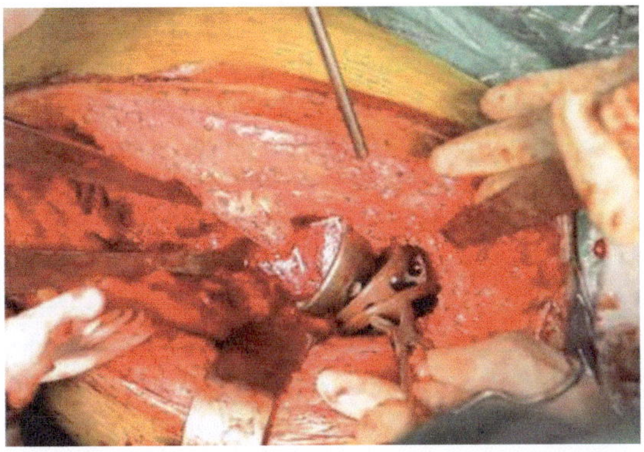

Fig. 4.28 Placing the augment

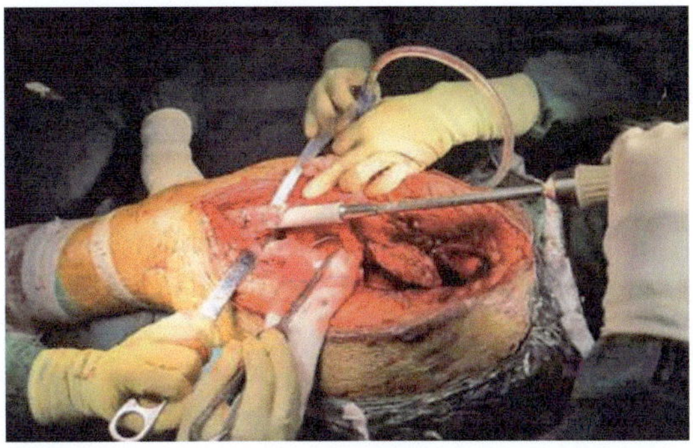

Fig. 4.29 Implanting the femur stem

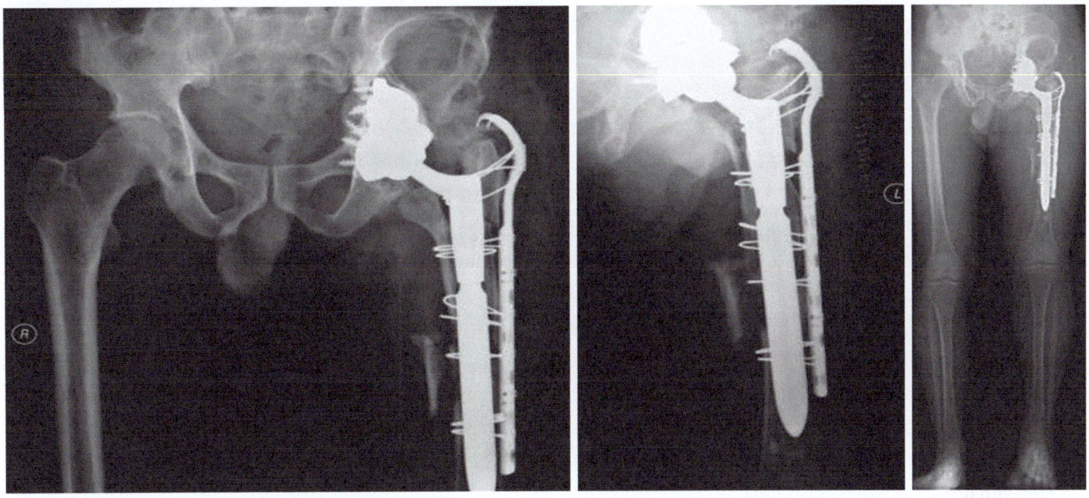

Fig. 4.30 Postoperative immediate X-rays

4.7.4 Postoperative Condition and Outcome

The overall principle of postoperative rehabilitation for this patient was early motion and late weight-bearing.

The patient was encouraged to start walking early without weight bearing between 3 weeks to 1 month after the operation. After 1.5 months, 15 kg weight was loaded walking flat-footed. The principles of rehabilitation could be more conservative, but staying in bed should be avoided as much as possible.

The postoperative immediate X-rays are shown in Fig. 4.30.

Postoperative follow-up examination after 5 years: Without attending to the hospital, the patient expressed great satisfaction with the hip functioning through telephone follow-up. Unfortunately, the patient did not provide imaging data.

4.7.5 Conclusion and Reflection

1. Preoperative evaluation: This case gave the authors a strong first impression. The radiographs revealed too many problems: massive bone defect on the acetabular side, periprosthetic comminuted fracture, and hip dislocation. In addition, it could also be seen that the

anteversion of the affected acetabulum was small, and an plus femur head was used, and so on.

There were some potential problems to be aware of: Although the patient stated "falling when getting off a bus," the comminuted fracture might not have been a low-energy injury. Associated injuries such as a history of coma, craniocerebral trauma, and damage of abdomen viscera should be screened to assess the systemic condition of the patient before making surgical decisions. It should be considered how much room was left for the operation. Besides, external infection should be eliminated in all PFF cases. Many fracture patients have high CRP and ESR. If the infection is not easy to eliminate, an aspiration test should be arranged. If the patients have experienced bone traction after injury, nail tract infection must be considered.

2. Key points of the reconstruction operation: Femoral stem retrieval was not required in the revision of this case, exposing along the osteotomy line was enough. There were relatively obvious bone blocks in the greater trochanter, which should be opened as early as possible to release the tension of the gluteus medius and lateral femur to prevent the avulsion of the gluteus medius. There was a large amount of cicatrix tissue during exposure. It could be seen that the points of the anteroinferior and inferoposterior acetabulum had abundant bone mass; thus, only the upper point required reconstruction.

   Our team conducted 3D printing of the patient's pelvis before the operation and conducted practice with a trial. Acetabular reconstruction was not as complicated as expected. Without a buttress augment at the time, two slope augments were applied, being stacked on top of each other. Bone cement connection was constructed between augments and between augment and bone, forming fixed rigid units with a large contact area. The surgeons also built mortise and tenon structures around the acetabulum, which, while not as elaborate as a carpenter's work, could also wedge the metal for better shear stress resistance. Bone cement was used for the fixation between the hemispherical acetabulum and augments; DBM and broken cancellous bone were mixed and filled into the frame-like structure of the augments. In fact, the augments were originally designed for bone grafting, while DBM has better bone-guiding and inducing effects.
3. Whether or not to employ allogeneic cortical bone plates: Many surgeons would choose allogeneic cortical bone plates for the revision of PFF with serious bone defects. The authors believed that the use of allogeneic cortical bone plates would require peeling off a lot of soft tissue and increase the risk of postoperative infection. It probably should have been used in this case, but it was not. If this case fails again after 10 years, revision of the femoral stem will not be too difficult.
4. Was a distal interlock nailing stem needed for the revision: It has been suggested in some literature that a stem with distal interlock nails can be employed for the revision of some PFF cases. From the author's point of view, if the initial stability of the stem is good, the interlock nail is not necessary; on the contrary, if the initial stability is poor, the use of interlocking nails does not make much sense. The biggest concern in cases like this was not the stem subsidence, but the torque due to the presence of the collodiaphyseal angle, which could affect fracture healing or even cause additional fracture. The cylindrical stem had poor resistance to rotation, and the interlocking nail could help with rotation stability, which would change the patient's rehabilitation pattern. Too early weight-bearing might cause rotation. Interlock nails only provide torsional stability in extreme circumstances and must be planned along with a postoperative rehabilitation strategy.
5. What was learned on postoperative radiograph viewing: according to postoperative radiographs, the position of the acetabular rotation center was generally ideal, which might be a little lower than the teardrop. The pelvic entrance plane fit, and the abduction angle and anteversion fit as well. The hemispherical cup made good contact with the medial dome and the inferior bone matrix. The reconstruction of the upper point was performed via augment, and the feedback in the

follow-up examination after 5 years was good. The stem revealed a bit of subsidence but was generally stable. The compact shadow in the distal stem was an antibiotic artificial bone used to prevent nail tract infection. Overall, the reconstruction on the femoral and acetabular sides was both successful.

A major regret in this case was leg length discrepancy; the affected extremity was notably shorter than the healthy side. The longest stem in the country was employed at the time of operation, and the condition of the soft tissue sleeve of the patient was not sufficient to stretch the leg any longer. It could also be seen that the sphenoid bone of the medial femur was not hooked by the cable. This would not affect the overall efficacy, but it had to be immediately explained to the patient and the family: In the future, the thigh could produce noise when in motion, and the bone blocks could undergo osseous healing or fibrous fixation. In such complicated cases, difficulty in bone piece restoration is a common issue.

4.8 Case 7

Yong Huang and Yixin Zhou

4.8.1 Case Summary

Medical History A 76-year-old female presented with an intertrochanteric fracture of the left hip caused by a fall 10 weeks ago. The patient received closed reduction and internal fixation for the fracture in another hospital. The wound healed well after the operation and was discharged normally. Left hip pain was developed after 3 weeks, and the left lower extremity was shorter than the healthy side. It was found in the re-examination that the internal fixation failed after left femur intertrochanteric fracture restoration. THA was performed in our hospital. A cable was applied to fix the intraoperative fracture.

Physical Examination Claudication; incision cicatrix could be seen on the posterolateral left hip, no redness or swelling; left hip greater trochanter tenderness (+); axial percussion pain (+); hip abductor force was normal; and severely limited mobility of the left hip.

Laboratory Examination No abnormality was detected in a routine blood test, ESR, and CRP.

Radiographic Data Preoperative X-ray of intramedullary nail internal fixation in the proximal femur (Fig. 4.31) showed an intertrochanteric fracture in the proximal femur.

Postoperative X-rays of the first intramedullary nail internal fixation in the proximal femur are shown in Fig. 4.32. The internal fixation failed after 3 weeks, with the head of the nail sticking out, as shown in Fig. 4.33. Intraoperative X-rays of initial THA are shown in Fig. 4.34.

P111

The AP and lateral X-rays 3 days after the initial THA showed subsidence and loosening of the femoral stem compared to the intraoperative radiographs, as well as forward migration of the greater trochanter, which can be seen in Fig. 4.35.

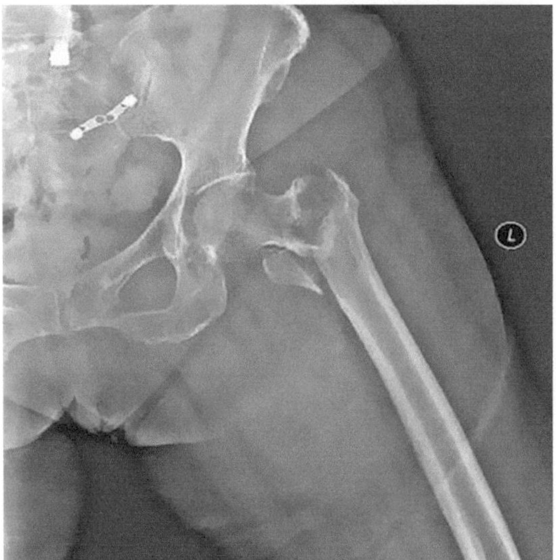

Fig. 4.31 Preoperative X-ray of intramedullary nail internal fixation in proximal femur

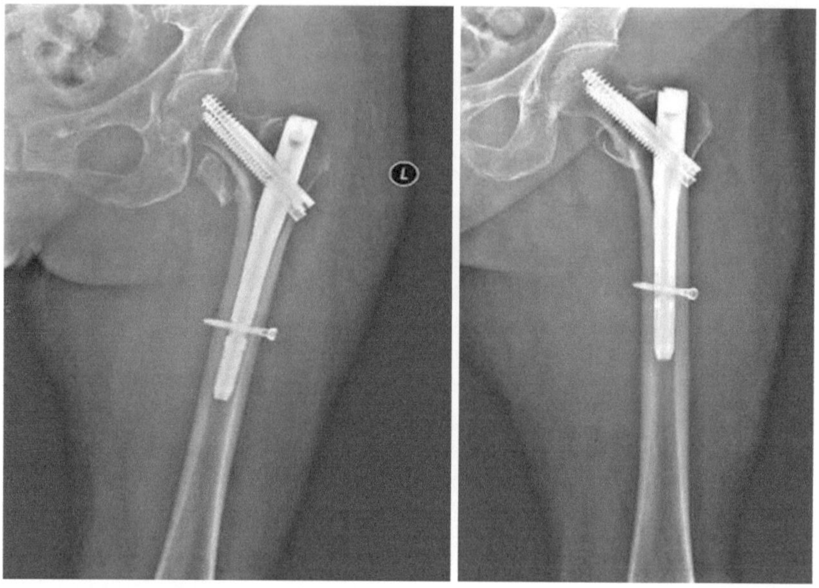

Fig. 4.32 Postoperative X-ray of the first intramedullary nail internal fixation in proximal femur

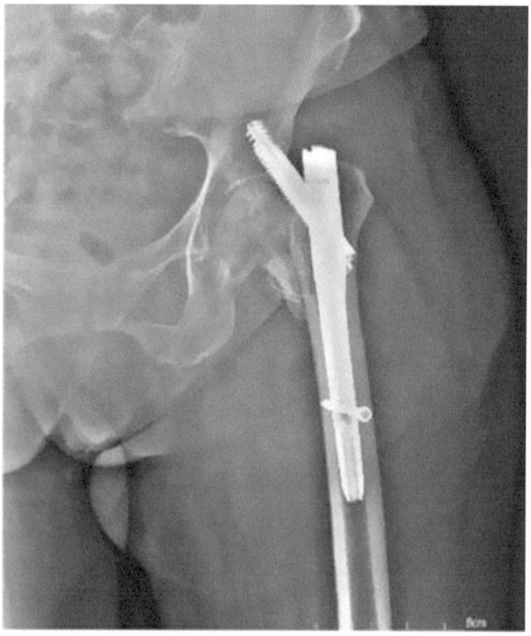

Fig. 4.33 Internal fixation X-rays after 3 weeks

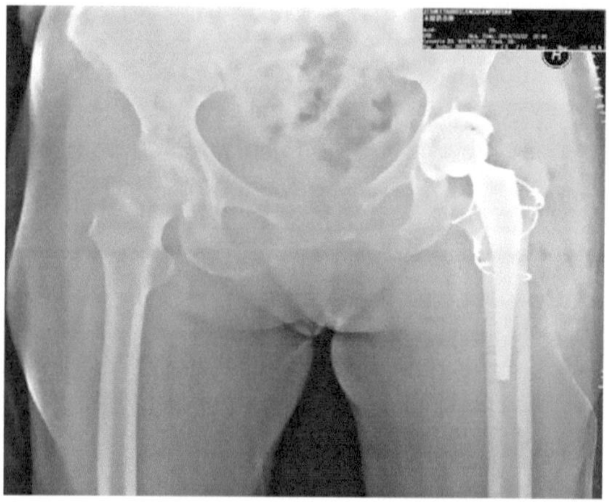

Fig. 4.34 Intraoperative X-rays of initial THA

4.8.2 Case Analysis and Surgical Planning

1. The reason for revision after THA: Femoral stem subsidence; greater and lesser trochanter migration, especially the forward migration of the greater trochanter; the greater trochanter was not firmly fixed; the embracement force of the cable was not sufficient to support the stem fixation; and insufficient initial stability of the stem. Without stem revision or an open working space, the greater trochanter was difficult to fix.
2. Treatment of PFF in the lesser trochanter: If the lesser trochanter had fracture without migration, it was usually not treated; If the fracture revealed migration, should it be treated? According to the authors' experience and opinion: There are fewer trochanter fracture patients without symptoms, and some

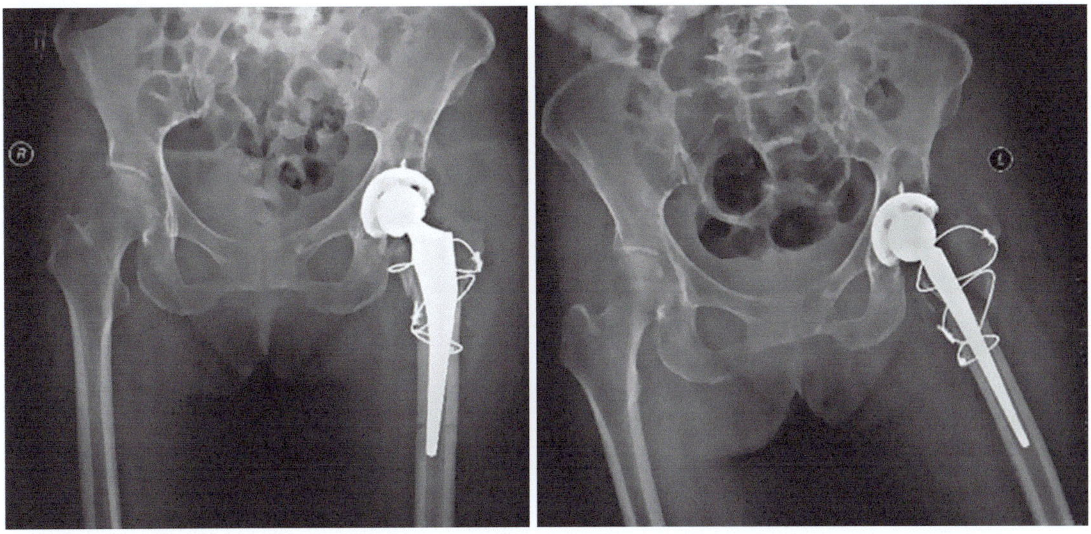

Fig. 4.35 AP and lateral X-rays 3 days after the initial THA

patients showed mild migration with minor symptoms. Local doctors usually recommend further operation when seeing the fracture line. The symptoms tended to last for 2–3 years after the operation, and the fracture subsequently healed itself and the symptoms improved.

3. Recommendations for initial THA in this patient: First, a femoral stem with distal fixation should be used. The femoral stem applied in this case was a proximal fixation, which required good proximal bone condition, continuity, and intactness. These conditions were obviously absent in this patient. Effective axial and torsional stability were hard to reach with the femoral stem of proximal fixation in this patient. The maximum rotation resistance wedge stems like this lie in the proximal end. Thus, they were not suitable for the initial THA of this patient in terms of either stability or torsional resistance. Second, the femoral stem should cross over the distal locking tack hole to avoid stress concentration. Moreover, the femur seemed to have some developmental problems. The CE angle was small, the medullary cavity was narrow, and the collodiaphyseal angle was large. The Wagner stem or modular stem with proximal porous coating could be selected so that bone growth could happen between the greater trochanter and the femoral stem, as shown in Fig. 4.36.

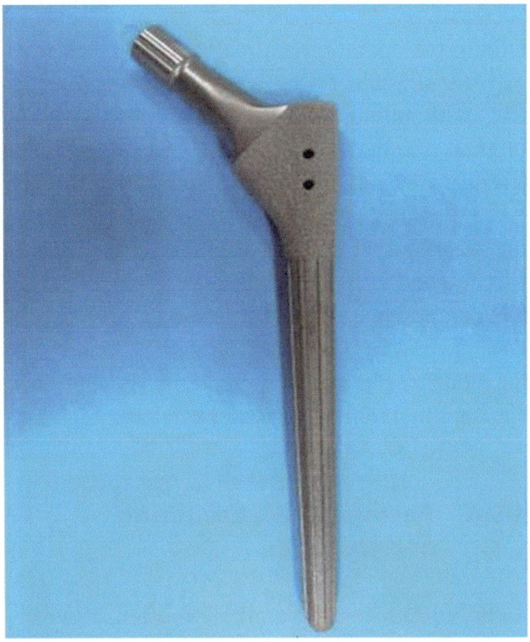

Fig. 4.36 Wagner stem with porous-surfaced shoulder

4. The tack hole left after the retrieval of the IMN distal cross-locking screw causes local weakness, and it usually takes about 4 months for normal human bones to repair and reconstruct. It has been reported in publications that with a diameter of 2–3 mm, a tack hole can

reduce the femoral energy absorption by 55%, while a 6-mm one can reduce the peak compressive stress of femur failure by 22%.
5. The THA of this patient was called conversion arthroplasty in foreign countries. It was different from the initial THA, but it was not a revision either. It was more complicated than the initial THA and simpler than the revision.
6. The lateral cortex of this patient was discontinuous with a small greater trochanter bone block and evident migration. Cable binding alone might not provide sufficient fixation. A greater trochanteric claw plate was required.

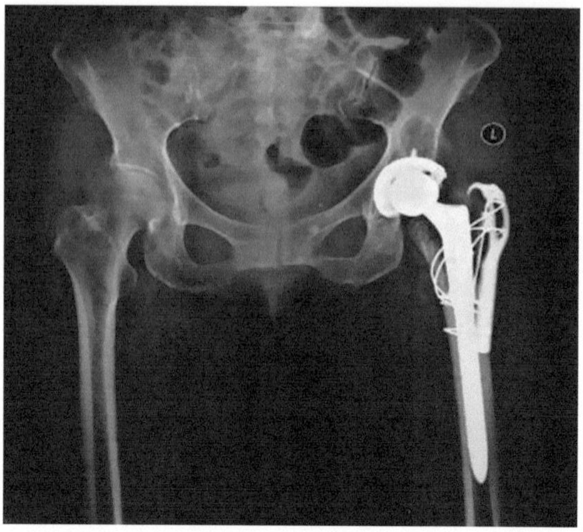

Fig. 4.37 Postoperative anteroposterior X-ray after 4 days

4.8.3 Surgical Procedure and Intraoperative Observation

During the operation, a greater trochanter proximal fracture was found when cleaning the cicatrix, with migration to the proximal end. The original fixing titanium cable was loose. The fracture area was unstable when moving the hip, and the contact area between the fracture end and the stem was small and unstable. Therefore, it was decided to replace the femoral stem.

Postoperative anteroposterior X-ray after 4 days is shown in Fig. 4.37. The distal fixation of the modular stem and the greater trochanter plate were applied to fix the greater trochanter.

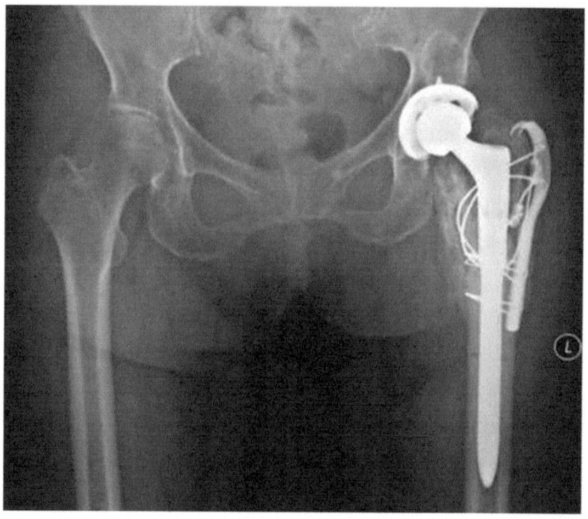

Fig. 4.38 Postoperative anteroposterior X-ray after 2 years

4.8.4 Postoperative Condition and Outcome

1. In the follow-up examination after 2.5 years, the Harris score was 78. The left side function was good, with stable femoral stem fixation and no subsidence (Fig. 4.38). However, the patient had a contralateral femoral neck fracture and a lumbar fracture later, with various complications and thus was long-term bedridden.
2. Postoperative and follow-up imaging evaluation: One regret was that the lesser trochanter was not fixed, but the area healed well.

Recommended Reading

1. Meek RMD, Norwood T, Smith R, et al. The risk of peri-prosthetic fracture after primary and revision total hip and knee replacement. J Bone Joint Surg Br. 2011;93-B(1):96–101.
2. Lindahl H, Malchau H, Herberts P, et al. Periprosthetic femoral fractures classification and demographics of 1049 periprosthetic femoral fractures from the Swedish national hip arthroplasty register. J Arthroplasty. 2005;20(7):857–65.
3. Ehlinger M, Delaunay C, Karoubi M, et al. Revision of primary total hip arthroplasty for peri-prosthetic

fracture: a prospective epidemiological study of 249 consecutive cases in France. Orthop Traumatol Surg Res. 2014;100(6):657–62.

4. Phillips JR, Moran CG, Manktelow AR. Periprosthetic fractures around hip hemiarthroplasty performed for hip fracture. Injury. 2013;44(6):757–62.
5. Fuchtmeier B, Galler M, Muller F. Mid-term results of 121 periprosthetic femoral fractures: increased failure and mortality within but not after one postoperative year. J Arthroplasty. 2015;30(4):669–74.
6. Marsland D, Mears SC. A review of periprosthetic femoral fractures associated with total hip arthroplasty. Geriatr Orthop Surg Rehabil. 2012;3(3):107–20.
7. Barenius B, Inngul C, Al Agic Z, et al. A randomized controlled trial of cemented versus cementless arthroplasty in patients with a displaced femoral neck fracture: a four-year fbllow-up. Bone Joint J. 2018;100-B(8):1087–93.
8. Lamb JN, Baetz J, Messer-Hannemann P, et al. A calcar collar is protective against early periprosthetic femoral fracture around cementless femoral components in primary total hip arthroplasty: a registry study with biomechanical validation. Bone Joint J. 2019;101-B(7):779–86.
9. Bigart KC, Nahhas CR, Ba GPR, et al. Does femoral morphology predict the risk of periprosthetic fracture after cementless total hip arthroplasty? J Arthroplasty. 2020;35(6):359–63.
10. Duncan CP, Masri BA. Fractures of the femur after hip replacement. Instr Course Lect. 1995;44(44):293–304.
11. Karam J, Campbell P, Desai S, et al. Periprosthetic proximal femoral fractures in cemented and uncemented stems according to Vancouver classification: observation of a new fracture pattern. J Orthop Surg Res. 2020;15:100.
12. Lee YK, Kim JT, Kim KC, et al. Conservative treatment for minimally displaced type B periprosthetic femoral fractures. J Arthroplasty. 2017;32(11):3529–32.
13. Buttaro MA, Farfalli G, Paredes Nunez M, et al. Locking compression plate fixation of Vancouver type-Bl periprosthetic femoral fractures. J Bone Joint Surg Am. 2007;89-A(9):1964–9.
14. Smitham PJ, Carbone TA, Bolam SM, et al. Vancouver B2 peri-prosthetic fractures in cemented femoral implants can be treated with open reduction and internal fixation alone without revision. J Arthroplasty. 2019;34(7):1430–4.
15. Zheng H, Gu H, Shao H, et al. Treatment and outcomes of Vancouver type B periprosthetic femoral fractures. Bone Joint J. 2020;102-B(3):293–300.
16. Patel NK, Whittingham-Jones P, Aston WJ, et al. Custom-made cement-linked mega prostheses: a salvage solution for complex periprosthetic femoral fractures. J Arthroplasty. 2014;29(1):204–9.
17. Zheng L, Lee WY, Hwang DS, et al. Could patient underwent surgical treatment for periprosthetic femoral fracture after hip arthroplasty return to their status before trauma? Hip Pelvis. 2016;28(2):90–7.

5 Periprosthetic Joint Infection

Yang Song and Hongyi Shao

5.1 Introduction

Hongyi Shao

Periprosthetic joint infection (PJI) is one of the most serious complications after total hip arthroplasty (THA). With the gradual popularization of THA, the rate and number of PJI have been increasing. Therefore, how to treat PJI after THA is also a key and difficult point in revision.

5.1.1 Epidemiology

The jury is still out on the incidence of PJI after THA. Pulido et al. examined nearly 10,000 patients who underwent initial total knee arthroplasty (TKA) or initial THA. Follow-up examination results showed an incidence of PJI of 0.7%. Therefore, with the continuous promotion and popularization of THA, the PJI rate has been increasing.

5.1.2 Risk Factors

PJI after THA is not caused by a single factor, but a combination of various factors. Literature has reported that patients with a previous medical history of diabetes, smoking, alcohol consumption, surgical history, and poor local soft tissue conditions are all risk factors for postoperative PJI. In addition, if wound exudation occurs continuously after the operation, the delay of wound healing is also correlated with PJI. When assessing the possibility of postoperative PJI after THA, the patient should be enquired in detail about the above risk factors.

5.1.3 Diagnosis and Evaluation

Up to now, there is no universal "gold standard" for the diagnosis of PJI. The diagnosis of PJI depends on the comprehensive judgment of the patient's local symptoms, signs, and laboratory examination. The most used diagnostic criteria for PJI to date are those set by the Musculoskeletal Infection Society (MSIS). For specific diagnostic criteria, see Table 5.1.

Therefore, if patients are suspected of PJI, it is necessary to conduct arthrocentesis to obtain white blood cells for preoperative cultures and synovial fluid analysis, so as to determine whether it is PJI.

5.1.4 Treatment Principle

The treatment principle of PJI after THA is to perform debridement thoroughly, control infection, and restore hip joint function. A

Y. Song · H. Shao (✉)
Department of Adult Joint Reconstructive Surgery, Beijing Jishuitan Hospital, Capital Medical University, Beijing, China

Y. Zhou (ed.), *Revision Total Hip Arthroplasty*, https://doi.org/10.1007/978-981-97-9804-9_5

Table 5.1 Diagnostic criteria for PJI (MSIS 2013 Edition)

Major diagnostic criteria	When a patient meets either of the following two diagnostic criteria, it is diagnosed as PJI positive: 1. Sinus tract which communicates with the articular cavity exists 2. Two cultures revealed positive and the same pathogenic bacteria were obtained
Secondary diagnostic criteria	When a patient meets three of the following five criteria, it is diagnosed as PJI positive: 1. Serum CRP and ESR both increased 2. White blood cell count increased or leukocyte esterase in synovial fluid is positive 3. Polymorphonuclear neutrophil percentage in synovial fluid increases 4. Histological analysis indicates infection 5. Single culture is positive
Note: Some patients with low virulence infection, clinically considered as PJI, can also be treated as an infection even if they do not meet the diagnostic criteria above	

thorough debridement requires evaluating the scope of infection, identifying the bacteria causing the infection, and the patient's systemic condition. The scope and method of debridement should be decided after comprehensive consideration. For cases with long-term infection, well-fixed prosthesis, and osteomyelitis, extensive resection can be considered for complete debridement. In some cases, prosthesis retrieval may be difficult, and extended trochanteric osteotomy (ETO) can be considered to increase the exposure. Good reconstruction is based on a successful debridement that lays a foundation for reconstruction.

To sum up, PJI after THA is a very typical condition that often requires comprehensive consideration and sometimes multi-department cooperation and comprehensive treatment. This chapter discusses the diagnosis and treatment of PJI after THA by reviewing some cases for readers.

5.2 Case 1

Yang Song and Hongyi Shao

5.2.1 Case Summary

Medical History A female, 76-year-old, patient underwent right THA after a right femoral neck fracture 6 years ago. Right hip pain was developed with no evident cause 4 months ago. The patient had hypertension for 15 years, undergoing oral drug control; daily blood pressure was stable. Total hysterectomy + pelvic lymph node dissection was performed for cervical cancer 8 years ago, and radiotherapy was performed on a regular basis. Before 6 years, a left femoral neck fracture occurred and was treated with THA. A left hip periprosthetic infection was discovered 5 years ago and treated with secondary revision.

Physical Examination The patient entered in a wheelchair; the body temperature was 36.4 °C; no abnormalities were detected; incision cicatrix of 15 cm was visible on both posterolateral hip joints; right hip area tenderness (+); no ulcer; no abnormal myodynamia in either lower extremity; slight edema was observed in the right lower extremity; no hypoesthesia; and pulse of bilateral dorsal artery of foot was palpable.

Laboratory Examination erythrocyte sedimentation rate (ESR): 61 mm/h; C-reactive protein (CRP): 72.1 mg/L; synovial fluid white blood cell (WBC) count: none; proportion of polymorphonuclear leukocyte (PMN) in synovial fluid: none; arthrocentesis liquid culture: oral streptococcus.

Radiographic Data See Fig. 5.1 for preoperative X-rays.

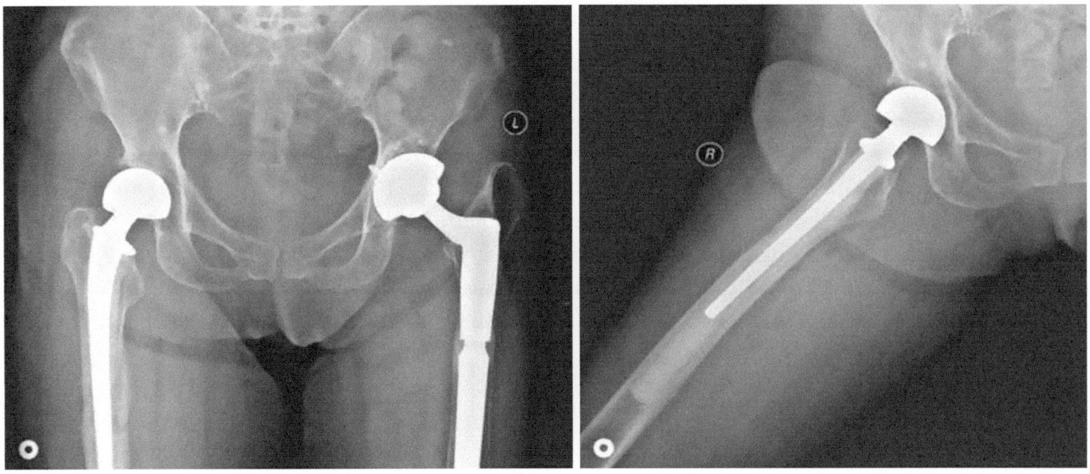

Fig. 5.1 Preoperative X-rays

5.2.2 Case Analysis

1. On reviewing the medical history of the patient, it was found that persistent pain existed, which was not clearly related to motion, and there was no obvious cause of trauma, so pathogeny such as periprosthetic infection, bone metabolic disease, and tumor should be considered. Meanwhile, conditions such as prosthesis loosening and periprosthetic fracture should be further screened.
2. The patient had a history of tumor as well as lymph node dissection after radical treatment of cervical cancer and had received abdominal radiotherapy for a period. Physical examination also showed slight swelling in the right limb. Considering that the patient's general condition was not excellent, and accompanied by right lower extremity lymphatic reflux disorder, the scale control of the following surgery should be relatively conservative.
3. Right hip AP X-rays showed an obvious periosteum reaction of the femur, which was irregular hyperplasia of the bone cortex. It was mostly manifested as osteomyelitis of infection, rather than erosive change of tumor. Thus, it was not mainly considered metastatic cancer. Moreover, it was observed that the filling bone cement was abundant, reaching distal femoral diaphysis. Removing bone cement while reserving the cortex would be an extremely complicated process.
4. Laboratory examination: Serological results showed that ESR and CRP were both relatively high. Combined with a medical history and radiographic data, it was more likely to be a periprosthetic infection. However, arthrocentesis was required for further determination.
5. Arthrocentesis: Arthrocentesis of the right hip joint was performed under the guidance of the C arm (a kind of X-ray perspective apparatus). The amount of aspiration fluid was limited, and thus saline solution was injected through the needle and then aspirated back out for culture. The culture result was oral streptococcus.
6. Diagnosis: Periprosthetic infection after right THA.

5.2.3 Preoperative Planning

1. The diagnosis of periprosthetic infection of this patient was confirmed. Considering that the patient had been suffering from pain for a long time and had developed an osteomyelitis infection, we believed that a two-stage operation should be performed to treat the periprosthetic infection, so as to maximize the success rate.

2. In order to increase the success rate, a two-stage operation was determined. However, during prosthesis retrieval and spacer implantation in the first stage, it should be taken into consideration that the patient had a medical history of radical treatment, radiotherapy, and lymphatic reflux disorders. In consequence, we performed the operation in a much faster manner, aiming to decrease the scale of the operation.

5.2.4 Operation Situation

1. During the incision, when reaching the lateral hip joint capsule, arthrocentesis was performed first. A large amount of purulent liquid was visible.
2. Due to good bone cement technique, the original prosthesis was well fixed, and in order to save time, ETO was performed to retrieve the stem directly.
3. After the stem was retrieved, it was found in the X-ray that the periosteum reaction part was a large area of dead bone. Similarly, in order to save the operation time, this part of the dead bone was resected and abandoned together with a large amount of bone cement covered on the surface.
4. Bone cement on the original greater trochanter was cleaned by ultrasonic osteotome, and thorough debridement was performed to the soft tissue of the acetabulum and femur. Hydrogen peroxide solution was employed to rinse the tissue repeatedly and the necrotic part was scraped off until the bleeding tissue surface appeared. Then the wound was rinsed with hydrogen peroxide, iodophor, and normal saline solution repeatedly.
5. After the debridement was completed, all surgical instruments were replaced and the sterile sheet was replaced. The spacer was made with bone cement mixed with vancomycin and a long stem. Subsequently, the incision was progressively closed.

The intraoperative observation is shown in Fig. 5.2.

5.2.5 Postoperative Condition and Outcome

1. Synovial fluid and tissue culture showed the same result as oral streptococcus. Therefore, it could be further confirmed for periprosthetic infection. We developed antibiotic therapy based on the results of pathogen susceptibility.
   (a) Intravenous use of second-generation cephalosporins within 1–2 weeks after operation.
   (b) After discharge from the hospital, oral intake of cefdinir + rifampicin was instructed for 3–6 weeks.
2. Two weeks after the antibiotic therapy, the patient visited our hospital again for laboratory and aspiration tests. ESR: 11.4 mm/h; CRP: 14 mg/L; synovial fluid WBC count: 509/mm^3; percentage of PMNs in synovial fluid: 53%; and aspiration liquid culture: negative.
3. Laboratory tests and aspiration results indicated that the infection was effectively controlled, and the patient underwent the second-stage revision surgery. Reconstruction of the affected extremity was performed using a tumor prosthesis. Postoperative 2-year follow-up examination showed that the patient could perform daily activities without reinfection.

The postoperative anteroposterior X-ray of the first-stage retrieval and spacer implantation is shown in Fig. 5.3.

The postoperative full-length film of the lower extremity of the second-stage revision is shown in Fig. 5.4.

5.2.6 Conclusion and Reflection

1. In clinical treatment, for arthroplasty patients without a sinus tract and no obvious manifestations of redness, swelling, or heat after the operation, we take the characteristics of pain as the main reference for patient classification. When does the pain

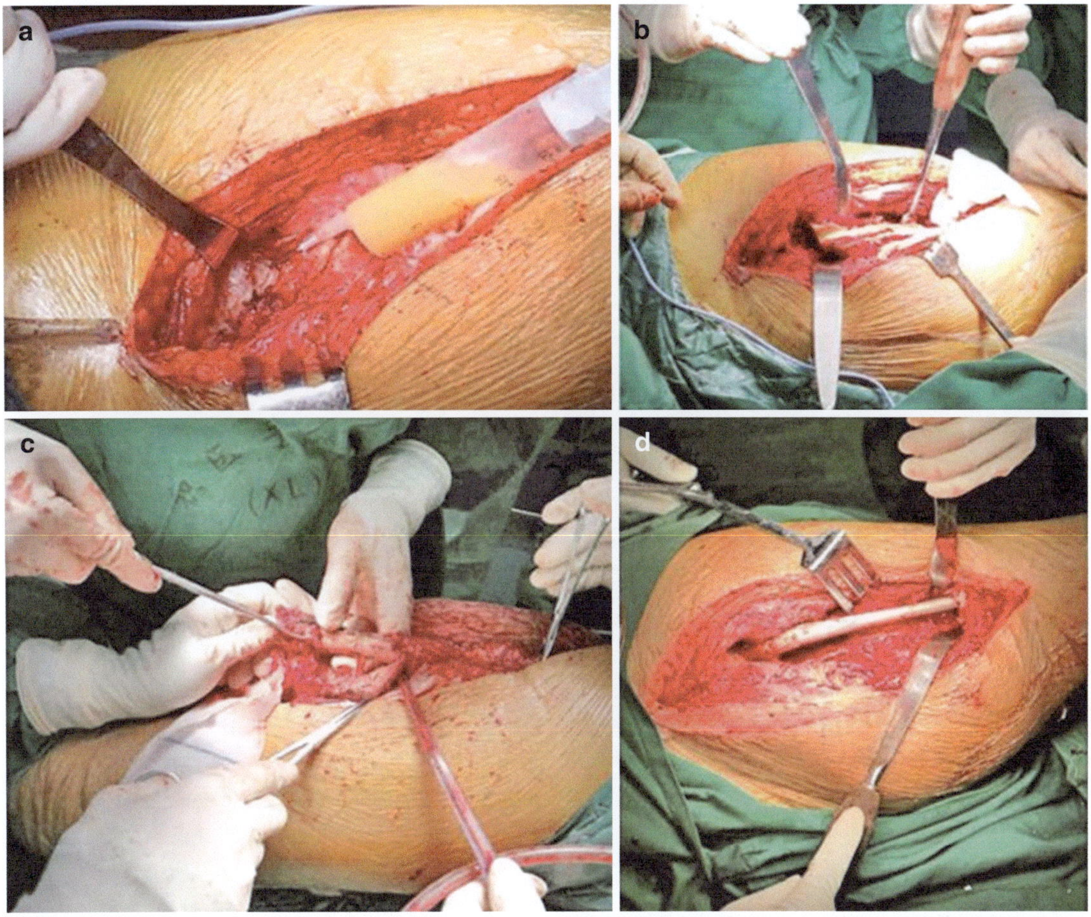

Fig. 5.2 Intraoperative observation. (**a**) The aspiration after cutting the skin. (**b**) A large amount of bone cement in femoral intramedullary after greater trochanter splitting. (**c**) Periosteum delamination of femoral periosteal reaction zone. (**d**) Long-stemmed bone cement femoral stem used as a temporary spacer

appear? How long does it last? Is it a resting pain or nocturnal pain? If chronic resting pain without trauma occurs, it should be considered for infections, tumors, or metabolic diseases; further combined with the patient's medical history, whether there has been recent infection in other parts of the body, previous tumors, or physical manifestations such as lymphatic edema; finally refer to the radiographs to check whether there is periosteum reaction, erosive changes, and so on. In the end, the next treatment plan should be formulated, either inviting the oncology department for consultation or performing aspiration synovial fluid for further analysis.

2. Clinical aspiration may encounter failure, that is, the synovial fluid cannot be collected or is insufficient for synovial fluid analysis in some patients. This situation is also graphically referred to as the "dry tap."
3. According to our experience and related literature reports, for periprosthetic knee infection patients, the elastic bandage is applied on the distal and proximal knee joints for pressure fix, so that the synovial fluid concentrates in the knee joint to improve the success rate of the aspiration test. For hip aspiration, we apply a guided aspiration test with a C-arm (a kind of X-ray perspective apparatus), and a special aspiration needle is employed. A lateral approach through a supe-

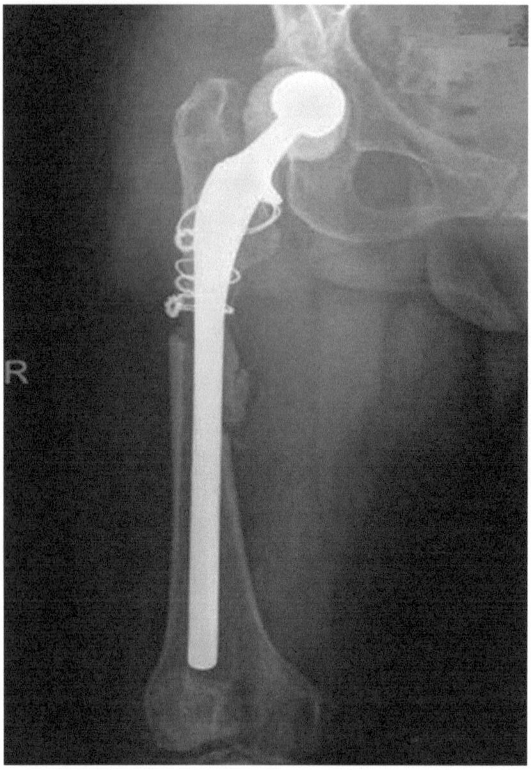

Fig. 5.3 Postoperative anteroposterior X-ray of the first-stage retrieval and spacer implantation

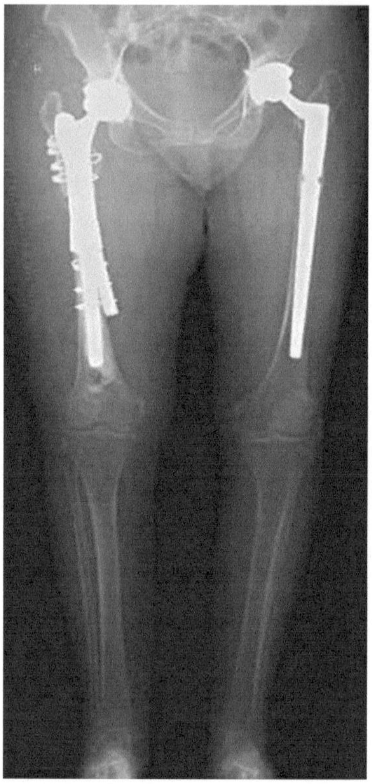

Fig. 5.4 Postoperative full-length film of lower extremity of second-stage revision

rior greater trochanter is adopted, and aspiration aims at the neck of the stem. The success rate of the aspiration test is improved by better accuracy, and after the aspiration test, the needle has reached the predetermined position, and hip flexion and extension can be applied to further improve the success rate. If the method above still fails to extract synovial fluid or for a sufficient amount, articular irrigation can be performed by injecting sterile normal saline solution via the aspiration needle. By extracting the cleaning fluid, we can obtain a culture sample.

4. Whether to apply a biopsy needle. Combined with clinical experience and previous literature reports, tissue biopsy is not suggested. We believe that tissue biopsy cannot collect infected tissue easily, and the positive rate of the collected articular tissue culture is lower. Meanwhile, the tissue biopsy itself causes greater damage and cost compared to the synovial fluid aspiration test. For the above reasons, we recommend a fine-needle synovial fluid aspiration test.
5. Tumor and infection should be distinguished. In clinical practice, for patients with suspected periprosthetic infection with previous tumor history, tumor metastasis or recurrence identification should be taken into consideration. Our institution will first strictly examine the radiographs for this type of patient. As bone destruction caused by tumors is mostly erosive, whereas periprosthetic infection is mostly manifested as osteomyelitis, it can be used as a reference for preliminary diagnosis. However, it is necessary to consult with the Department of Bone Oncology and their consultation advice should be included as the basis for the final treatment.
6. The selection of surgery among debridement, first stage, and second stage. The bone cement of this patient was extremely thick, which was

very difficult to remove. In order to shorten the operation time and control the operation scale, greater trochanter splitting was adopted to directly section and retrieve the stem, and the necrotic bone part was excised. It saved the process of bone cement removal and only the greater trochanter was retained for later reconstruction, followed by thorough debridement.

No matter what kind of treatment is used, the purpose is to control infection, reduce recurrence, and rebuild function. At the same time, comprehensive consideration should be given to the patient's physical conditions, personal needs, financial status, and many other factors to develop a tailored strategy that meets the patient's personal needs.

7. The selection of a spacer should also be made based on the actual situation of the patient. A good spacer can provide better motion function and help the reconstruction in the future. Previous literature showed no significant difference between mobile spacers and static spacers in terms of motor function in secondary follow-up examinations. However, a short-term follow-up examination showed that a mobile spacer was better for articular motion maintenance. The second-stage revision courses we performed were all within 6 months; thus, our institution applied mobile spacers to patients with appropriate conditions in order to reach better motor function after the second-stage revision and reconstruction.

5.3 Case 2

Yang Song and Hongyi Shao

5.3.1 Case Summary

Medical History Male, 49 years old, suffered from left hip pain caused by an accidental fall 9 years ago, which was not immediately diagnosed and treated. After 20 days, no obvious abnormality was found when attending a local hospital, and symptomatic treatment was given. After a bedridden rest at home, the patient recovered and had limited mobility. Left THA was performed at a local hospital 7 years ago. Before 6 years, the patient received second-stage revision for periprosthetic infection in another hospital. The sinus tract occurred at the incision of the left hip 2 years ago, and debridement was performed at a local hospital. The sinus tract appeared again in the same location 1 year ago. The patient attended our institution for further treatment. He had suffered a traumatic brain injury and fracture of multiple ribs caused by a car accident 9 years ago. Left femoral deep vein thrombosis (DVT) was developed 1 year ago, and the inferior vena cava filter implantation was performed, which was retrieved after 2 weeks. Oral administration of warfarin lasted for 6 months.

Physical Examination Walked in with crutches; the temperature was 36.4 °C; the examination results of all systems were normal; a previous incision scar was seen on the posterolateral skin of the left hip; a sinus tract was in the middle of the scar with exudation; skin temperature was normal; left hip tenderness (−); limited mobility of left hip; Patrick's sign of left hip (+); Thomas sign of left hip (+); Trendelenburg sign of left hip (unidentified); mild edema in the left lower extremity; left knee mobility (0–30°); no hypoesthesia; the pulse of bilateral foot dorsal artery was palpable; grade IV myodynamia of left quadriceps, grade II myodynamia of iliac psoas; bilateral knee and Achilles tendon reflexes were normal; and bilateral Babinski sign (−).

Laboratory Examination ESR: 19 mm/h; CRP: 17.4 mg/L; synovial fluid WBC count: none; percentage of polymorphonuclear leukocytes in synovial fluid: none; and aspiration liquid culture: *Staphylococcus aureus* and *Acinetobacter baumannii*.

Radiographic Data See Fig. 5.5 for the preoperative X-rays.

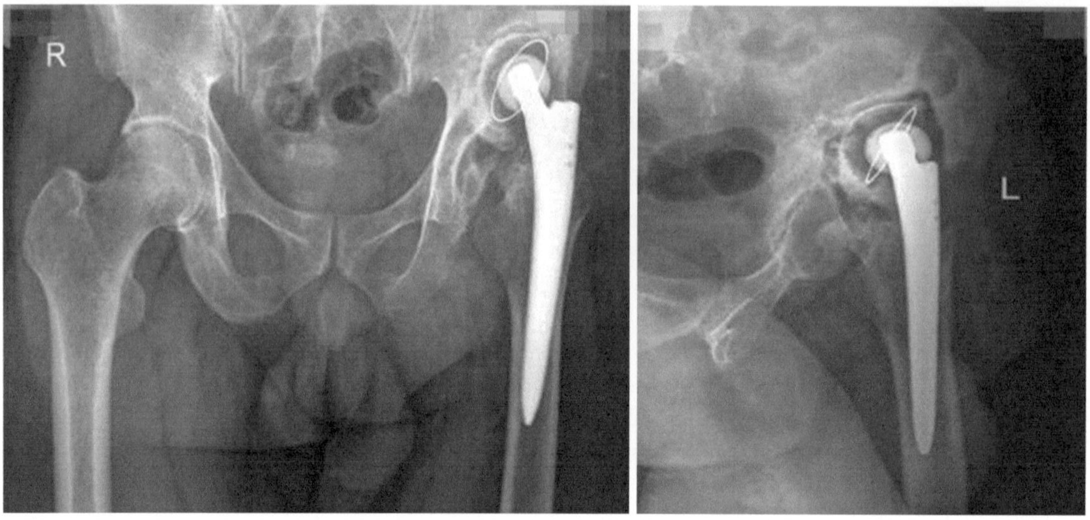

Fig. 5.5 Preoperative X-rays

5.3.2 Case Analysis

1. Medical history showed that the patient had undergone multiple surgeries for the left hip and had a long-term sinus tract. At the same time, limited mobility of the left hip due to trauma had already existed before the initial arthroplasty. A preoperative physical examination showed limited mobility in the left hip. Therefore, it should be fully considered that the left hip soft tissue compliance could be extremely poor, which was likely to greatly influence the operation.
2. X-rays: It could be seen that the cup was placed in the superior of the true acetabulum which was intact without any traces of surgical treatment. Therefore, it could be inferred that the acetabulum was placed in the false acetabulum during the initial arthroplasty. It could be seen that the poor compliance of the joint soft tissue had a significant impact on the first operation.
3. Laboratory test: Serological examination results showed slightly higher ESR and CRP, and periprosthetic joint infection was diagnosed in combination with the sinus tract, physical examination, and radiographic data.
4. Aspiration test: The aspiration of the right hip was performed under C-arm (a kind of X-ray perspective apparatus) guidance. The amount of aspiration liquid was limited. Thus, the culture sample was collected by injecting normal saline. The culture results were *Staphylococcus aureus* and *Acinetobacter baumannii.*
5. Diagnosis: Left hip periprosthetic joint infection.

5.3.3 Preoperative Planning

1. Periprosthetic joint infection was confirmed. Due to the repeated operations on the left hip joint, the long-term presence of the sinus tract, as well as the preoperative culture result of multiple bacterial infections, it indicated that this patient was a refractory infection case. We believe that a two-stage surgery should be selected to treat the periprosthetic joint infection, so as to improve the success rate as much as possible.

In order to improve the success rate of the treatment, two-stage surgery was decided. During the first stage, we selected an appropriate antibiotic to make the antibiotic cement spacer according to the preoperative drug sensitivity. And we made a further soft tissue release for the poor compliance. The spacer was placed above the true acetabulum for full preparation for the second-stage revision.

5.3.4 Operation Situation

1. During the operation, when reaching the hip joint capsule, we first performed aspiration. Only a small amount of fluid was collected, which was not enough for routine examination. Thus, culture examination was employed. At the same time, the sonication fluid of the spacer was collected and cultured. The sonication process is shown in Fig. 5.6.
2. Due to the poor compliance of the periprosthetic soft tissue, articular dislocation was not available, and ETO was performed intraoperatively to retrieve the femoral stem.
3. After the femoral stem removal, the soft tissue around the hip joint was further loosened for sufficient operating space, so that the acetabular component could be retrieved.
4. During the release step, the sinus tract approach was discovered in the anterior joint capsule. Resection of the soft tissue was performed when cutting along the sinus tract. And acetabular and femoral soft tissue was thoroughly debrided at the same time. Hydrogen peroxide was used to irrigate the tissue repeatedly and the necrotic tissue was scaled off until the bleeding tissue surface appeared. Then the wound was repeatedly washed with hydrogen peroxide, iodophor, and normal saline solution. We did this irrigation three times with a consumption of brine 9000 mL at least.
5. After completing the debridement, the full set of surgical instruments and the sterile sheet were replaced. A temporary spacer was made with cement mixed with vancomycin and a long stem on the femur side. The polyethylene liner was also fixed on the acetabular side using cement mixed with vancomycin. Subsequently, the incision was sealed layer by layer with a drainage implantation.

Intraoperative observation is shown in Fig. 5.7.

5.3.5 Postoperative Condition and Outcome

1. Intraoperative retention of tissue and synovial fluid for culture: *Staphylococcus aureus*, penicillase (+), MLSb resistant; intraoperative

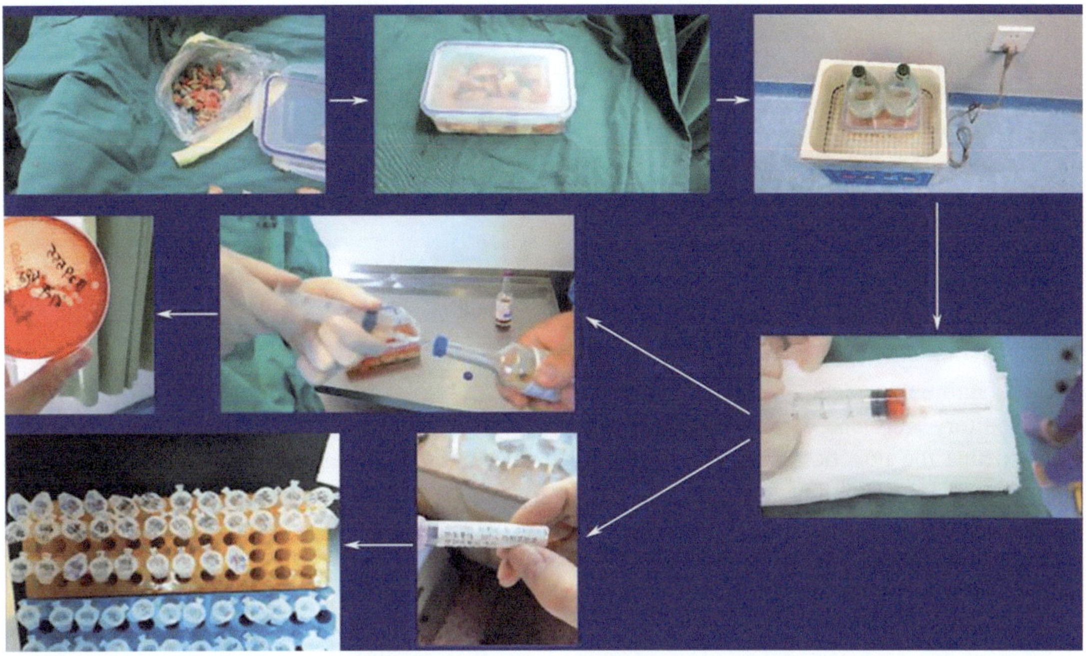

Fig. 5.6 Sonication process

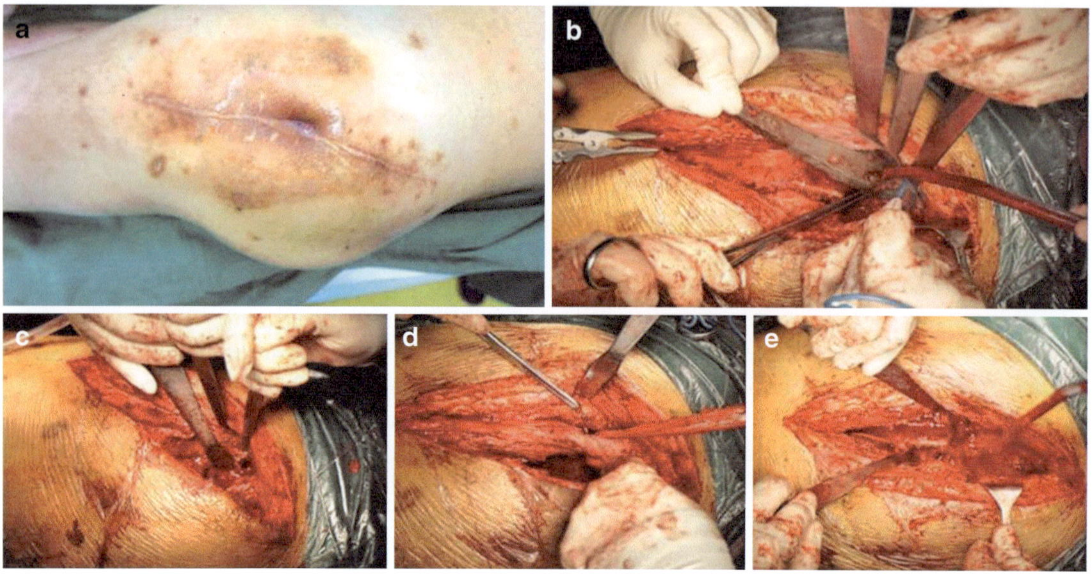

Fig. 5.7 Intraoperative observation. (**a**) Preoperative sinus tract formation, serious cicatrix from multiple operatives. (**b**) The femoral stem was first retrieved through extended trochanteric osteotomy. (**c**) The acetabular component could be seen buried deep within the false acetabulum. (**d**) Thorough cleaning of the anterior sinus tract. (**e**) The true acetabulum was filed for the spacer implantation

ultrasonic culture: *Staphylococcus aureus*, penicillase (+), MLSb.

2. Based on the drug sensitivity results preoperation, the intraoperative spacer should be constructed with vancomycin mixed with bone cement (12.5%). Vancomycin sodium was administered intravenously for 2 weeks after the operation. Subsequently, cefdinir + rifampicin was taken orally for 4 weeks.
3. Two weeks after the antibiotic treatment, the patient attended our hospital for laboratory and aspiration tests. ESR: 7 mm/h; CRP: 3.4 mg/L; synovial fluid WBC count: 122/mm^3; percentage of polymorphonuclear leukocytes in synovial fluid: 40%; aspiration fluid culture: negative.
4. Laboratory tests and aspiration results indicated that the infection was effectively controlled, and the patient was provided with second-stage revision. The affected extremity was reconstructed on the femoral side with a long modular stem, and the acetabular side was reconstructed using acetabulum + augment in the true acetabulum. Postoperative follow-up examination after 2 years showed that the patient could perform daily activities without recurrence of infection.

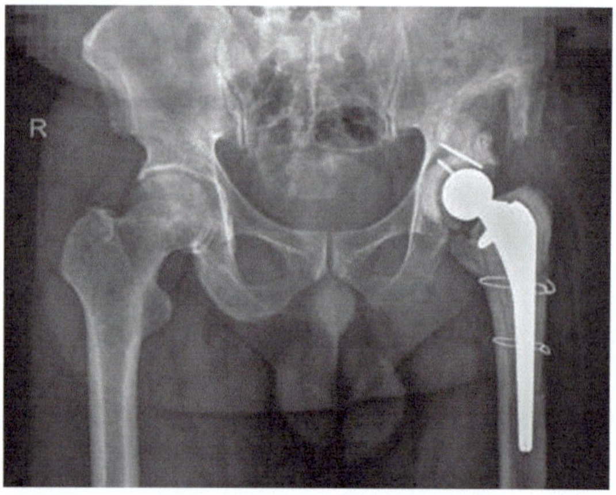

Fig. 5.8 Postoperative anteroposterior hip X-ray of first-stage retrieval and spacer implantation

The postoperative anteroposterior hip X-ray of first-stage retrieval and spacer implantation is shown in Fig. 5.8.

The postoperative anteroposterior hip X-ray of the second-stage revision is shown in Fig. 5.9.

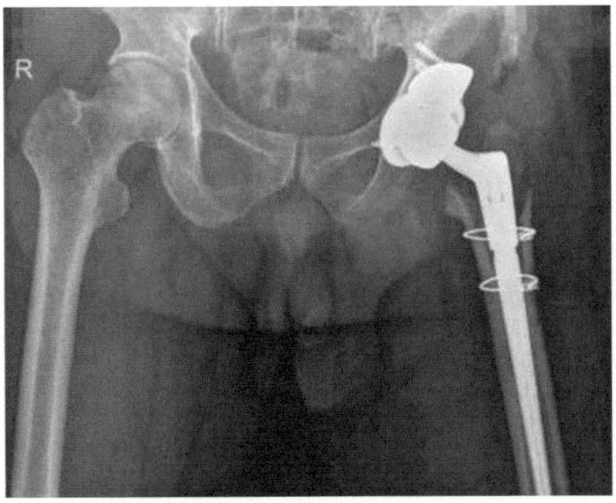

Fig. 5.9 Postoperative anteroposterior hip X-ray of second-stage revision

1. Diagnosis should not be given on assumption without verification. In this case, the patient had a long-term sinus tract, which was consistent with the main diagnostic indicators of periprosthetic infection. However, in the process of diagnosis and treatment, it is still necessary to refer to examinations such as hematological indicators, synovial fluid routine tests, and synovial fluid cultures, so as to confirm the diagnosis. Even if the diagnosis seems to be clear, it is important to follow a step-by-step approach to avoid missing the presence of other diseases.
2. The patient's medical history and previous radiographs showed that the hip dislocation was not congenital but caused by a contracture around the hip joint due to post-traumatic non-surgical treatment. Moreover, the initial arthroplasty and the revision after the primary THA did not reconstruct the acetabulum in its true position. The false acetabulum position indicated poor compliance of the periprosthetic soft tissue of the patient's left hip joint.

   At the same time, it could also be seen from the radiographs that the true acetabulum was relatively well preserved and reconstruction of the acetabulum would not be too difficult. In addition, the distal fixation stem could be applied as the femoral side tubular bone was intact. Therefore, the difficulty of this operation lay in the soft tissue around the hip joint. Extended trochanteric osteotomy was decided to retrieve the stem to reduce the operation time for the solid cement fixation. Soft tissue was released in these two stages. A mobile spacer was implanted to allow the joint to move between the first and second stages of surgery, which aimed to further release soft tissue.
3. According to the medical history, the left hip sinus tract of the patient existed for many years. The possibility of multiple bacterial infections should be considered in such situations. Long-term sinus tract formation generates a channel between the prosthesis and the environment; many opportunistic pathogens in various environments will become pathogens of periprosthetic infection.

   The preoperative culture results of this case were multi-sensitive *Staphylococcus aureus*, as well as *Acinetobacter baumannii*. Although the intraoperative culture result showed only multi-sensitive *Staphylococcus aureus*, when applying antibiotics treatment, it should be considered to cover both preoperative pathogens.
4. The sinus tract multi-existed for the pathogens expanding along the intramuscular space. It should be specially considered during the debridement, in which all potential sinus tract and dead space should be cleaned. In this case, it was found that the long-standing sinus tract protruded from the anterior gluteus medius; thus, the gluteus maximus and gluteus medius space was widened and separated for complete debridement. For other patients with more complex conditions, even though the sinus tract protrudes anteriorly, thorough cleaning must be performed. Despite double or multiple incisions of the anterior and posterior approach, a thorough resection of the soft tissue surrounding the sinus tract is necessary.
5. The treatment of periprosthetic joint infections is often compared to tumor treatment, both of which share many common characteristics. First, it is difficult to cure. What we can provide for patients is a functional joint without periprosthetic joint infection symptoms

and recurrence. However, there is no proof that all the pathogens are wiped out. This is also illustrated in the latest definition of successful treatment of periprosthetic joint infections by the Muscularskeletal Infection Society (MSIS), which is to guarantee a state with no symptoms of Infection, recurrence, or more operation, rather than claim cure of the periprosthetic infection.

Second, the recovery of periprosthetic joint infection, like a tumor, is also the result of multiple factors. For tumors, it is the interaction between host and tumor types, whereas, for periprosthetic joint infection, it is the interaction between host, pathogen, and the implant. When the host is in a good state, the pathogen is sensitive to antibiotics, and the infection is easier to control when there are fewer implants; otherwise, it is difficult to control. Before treatment, these three factors should be fully considered, and adequate thinking and preparation should be conducted.

Finally, just like tumor treatment, the treatment of periprosthetic joint infections is also a team effort. Tumor treatment is not simple resection; both early-stage diagnosis and late-stage radiotherapy and chemotherapy are equally important. The same principle applies to periprosthetic joint infections. Pathogen characteristic identification by microbiologists and pathologists, corresponding antibiotic solutions provided by pharmaceutical experts, and postoperative functional exercise for recovery by rehabilitation physicians are all required. The successful treatment of a patient with periprosthetic joint infection cannot be achieved without the full cooperation of a team, in which the surgeons play the central role. In addition to performing surgery, team building is also of great significance for better treatment of the periprosthetic joint infection.

Recommended Reading

1. Permkumar A, Kolin DA, Farley KX, et al. Projected economic burden of periprosthetic joint infection of the hip and knee in the United States. J Arthroplast. 2021;36(5):1484–9.
2. Kurtz SM, Lau E, Watson H, et al. Economic burden of periprosthetic joint infection in the United States. J Arthroplast. 2012;27(8 Suppl):61–5.
3. Barton CB, Wang DL, Qiang AN, et al. Two-stage exchange arthroplasty for periprosthetic joint infection following total hip or knee arthroplasty is associated with high attrition rate and mortality. J Arthroplast. 2020;35(5):1384–9.
4. Pulido L, Ghanem E, Joshi A, et al. Periprosthetic joint infection: the incidence, timing, and predisposing factors. Clin Orthop Relat Res. 2008;466(7):1710–5.
5. Kremers K, Leijtens B, Camps S, et al. Evaluation of early wound leakage as a risk factor for prosthetic joint infection. J Am Assoc Nurse Pract. 2019;31(6):337–43.
6. Parvizi J, Gehrke T. Definition of periprosthetic joint infection. J Arthroplast. 2014;29(7):1331.

6 Dislocation Following Total Hip Arthroplasty

Hao Tang, Zhuyi Ma, and Shengjie Guo

6.1 Introduction

Hao Tang

Dislocation following total hip arthroplasty (THA) is one of the main reasons for revision. Currently, 11–24% of patients with revision total hip arthroplasty undergo dislocation following THA. The annual dislocation rate after initial THA in the International Society of Arthroplasty Registries is 0.2–10%. Data from the National Arthroplasty Register of Scotland showed that between 1996 and 2004, the dislocation rate among 14,314 THA patients was 1.9%, which was 28% in the revision patients. Early-stage dislocation within 3 months accounted for 55–77%, while 32% of patients showed late-stage dislocation within more than 5 years after the operation, in which the recurrent dislocation rate was 55%.

The mechanical stability of THA relies on appropriate prosthesis positioning, soft tissue tension, muscle function, and harmony in biomechanics such as spinal–pelvic motion. Failing to meet these mechanical requirements may result in the instability of hip arthroplasty. In the case of dislocation following THA, it is essential to distinguish the cause between traumatic and non-traumatic, the latter of which often indicates the lack of tissue tension or malposition. Dislocation can be divided into anterior and posterior dislocation according to the direction. The causes of hip joint dislocation can be classified into three categories: patient factors, prosthesis factors, and surgical factors.

6.1.1 Patient Factors

1. Soft tissue factors: Joint muscle and capsule weakness are common mechanisms for hip joint stability in hip arthroplasty. Therefore, in patients with neuromuscular diseases (such as cerebral palsy, adverse muscular nutrition, dementia, and Parkinson's disease), the annual dislocation rate is high, ranging from 5% to 8%. Patients with a previous hip fracture or surgical history are at increased risk of dislocation. For patients with severe soft tissue trauma, extensive cicatrix, and ectopic ossification, the dislocation rate can be as high as 28%.
2. Spinal–pelvic motion factors: Dislocation usually attacks during postural changes in daily activities (e.g., standing and sitting in a chair and picking up objects from the floor). Therefore, the impact of spine–pelvic interactions during postural changes should be considered when discussing a dislocation following THA. According to Schwab et al., a balanced spine–pelvis relationship should be lumbar lordosis = pelvic incidence (PI) ± 10°

H. Tang (✉) · Z. Ma · S. Guo
Department of Adult Joint Reconstructive Surgery, Beijing Jishuitan Hospital, Capital Medical University, Beijing, China
e-mail: 1510122417@pku.edu.cn

Y. Zhou (ed.), *Revision Total Hip Arthroplasty*, https://doi.org/10.1007/978-981-97-9804-9_6

in a standing position. Lumbar lordosis reduction, thoracic kyphosis deformity, and hip/knee joint contracture may result in sagittal disequilibrium. Compensatory pelvic motion can occur through the spine, pelvis, and lower extremity region. As a compensatory mechanism for the loss of lumbar lordosis, different changes such as posterior rotation of the pelvis, posterior hip extension, knee flexion, and ankle flexion may occur to maintain the overall balance of the sagittal position.

When moving from standing upright to sitting, the lumbar lordosis is reduced, the pelvic posteriorly tilts 20°, and the hip flexion is about 55–70° instead of 90°. As part of the pelvis, the acetabulum also tilts posteriorly along with the pelvis when sitting, resulting in an increased anteversion and abduction angle. This change occurs to accommodate the flexion and internal rotation of the hip, as well as the flexion of the anterior hip, to avoid impingement. An increase of 1° in pelvic tilt (PT) increases approximately 0.7° in the acetabulum anteversion. Spinal–pelvic rigidity is defined as an increase in PT of less than 10° when changing from an upright position to a sitting position. This rigidity is usually associated with lumbar disc degeneration or lumbar fusion surgery. Patients with degenerative changes in both spine and hip arthritis are prevalent. Up to 40% of patients receiving THA have degenerative diseases in the lumbar spine.

Phan et al. divided spinal–pelvic motion into four types and proposed solutions for each class:

(a) Soft-balanced, considered normal spinal–pelvic motion. The cup can be placed in a traditional safe zone because it can flexibly compensate for postural changes.
(b) Rigid-balanced, spinal–pelvic rigidity that occurs after severe degenerative changes in spinal or lumbar fusion. A sitting-compensatory anteversion of the acetabulum does not happen, which can lead to anterior impingement and posterior dislocation. In this case, fixing the cup in a more anteverted position is more favorable.
(c) Flexible-unbalanced, classified as excessive motion. In this type, the anteversion of the acetabulum excessively increases when standing, and there is a potential risk of anterior dislocation due to posterior impingement during hip extension.
(d) Rigid-unbalanced, characterized by severe spinal rigidity and unbalanced standing posture. The coexistence of rigidity and imbalance renders an extremely narrow safe zone, or even no safe zone exists, and arbitrary general recommendations on cup anteversion become pointless and detrimental. Patients with this pattern may develop spinal kyphosis or flat back deformity with an increased PT in the standing posture for compensation for the imbalance. The risk of anterior dislocation also increases due to posterior impingement. On the contrary, rigidity leads to a lack of compensation and an increased risk of posterior dislocation in sitting posture. This contradictory dilemma requires a comprehensive quantitative analysis to reduce the dislocation hazard.

6.1.2 Surgical Factors

1. Surgical approach: Numerous studies have shown a higher risk of dislocation with a posterior hip approach where the external rotation muscle and the posterior joint capsule were damaged, compared to the lateral, anterior, or anterior approach. A meta-analysis involving more than 13,000 primary THA with postoperative follow-up examinations within at least 12 months has reported posterior approach dislocation rates of 3.23%, compared with 0.55% and 2.18% for lateral and anterolateral approaches. However, anatomic repair of the posterior joint capsule and the external rotation muscle can significantly reduce the posterior approach dislocation rate to 0.7%. In contrast, the lateral hip approach through the gluteus medius increases the risk of reduced abductor function due to partial

dissection of the gluteus medius or fracture of the greater trochanter.

2. Prosthesis positioning: The orientation of the implant during hip arthroplasty is particularly important for the stability of total hip arthroplasty. Lewinnek's safe zone theory of 40° ± 10° abduction and 15 ± 10° anteversion has recently been proven ineffective in predicting postoperative dislocation. Growing evidence suggests that the angle of the prosthesis should be tailored to the patient's overall balance, as well as the functional posture of the pelvis.

6.1.3 Prosthesis Factors

Prosthesis impingement is one of the main mechanisms of hip dislocation. The prosthesis design may result in a non-mechanically good hip joint, and the head–neck ratio of the stem is particularly important for the prosthesis's stability impingement-free range of motion. A giant femoral head (36 mm) allows a broader range of mechanical motion than a femoral head with a smaller diameter (28 mm). A big femoral head requires a longer jump distance away from the center of the acetabulum before migrating over the cup margin. Therefore, a larger diameter of the head can better prevent dislocation. However, the diameter of the femoral head cannot be increased indefinitely: The thickness of the liner decreases with the increase of head diameter; wear at the head and neck connection increases; and expanding the range of motion promotes secondary impingement, resulting in contact between the proximal femur and the pelvis. Due to the reasons above, femoral heads larger than 40 mm are usually not applicable in THA. A design with a metal extension head with a skirt may severely reduce the stem's head–neck ratio and is a high-risk factor for the impingement-dislocation mechanism. In addition, the bearing surfaces of THA are available in various options such as ceramic on ceramic, ceramic on polyethylene, metal on metal, and metal on polyethylene, among which wear of the polyethylene liner is one of the main factors causing late-stage dislocation.

6.1.4 Patient-Specific Safe Zone (PSSZ)

An appropriate orientation between the cup and femoral stem is critical to avoid post-THA impingement, wear, dislocation, liner fracture, and other complications caused by malpositioned components. Nevertheless, traditional safe zones have been found to be ineffective in predicting dislocation. The pelvic tilt is considered a vital cause of the failure of Lewinnek's safe zone, as it affects the functional orientation of the prosthesis after implantation. Lumbar pelvic rigidity and sagittal imbalance significantly increase the risk of dislocation and wear after THA. As a result, the safe zone should be personalized rather than based on general criteria.

To solve this problem, Tezuka et al. proposed a new functional safe zone, the Combined Sagittal Index, which incorporated the sagittal tilt angle of the acetabular and the pelvic–femoral motion into the parameters guiding the positioning of the THA prosthesis. Phan et al. recommended that patients be classified according to the degree of spinal rigidity and imbalance to help surgeons choose an appropriate cup anteversion (see above). Although these qualitative methods provide recommendations for cup positioning, the specific target angle of the cup remains challenging to personalize for surgeons who wish to minimize dislocation and wear for each particular patient.

Impingement is one of the fundamental mechanisms leading to dislocation, liner fracture, and loosening. Hsu et al. reported a mathematical algorithm that uses the formula published by Yoshimine and Ginbayashi to calculate the angle of an impingement-free prosthesis based on PT. Thus, PT can be quantitatively integrated into the THA safe zone. However, due to the dynamic motion of the pelvis, the PT-based safe zone based on a single posture may not meet the functional requirements of other pelvic postures. To solve this problem, we designed a new strategy to establish PSSZ. By calculating the intersection of the safe zone under different poses, such as standing and sitting, an impingement-free safe zone that covers functions such as walking, sitting, and squatting can be shaped.

Meanwhile, Esposito et al. reported that the edge loading of the anterosuperior cup while standing is more harmful than the posterior edge loading while sitting because of higher local stresses. Scholars such as Leslie and Callanan suggested that the upper limit of cup abduction should be 45° to reduce the wear rate of polyethylene. Therefore, we adopted the functional abduction <45° while standing as the limitation of abduction angle to obtain a PSSZ that is impingement-free and edge-loading-free. This safe zone is used not only for preoperative planning of initial THA or revision patients but also for quantitative dynamic analysis of the functional cup position for patients with dislocation following THA. PSSZ can provide accurate cup positioning for robot-assisted THA, aiding personalized and functional THA.

6.2 Case 1

Hao Tang and Zhuyi Ma

6.2.1 Case Summary

Medical History A 74-year-old male patient fell at home 1 year ago and had a left femoral neck fracture. He had conservative treatment at home, while his recovery was poor. He received a femoral hemiarthroplasty at another local hospital 1 month before admission. Ten days after the surgery, the patient discovered limited mobility in off-bed activities; X-ray examinations were performed, and it was diagnosed as "left hip joint dislocation after hemiarthroplasty." His medical history was remarkable for a previous Parkinson's disease of 10 years.

Physical Examination The patient was pushed into the ward on a gurney. No pelvis tilt; flexion of left hip, with external rotation deformity; and limited flexion, abduction, and internal rotation.

Laboratory Examination No abnormality was detected in the routine blood test, erythrocyte sedimentation rate (ESR), or C-reactive protein (CRP).

Radiographic Data Preoperative X-ray is shown in Fig. 6.1.

6.2.2 Case Analysis

1. Preoperative X-ray showed abnormal enlargement of the lesser trochanter, with the femoral head lateral facing and external rotation position of the left leg. Hyperplasia and ossification were observed in the gap between the acetabulum and femur, suggesting two possibilities: (1) long history of dislocation, resulting in heterotopic ossification (HO), and (2) the patient had a neuromuscular disease and adverse neural innervation, resulting in HO. Considering that the patient had an operation 1 month ago and the dislocation only 10 days after the index surgery, it was consistent with the second possibility, i.e., Parkinson's disease triggered the dislocation.
2. From the perspective of surgery: (1) there were obvious errors in the operation; the anteversion of the stem was excessively large; (2) without surgical treatment, the dislocation could not be reduced; or even reduced, the mechanical stability of the hip could not be

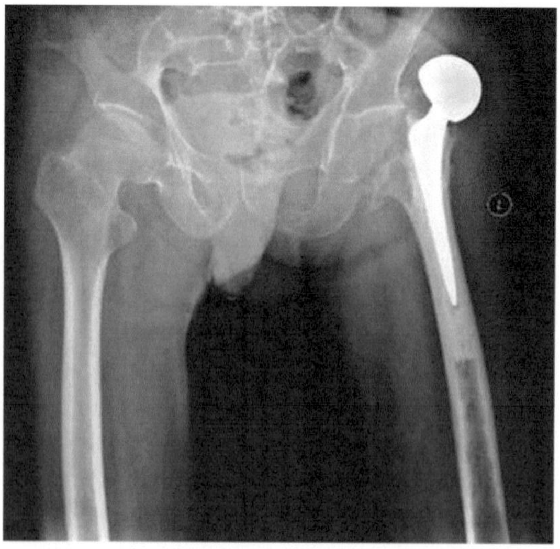

Fig. 6.1 Preoperative X-ray

maintained. Elderly patients with hip dislocation lose the ability to walk. Long-term bed-ridden may cause complications such as systemic pneumonia, pressure ulcers, and lower extremity thrombosis. The mortality rate is as high as 20% within 1 year, and the complication rate of conservative treatment is high. Therefore, the indications for revision surgery were clear.

3. Diagnosis: anterior dislocation following left hemiarthroplasty.

6.2.3 Preoperative Planning

1. Conversion to THA: (1) Hip arthritis already existed because of lesions and wear of the joint cartilage; (2) anteversion of the cup could be adjusted to improve joint stability. The stability advantage of the large femoral head in hemiarthroplasty could be further enhanced with a bipolar femoral head; (3) hemiarthroplasty was not necessarily more stable than THA. The upper margin of the acetabulum can be seen at around 40° abduction in THA, and the abduction of THA is smaller than that of the original abduction in the bony acetabulum. In contrast, the femoral head in hemiarthroplasty is less covered than in THA.
2. Stem revision: The preoperative radiograph showed a large amount of cement around the femoral stem with intact cement shells, indicating good cement technique used by the prior surgeon. From the damage control perspective, cement in cement was an ideal choice for revision, which could shorten the operation time and reduce the systemic damage to the elderly patient. At the same time, the application of a cemented stem would allow more freedom to adjust its anteversion and improve its stability.
3. What type of femoral head to choose: According to the literature, there has been increasing use of dual mobility (DM) femoral heads globally. First, there was no ready-for use DM head with a ceramic-polyethylene-metal bearing surface for THA for the authors' team. The implant of a DM head in a 40-mm polyethylene liner would increase the jump distance, and the mismatch between the head and socket would be reduced, which was of great help to dislocation control. If any further instability occurred, it could also be revised into a constraint liner. According to the literature, monoblock femoral head sizes above 40 mm are less rewarding for dislocation prevention. To sum up, we decided to use the original 40-mm DM head.
4. Why the constraint liner was not considered:
   (a) A constraint liner would increase the risk of loosening.
   (b) The size of the external cup had to be above 52 mm.
   (c) Handling the possible dislocation without open reduction would be difficult.

   To sum up, the constraint liner cup should be the last resort for revision.
5. Special notes regarding soft tissue: The patient had a long history of Parkinson's disease. Thus, there was a potential for dislocation due to imbalanced muscle tension. In addition, gluteus medius injury was possibly present. Therefore, before surgery, gluteus medius restoring materials (synthetic mesh or ligament) should be prepared.

6.2.4 Operation Process

A small skin incision was made during the operation. Torsion in the proximal femur, stem malposition (femur anteversion 100°), and visible gluteus medius tear were observed. It was speculated that the gluteus medius was ruptured with scars and atrophy, possibly due to severe damage in the previous surgery.

The original DM head and femoral stem were retrieved with suitable tools. Some of the cement blocking the stem entrance was removed with devices such as a grinder and piezoelectric osteotome. The minimum EXTER femoral stem was selected, with a reduced anteversion to 10°, and was fixed with low-viscosity cement using a cement-in-cement technique. A 40-mm DM head was used.

The acetabular reamer was used from small to large to expand the acetabulum to 56 mm in diameter. A 56-mm non-cement cup was implanted with a good press fit, aiming at 40°

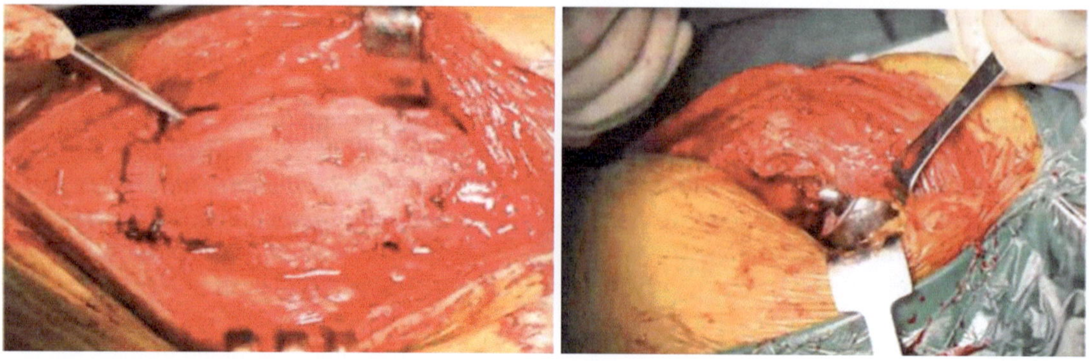

Fig. 6.2 Intraoperative repair of the gluteus medius muscle

extraversion and 20° anteversion, and an inner liner was inserted.

The posterior half of the gluteus medius had an old avulsion, which was strengthened with an artificial mesh ligament.

The intraoperative observation is shown in Fig. 6.2.

6.2.5 Postoperative Condition and Outcome

Postoperative X-ray taken 3 days after the operation is shown in Fig. 6.3.

According to the follow-up, the patient died 2 years after the surgery. His family suggested that the condition after the revision was satisfactory before his death, and no dislocation occurred again.

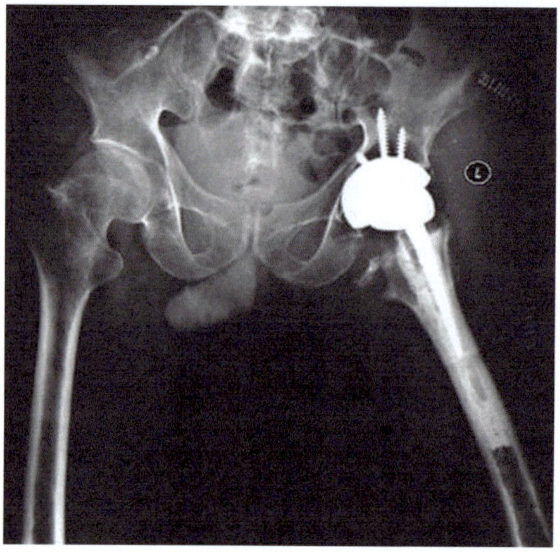

Fig. 6.3 Postoperative X-ray on day 3

6.2.6 Conclusion and Reflection

This case covered almost all causes of hip joint dislocation, including malposition, poor soft tissue conditions, and neuromuscular diseases. Each etiology was treated accordingly in operation.

1. During the exposure, suture knots were visible in the muscle belly of the gluteus medius with severe fatty infiltration. The transition area between the greater trochanter and gluteus medius tendons was attenuated, revealing an hourglass-like shape. We used mesh augments to strengthen the connection, drilled holes in the posterior edge of the greater trochanter with a lumbar puncture needle, repaired the posterior joint capsule with a thick non-absorbable suture, and strengthened the gluteal muscle fascia with a mesh.
2. All potential problems leading to dislocation need to be adjusted, including soft tissue balance, position adjustment, and DM head application.
3. Postoperative radiographs of the patients indicated that the affected extremity was still in external rotation, which was possibly related to the following reasons:
   (a) Treatment for the previous dislocation was performed 10 days after it occurred, and the soft tissue tension was not recovered.

(b) Hemiarthroplasty was performed 1 year after the hip fracture. The preoperative situations were unknown, yet it was speculated that external rotation deformity might have occurred due to long-term immobilization.
(c) The external rotation was not corrected after the operation, indicating a fixed rotational deformity.

6.3 Case 2

Hao Tang, Shengjie Guo, and Zhuyi Ma

6.3.1 Case Summary

Medical History A 52-year-old female patient underwent THA for left hip stunting 11 months ago. The surgery was successful, and the patient recovered. The functional exercise was intensified after discharge. Ten days after the operation, the patient reported sudden snapping of the left hip when sitting on the edge of the bed, accompanied by local pain and limited mobility. When arriving at another hospital, it was discovered in physical examination that left lower extremity discrepancy, flexion, adduction, and internal rotation occurred. Radiography showed total left hip dislocation. Symptomatic treatments such as manipulative reduction, immobilization of the affected extremity, and pain relief were performed. One week later, the patient reported sudden left hip pain when leaving the bed. X-ray showed dislocation following left THA. Closed reduction was applied again but failed. The patient subsequently presented sudden pulmonary embolism symptoms, dyspnea, and decreased oxygen saturation and was transferred to the intensive care unit (ICU) for further treatment. Due to the concern about pulmonary embolism recurrence, the patient refused a second close reduction or surgical treatment and requested discharge.

Physical Examination The patient entered with double crutches; the pelvis tilted to the right; and limited internal/external rotation in the left hip, with a leg length discrepancy of 5 cm.

Laboratory Examination No abnormality was detected in a routine blood test, ESR, or CRP.

Radiographic Data See Fig. 6.4 for preoperative X-rays of the initial left THA.

Preoperative EOS X-rays of the standing and squatting positions after the initial right THA are presented in Fig. 6.5.

One week after the initial left THA, the patient presented dislocation when sitting, which relapsed after closed reduction. Due to lower extremity DVT and pulmonary embolism, the patient was

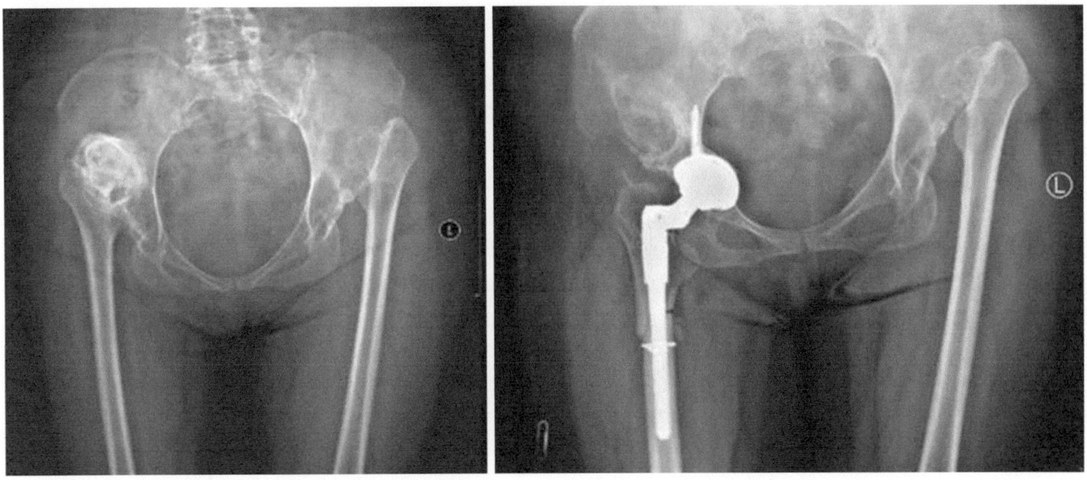

Fig. 6.4 Preoperative X-rays of the initial left THA

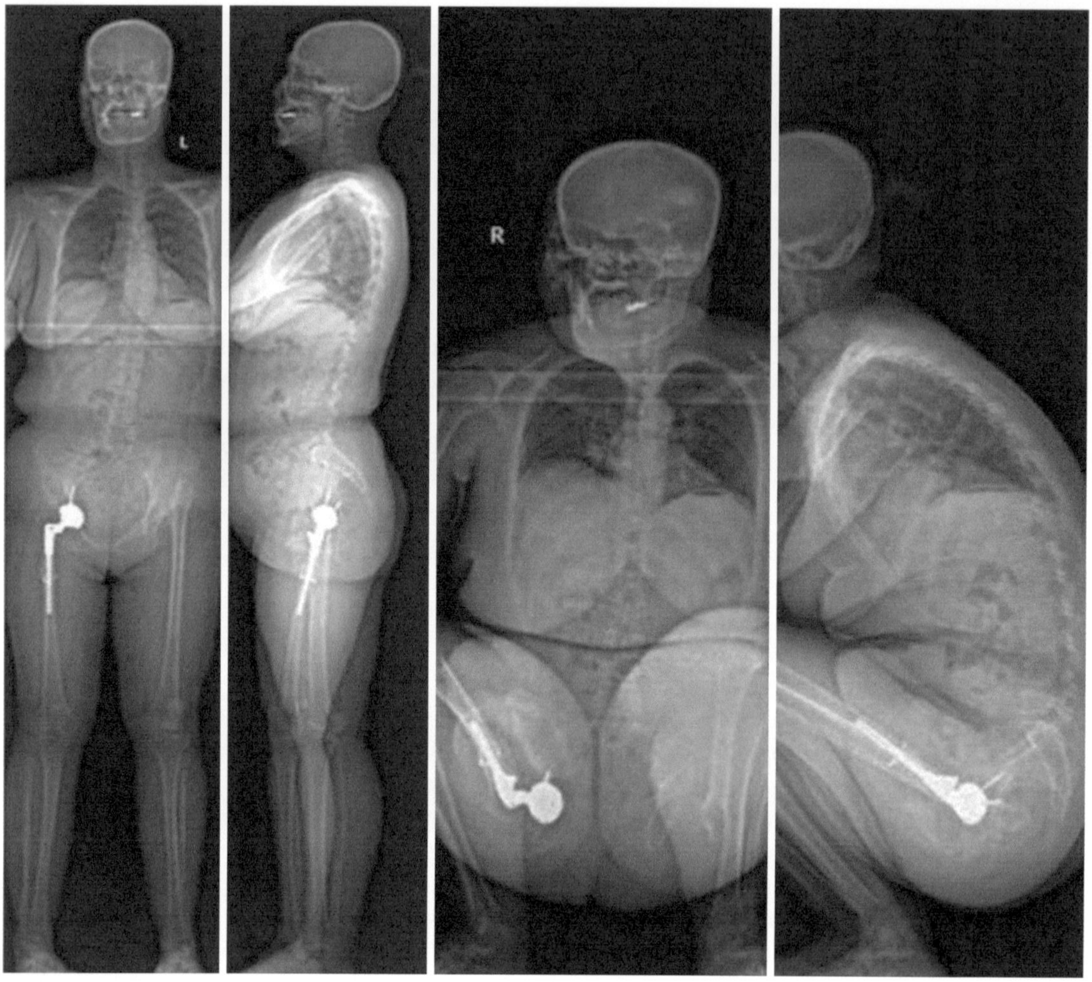

Fig. 6.5 Standing and squatting preoperative EOS functional images on the left side

treated in ICU for 1 week. Closed reduction and open reduction were both refused. She came back to our hospital 1 year later for further treatment.

Preoperative radiographs showed changes after the left THA, in which the posterolateral femoral head dislocation was visible. For the preoperative X-ray, see Fig. 6.6.

Preoperative position views (Fig. 6.7) suggested good mobility; no evident flexion deformity was seen.

6.3.2 Case Analysis

The dislocation rate following THA in patients with high riding hip dislocation is 5–10 times higher than that of typical patients for the following reasons:

1. Acetabular bone structural factors: Surgeons tend to compromise on cup placement considering the bone mass and deformity.
2. Femur side bone factors: This patient had subtrochanteric shortening osteotomy. On the one hand, too much shortening led to the loosening of the outer sleeve of the soft tissue. On the other hand, poorly controlled rotation of the proximal femur could result in the greater trochanter tilting forward or backward, which restrains the function of the gluteus medius.
3. Soft tissue factors: Adequate soft tissue release was performed for reduction; the increase in dislocation rate could be caused by either excessive or insufficient release in which the excessive strain led to fixed hip flexion contracture.

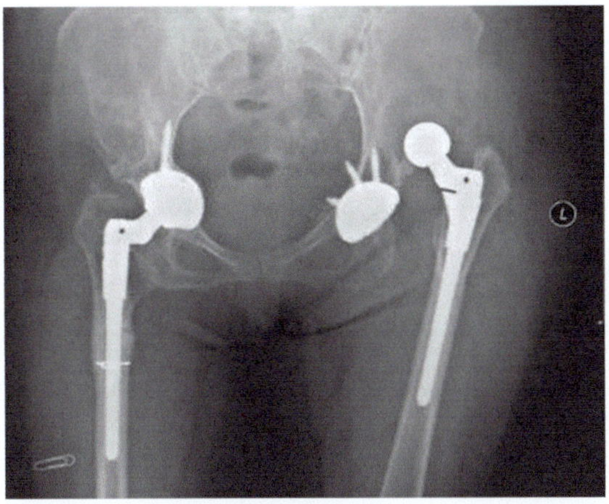

Fig. 6.6 Preoperative X-ray image for revision

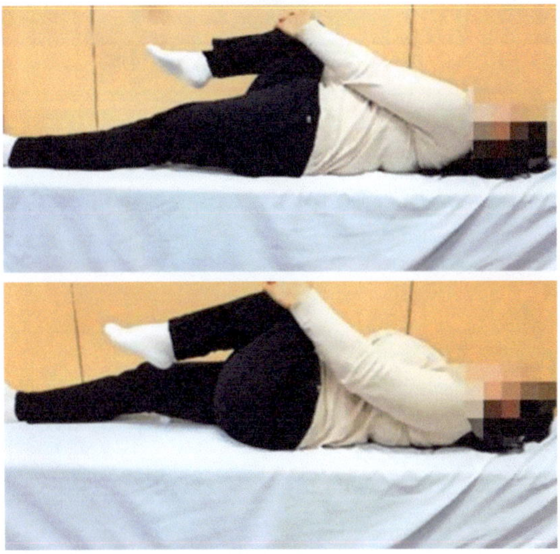

Fig. 6.7 Preoperative positioning image

4. Overall deformity of the lower extremity: It could be associated with lower limb deformities, namely, hip joint adduction due to a valgus knee joint.
5. Lumbopelvic motion factors: With increased lordosis, the patient could present with degeneration and rigidity of the lumbar spine, significantly reducing the safe zone of THA.
6. Acetabular prosthesis: Due to the low bone stock, small cup diameter, and small femoral head diameter, the head-to-neck ratio and jump distance were significantly reduced, resulting in a reduction of the safe zone.
7. Femoral prosthesis: Valgus knee with loose soft tissue occurred due to subtrochanteric osteotomy. This makes the intraoperative control of the femoral stem anteversion difficult, either too large or too small, which could lead to a femoral stem–acetabular angle mismatch.

Interestingly, the patient had no dislocation on the right but posterior dislocation on the left after bilateral THA. However, according to the X-ray (Fig. 6.6), there was no significant difference in the anteversion of both cups, which could not explain the dislocation on the left but not on the right. Therefore, it was easy for surgeons to consider the dislocation caused by soft tissue factors alone.

Measurement of the anatomical anteversion was 25° of the right cup and 24° on the left, according to the preoperative CT; left femoral anteversion was 13° on the right side and −1° on the left side, as shown in Fig. 6.8.

The angles of bilateral femoral stems revealed significant differences, but a difference of 14° is prevalent clinically and could not be identified as the cause of the hip dislocation.

Therefore, we collected preoperative EOS functional images of patients in standing and sitting positions before the revision to analyze spine-pelvic movement, as shown in Fig. 6.9.

6.3.3 Preoperative Planning

1. The patient had a history of high-riding DDH, spine and lower extremity deformity, and excessive soft tissue release. Since the patient had dislocation for 1 year, it should be considered how the soft tissue could be balanced and whether there would be partial release and contracture around the hip joint.
2. Compared with merely stem revision, a combined acetabulum revision could improve factors such as the center of rotation and unsatisfactory anteversion. Still, the reconstruction of the rotation center and cup anteversion in the primary THA was acceptable and comparable to the right side. Meanwhile, the bone stock of the acetabular side was so small (a 46-mm cup) that revision would be complex after cup removal.

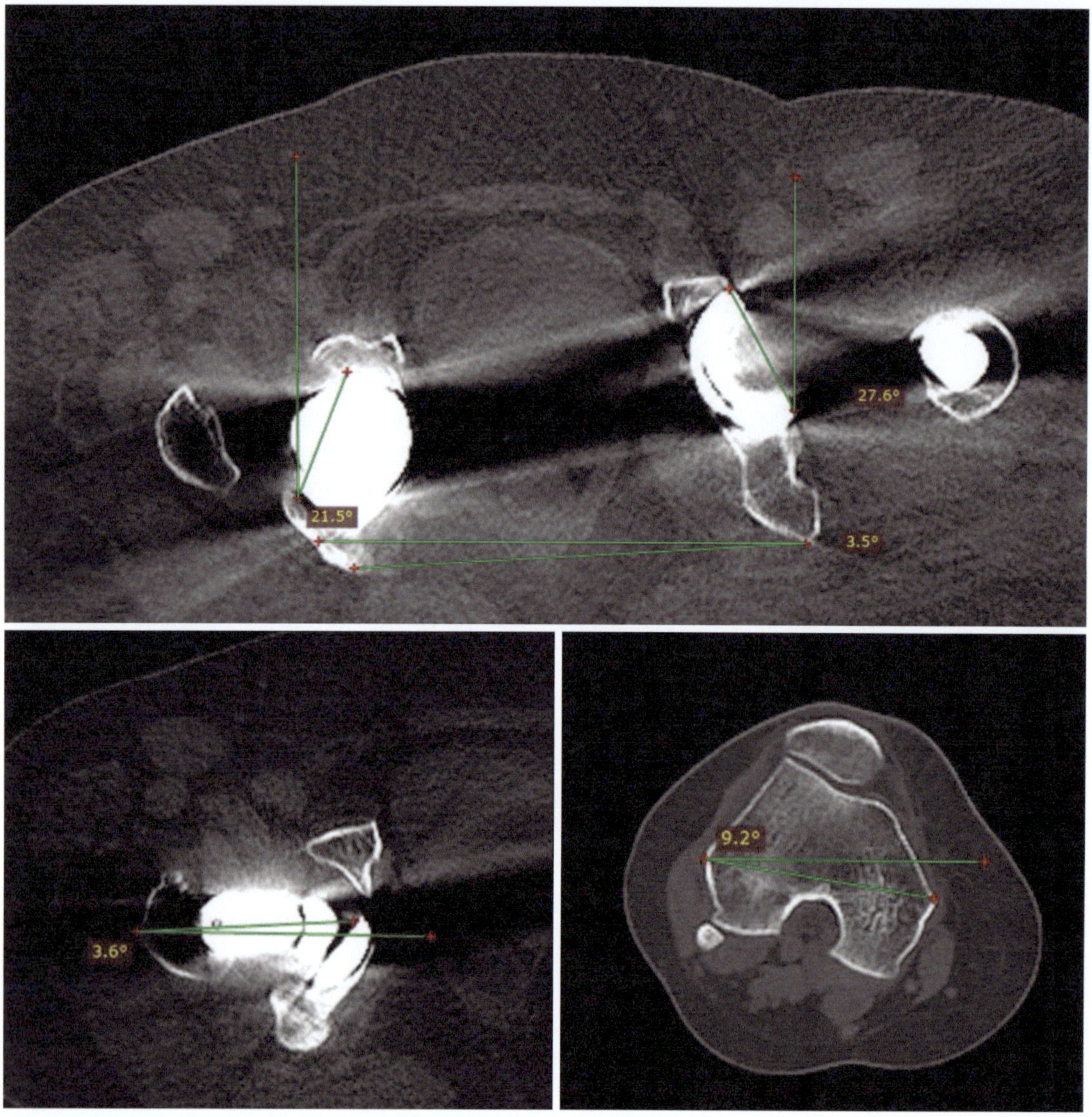

Fig. 6.8 Preoperative CT scan and measurement of components anteversion

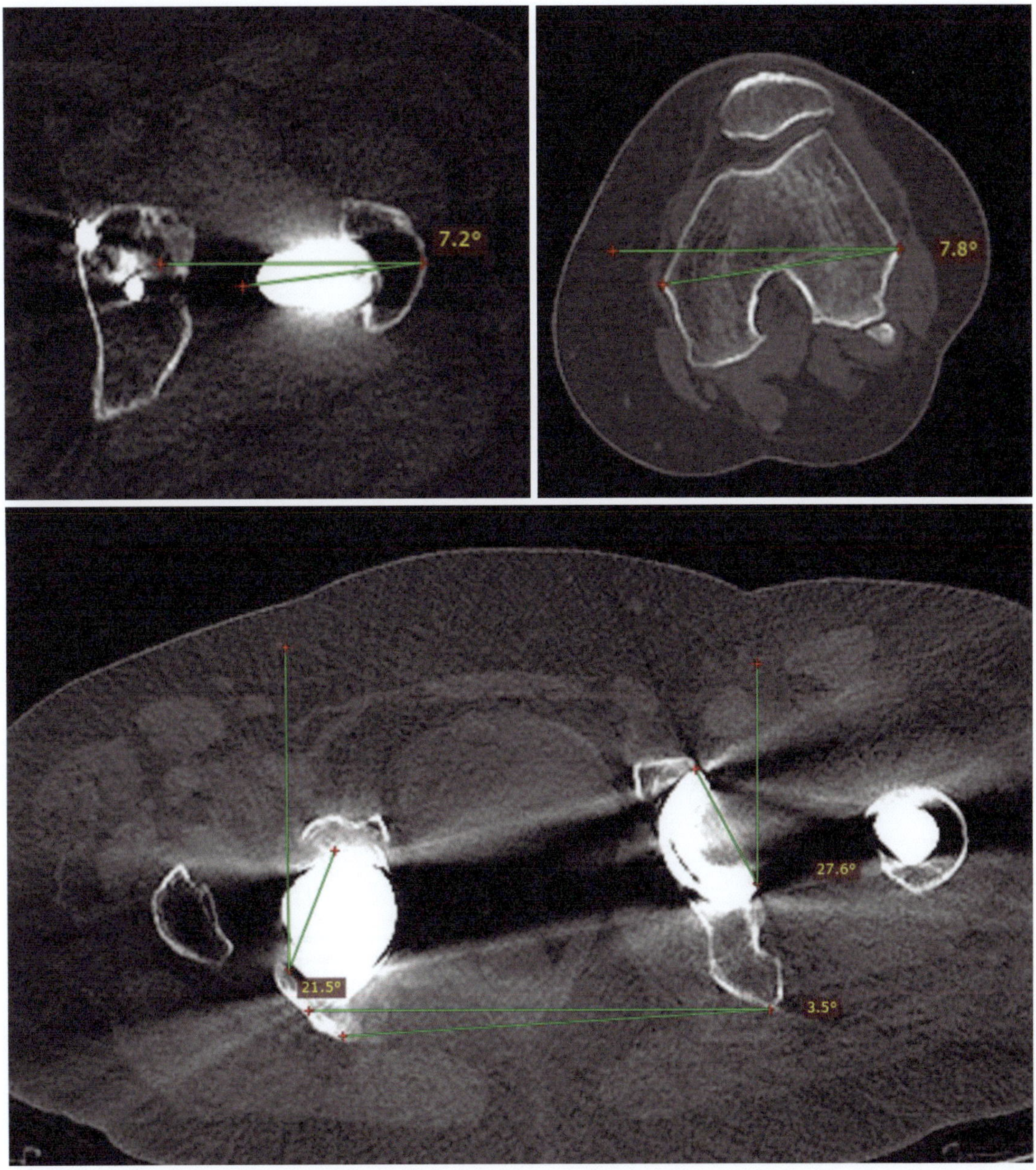

Fig. 6.8 (continued)

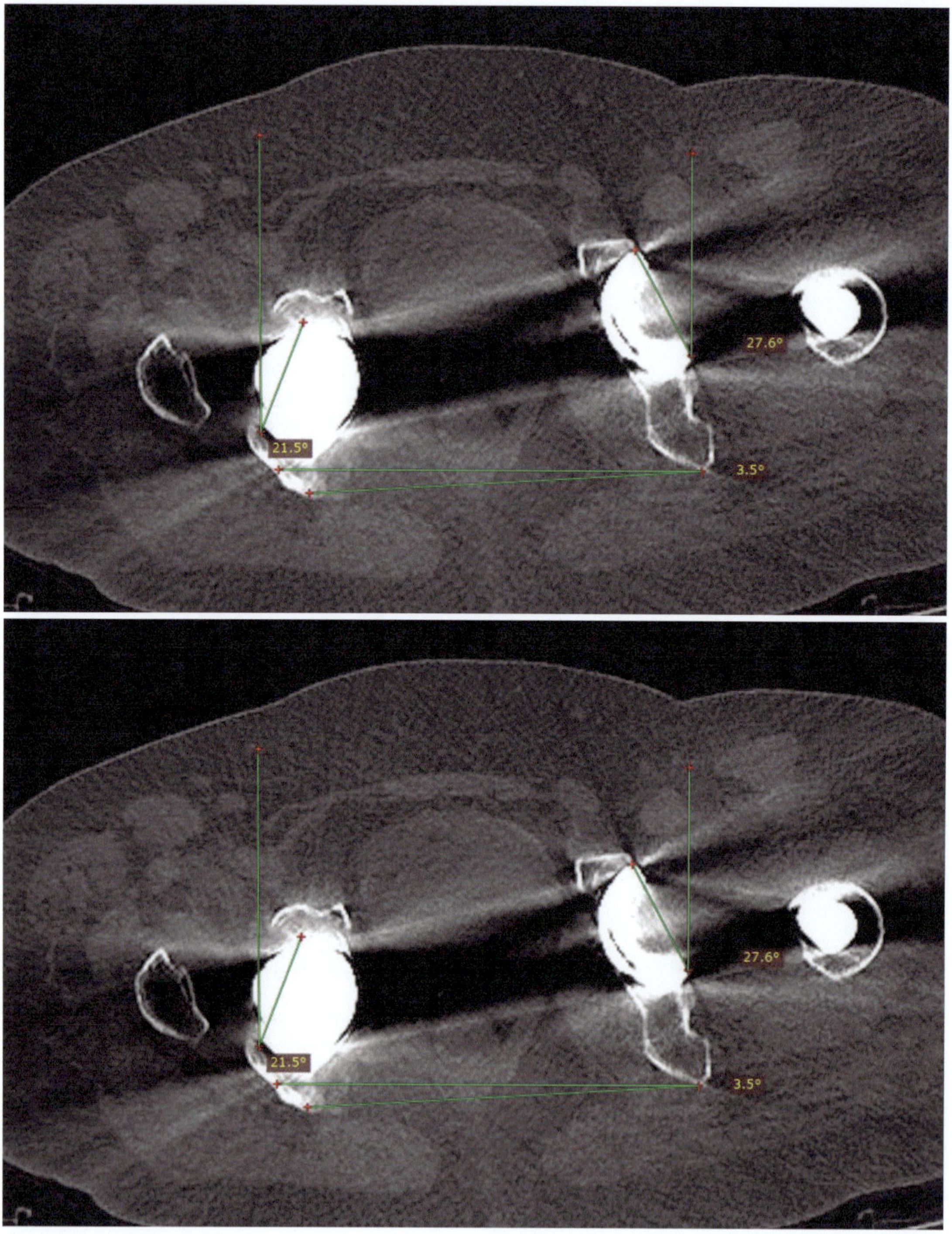

Fig. 6.8 (continued)

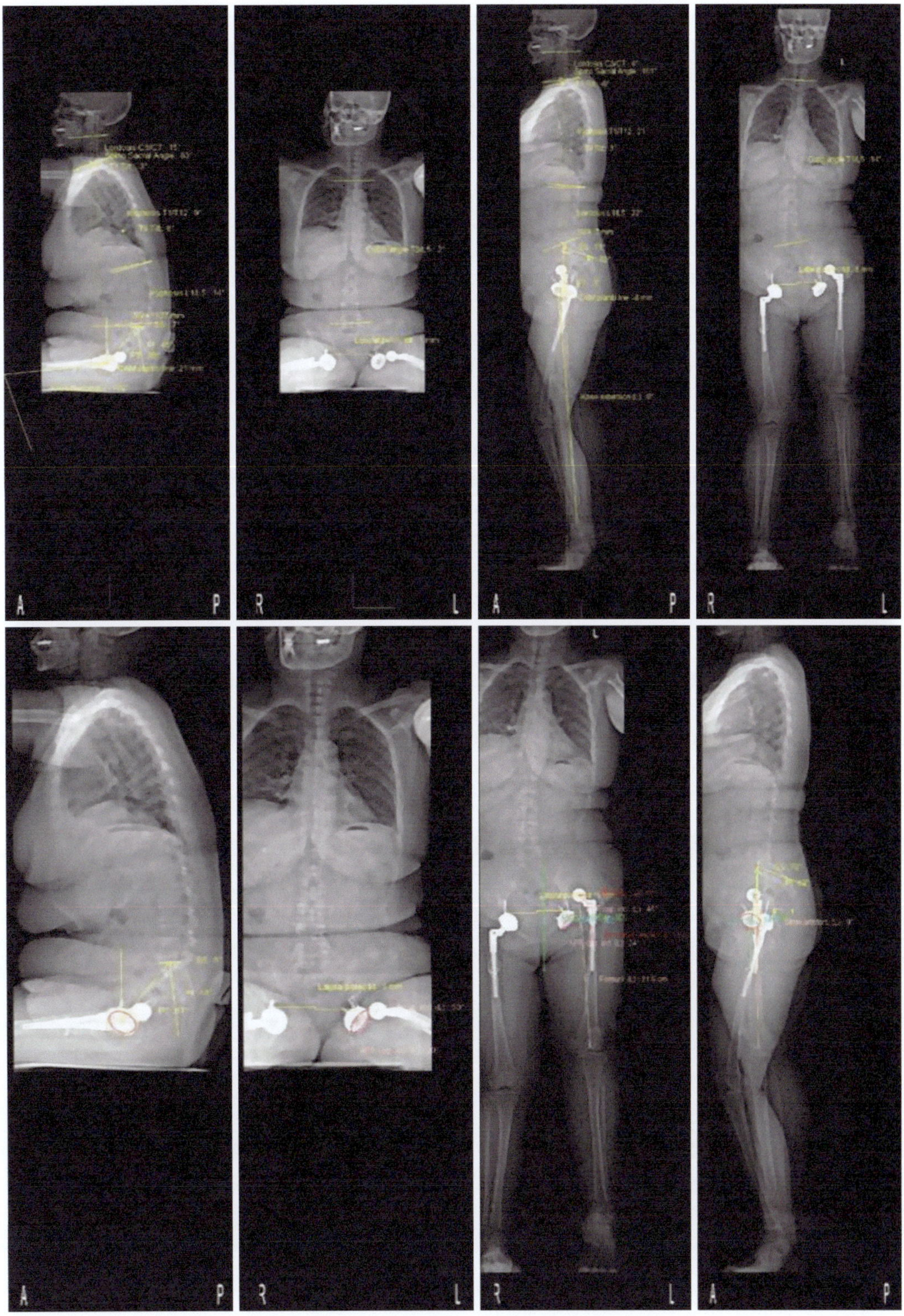

Fig. 6.9 Preoperative EOS functional images of standing and sitting position

3. Revising the stem could help adjust the joint tension by increasing the offset in case of inadequate soft tissue tension. If the soft tissue tension is adequate and the proximal sleeve is stable, we can use a new Stability and Range of Motion (S-ROM) stem to revise the stem version. A fully coated modular revision femoral stem must be prepared to stand by in case of a damaged proximal sleeve.
4. To identify the cause of the dislocation and determine whether there was functional malposition of the prosthesis, the patient-specific safe zone (PSSZ) method was applied for quantitative analysis: in the setting of 0° stem anteversion, the 47°/17° cup position fell outside the PSSZ (the green zone); if the stem anteversion was adjusted to 15°, then the 47°/17° cup position fell within the PSSZ (the green zone), as shown in Fig. 6.10. Therefore, we planned to revise the femoral stem only before the operation.

6.3.4 Operation Situation

No apparent soft tissue laxity was seen during the operation. The Mako robot was employed to examine and adjust the anteversion of the femoral stem. The S-ROM stem was removed, and the sleeve was retained. A new S-ROM stem was placed in and changed to 26° anteversion, a trial head was used to test the stability in all directions, and torsion tests were negative. A 28-mm fourth-generation ceramic femoral head was applied. See Fig. 6.11 for intraoperative registration.

Intraoperative verification of the acetabular angle is shown in Fig. 6.12. It was validated as 47°/17° of acetabulum, with 1° femoral stem anteversion.

Intraoperative verification of the femoral anteversion is shown in Fig. 6.13

The revision was only performed on the stem side; the anteversion was adjusted to 26°, as shown in Fig. 6.14.

6.3.5 Postoperative Condition and Outcome

The patient's femoral stem anteversion was 1°. To avoid further postoperative dislocation, we enlarged the anteversion of the femoral stem to 26° during the revision, compared with the estimated 15°. The overall joint anteversion was 43°.

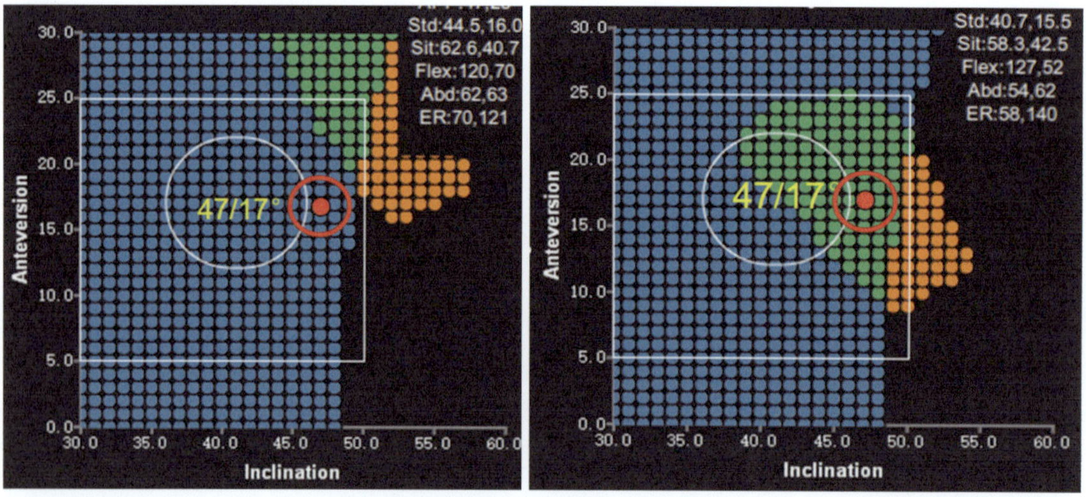

Fig. 6.10 Quantitative analysis of PSSZ. Abscissa: Acetabular abduction; Ordinate: acetabular anteversion. (**a**) With 0° anteversion of the stem, the 47°/17° cup position fell outside the PSSZ. (**b**) With a 15° anteversion of the stem, the 47°/17° cup angle fell within the PSSZ

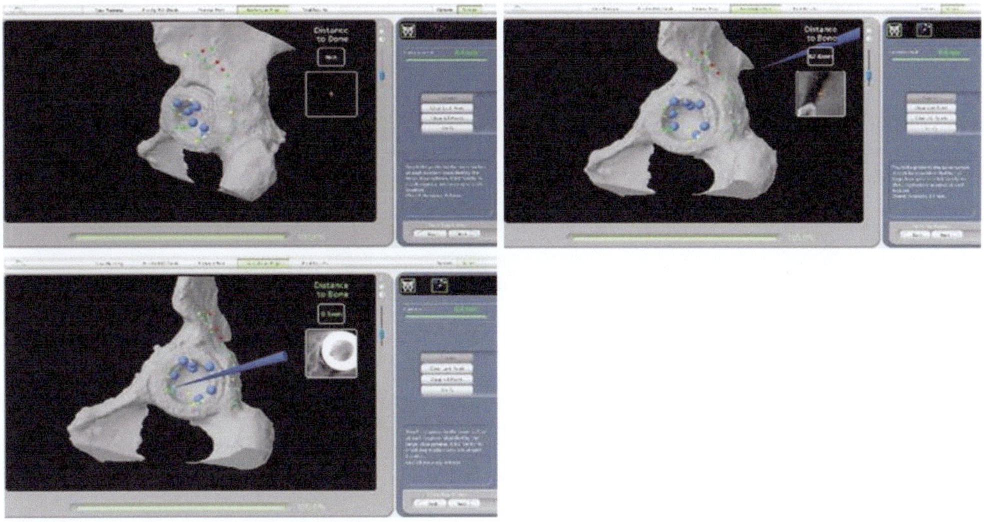

Fig. 6.11 Intraoperative registration

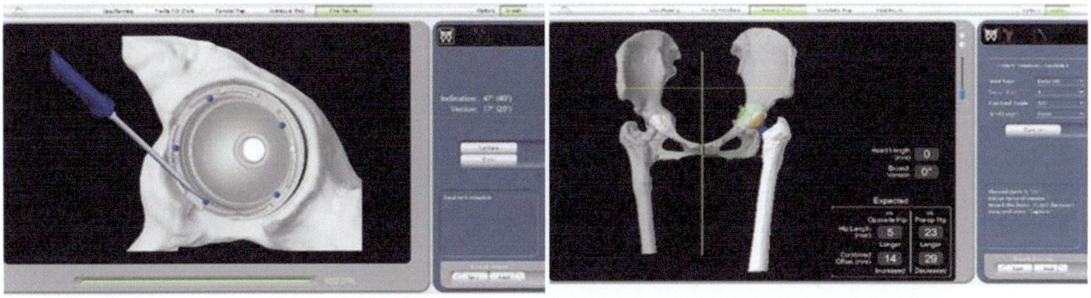

Fig. 6.12 Verification of the acetabular angle using the robot system

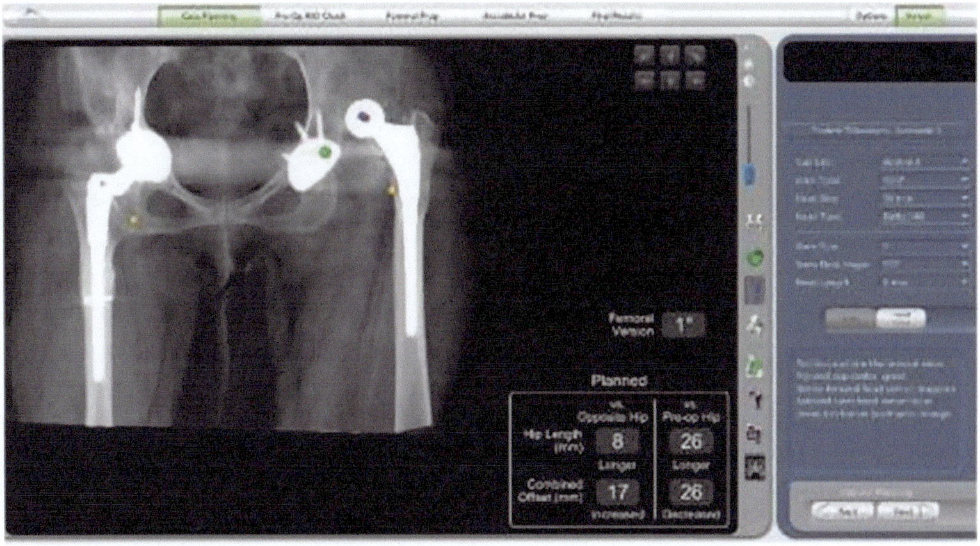

Fig. 6.13 Verification of the femoral anteversion using the robot system

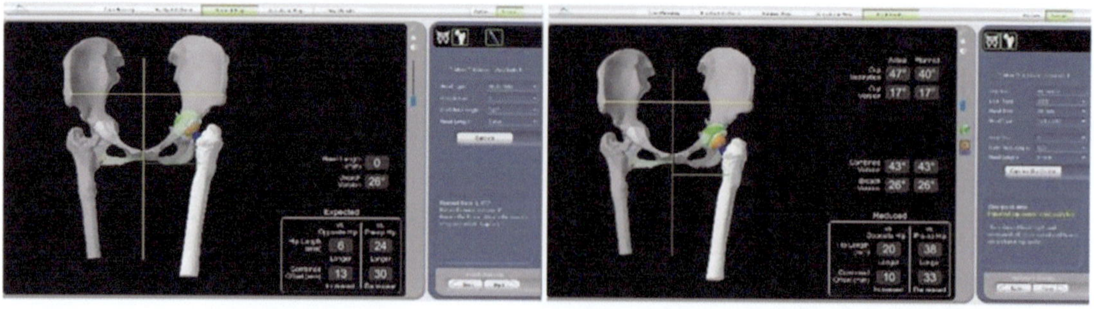

Fig. 6.14 Intraoperative operation interface

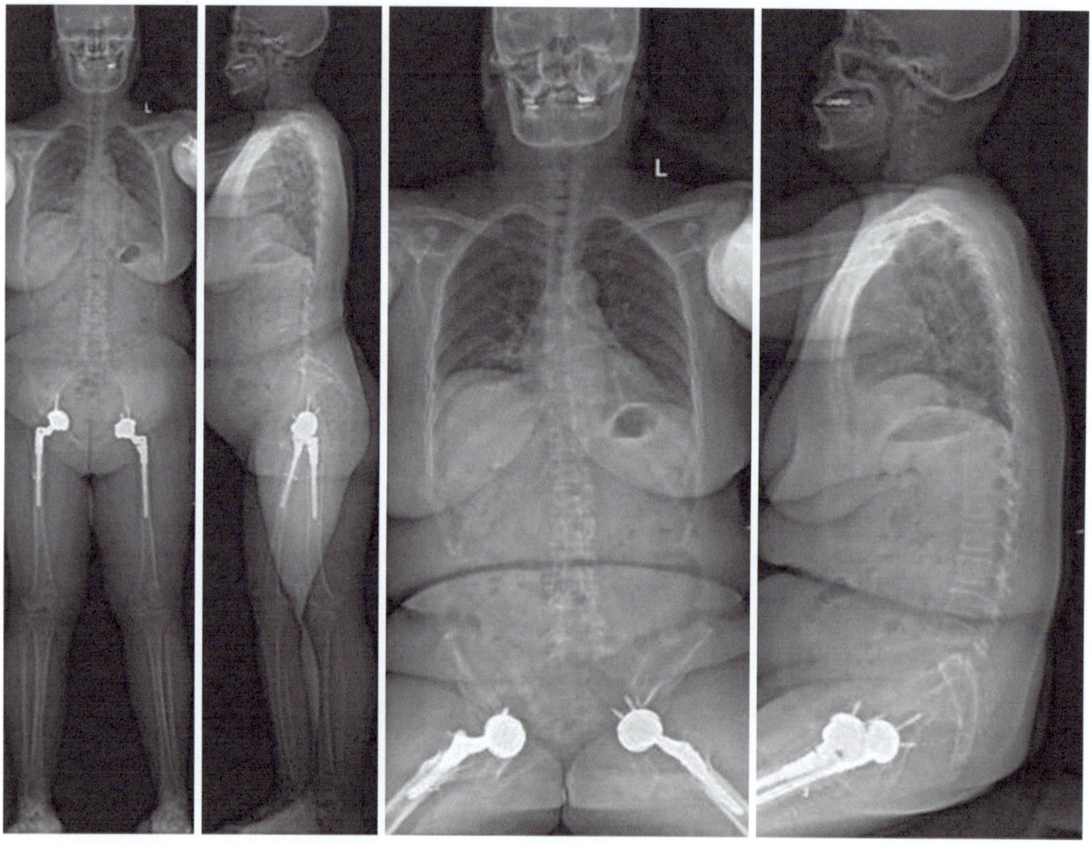

Fig. 6.15 Postoperative X-rays 5 days after revision

Postoperative X-rays after 5 days are shown in Fig. 6.15.

However, 17 days after the revision, the patient reported left hip pain again after trying to push her pelvis forward in the bed and suddenly lost mobility in the left hip. An X-ray showed anterior dislocation in the left hip. She was treated with a closed reduction in our emergency department. X-rays before removal are shown in Fig. 6.16.

Physical examination: lower extremity discrepancy, external rotation, and limited internal rotation.

PSSZ quantitative analysis: The cup position was at the edge of the current PSSZ after revision with the stem version adjusted to 26° (see Fig. 6.17). Thus, we consider the change of posterior dislocation to anterior dislocation for this patient was due to the excessive increase in femo-

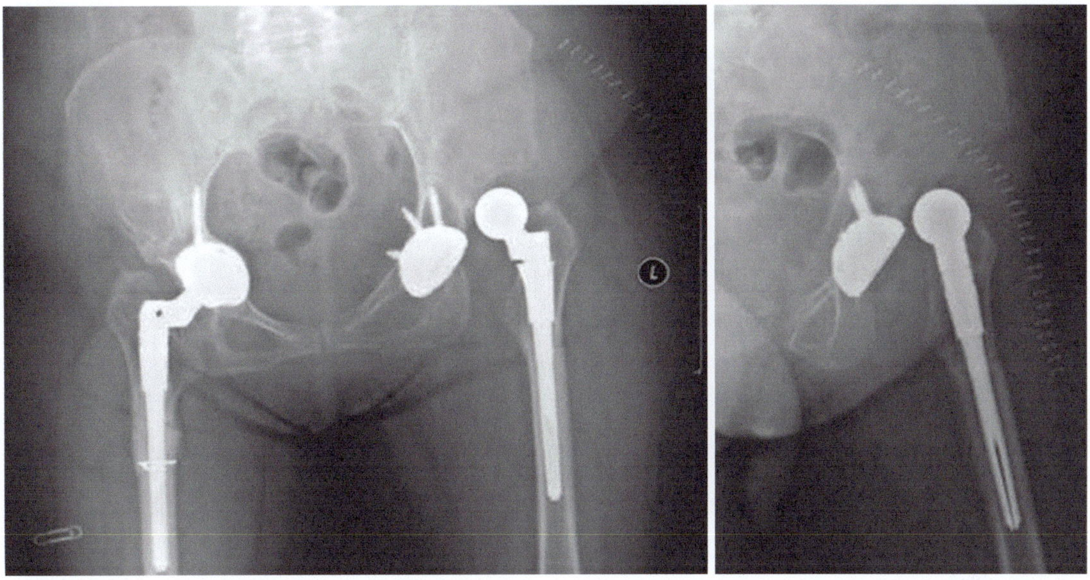

Fig. 6.16 X-rays before the close reduction showing anterior dislocation. The patient pushed her pelvis forward in the bed when the dislocation happened

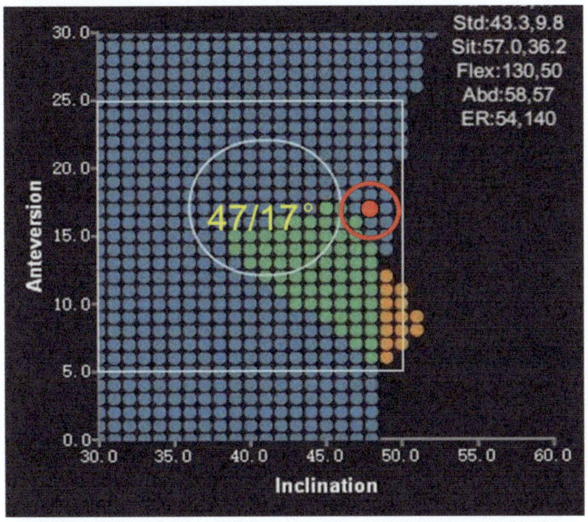

Fig. 6.17 Quantitative analysis of PSSZ (before reduction)

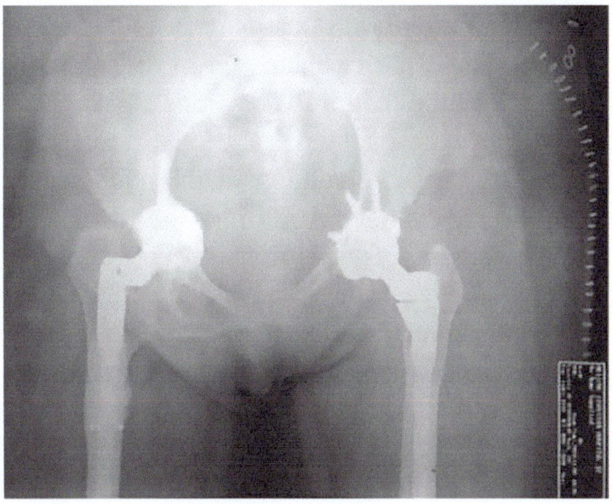

Fig. 6.18 X-ray after close reduction

ral stem anteversion to 26° instead of the predesigned 15°. Since the deviation of the cup orientation from the PSSZ was not far away, and the anterior soft tissue of the hip had not healed at the early postoperative stage, we conducted a closed reduction for the patient without doing a second revision, expecting the joint stability to improve after soft tissue healing.

The dislocation reduction in the emergency department was successful, and the X-ray after revision is shown in Fig. 6.18.

See Fig. 6.19 for X-rays of reexamination at 12 months.

6.3.6 Conclusion and Reflection

1. The patient had an early dislocation after the revision THA, but no dislocation occurred after closed reduction. We learned great lessons from this case: (1) the joint stability of high-riding DDH patients is very sensitive to com-

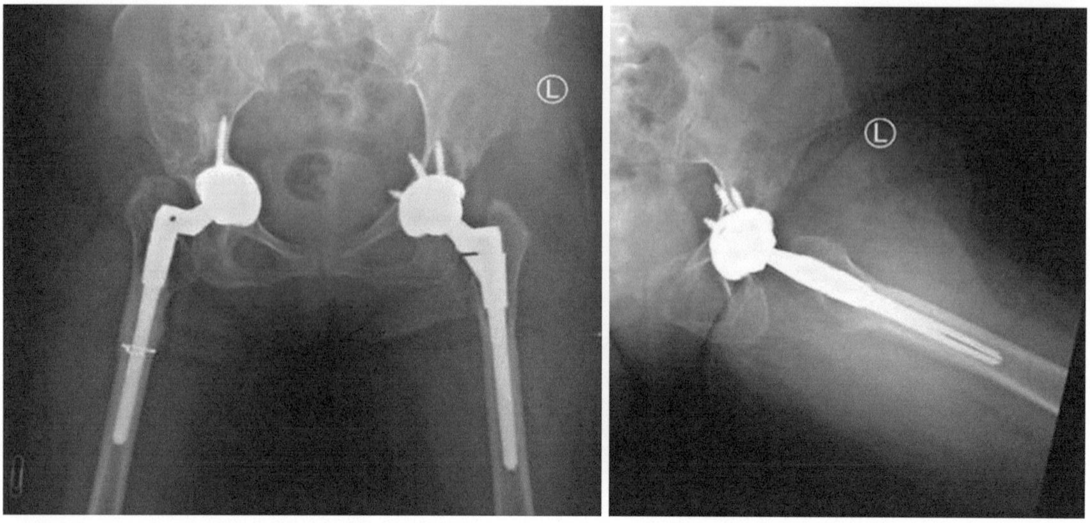

Fig. 6.19 Postoperative X-rays after 12 months

ponent misorientation; (2) the stem version played a vital role in the joint stability; and (3) even in posterior dislocation, the stem anteversion should not be increased too much, as it may lead to anterior dislocation, especially in patients with small femoral head diameters.

The soft tissue condition of this patient surprised the surgeons during the operation. Although the dislocation had been presenting for over a year, there was no significant soft tissue contracture, and it was not challenging to reduce. In the authors' opinion, one of the most important reasons was that the patient walked with crutches, possibly as a stretch on soft tissue. Preoperative physical examination showed a certain degree of mobility (abnormal motion) in the affected hip. Since it could perform flexion, the movement of sitting down and standing up again could be instructed for the patient to stretch soft tissue.

The postoperative soft tissue reconstruction after THA is time-consuming for patients with high DDH. The risk of dislocation was further increased as the patient was in a chronic twisted condition and with a relaxed lateral sleeve due to discrepancy osteotomy.

2. The cause of dislocation following THA is multi-factorial. Accurate identification of the cause of dislocation allows a targeted revision to correct the precise cause and prevent further dislocation. The method of PSSZ enabled us to accurately judge whether the functional position meets the needs of daily activity and quantitatively diagnose the contribution of malposition to the dislocation in a personalized way.
3. Despite the anterior dislocation after revision, the PSSZ method guided our confidence in the decision of conservative treatment. This case was an early case of our team applying PSSZ for dislocation revision. For the subsequent patients with dislocation revision, the quantitative analysis of PSSZ was strictly followed to guide the revision strategy.
4. In this case, it can be seen that quantitative diagnosis of the causes of dislocation can help the decision-making in revision surgeries and minimize surgical trauma and complications.

Recommended Reading

1. Wetters NG, Murray TG, Moric M, et al. Risk factors for dislocation after revision total hip arthroplasty. Clin Orthop Relat Res. 2013;471(2):410–6.
2. von Knoch M, Berry DJ, Harmsen WS, et al. Late dislocation after total hip arthroplasty. J Bone Joint Surg Am. 2002;84(11):1949–53.

3. Meek RM, Allan DB, McPhillips G, et al. Epidemiology of dislocation after total hip arthroplasty. Clin Orthop Relat Res. 2006;447:9–18.
4. Terran J, Schwab F, Shaffrey CI, et al. The SRS-Schwab adult spinal deformity classification: assessment and clinical correlations based on a prospective operative and nonoperative cohort. Neurosurgery. 2013;73(4):559–68.
5. Lazennec JY, Charlot N, Gorin M, et al. Hip-spine relationship: a radio-anatomical study for optimization in acetabular cup positioning. Surg Radiol Anat. 2004;26(2):136–44.
6. Wan Z, Malik A, Jaramaz B, et al. Imaging and navigation measurement of acetabular component position in THA. Clin Orthop Relat Res. 2009;467(1):32–42.
7. Phan D, Bederman SS, Schwarzkopf R. The influence of sagittal spinal deformity on anteversion of the acetabular component in total hip arthroplasty. Bone Joint J. 2015;97-B(8):1017–23.
8. Masonis JL, Bourne RB. Surgical approach, abductor function, and total hip arthroplasty dislocation. Clin Orthop Relat Res. 2002;405:46–53.
9. Abdel MP, von Roth P, Jennings MT, et al. What safe zone? The vast majority of dislocated THAs are within the Lewinnek safe zone for acetabular component position. Clin Orthop Relat Res. 2016;474(2):386–91.
10. Lewinnek GE, Lewis JL, Tarr R, et al. Dislocations after total hip-replacement arthroplasties. J Bone Joint Surg Am. 1978;60(2):217–20.
11. Yoshimine F. The influence of the oscillation angle and the neck anteversion of the prosthesis on the cup safe-zone that fulfills the criteria for range of motion in total hip replacements. The required oscillation angle for an acceptable cup safezone. J Biomech. 2005;38(1):125–32.
12. Widmer KH, Zurfluh B. Compliant positioning of total hip components for optimal range of motion. J Orthop Res. 2004;22(4):815–21.
13. Esposito CI, Gladnick BP, Lee YY, et al. Cup position alone does not predict risk of dislocation after hip arthroplasty. J Arthroplasty. 2015;30(1):109–13.
14. Tezuka T, Heckmann ND, Bodner RJ, et al. Functional safe zone is superior to the Lewinnek safe zone for total hip arthroplasty: why the Lewinnek safe zone is not always predictive of stability. J Arthroplasty. 2019;34(1):3–8.
15. Ike H, Bodner RJ, Lundergan W, et al. The effects of pelvic incidence in the functional anatomy of the hip joint. J Bone Joint Surg Am. 2020;102(11):991–9.
16. Ike H, Dorr LD, Trasolini N, et al. Spine-pelvis-hip relationship in the functioning of a total hip replacement. J Bone Joint Surg Am. 2018;100(18):1606–15.
17. Yoshimine F. The safe-zones for combined cup and neck anteversions that fulfill the essential range of motion and their optimum combination in total hip replacements. J Biomech. 2006;39(7):1315–23.
18. Hsu J, de la Fuente M, Radermacher K. Calculation of impingement-free combined cup and stem alignments based on the patient-specific pelvic tilt. J Biomech. 2019;82:193–203.
19. Yoshimine F, Ginbayashi K. A mathematical formula to calculate the theoretical range of motion for total hip replacement. J Biomech. 2002;35(7):989–93.
20. Esposito CI, Walter WL, Roques A, et al. Wear in alumina-on-alumina ceramic total hip replacements: a retrieval analysis of edge loadinging. J Bone Joint Surg Br. 2012;94(7):901–7.
21. Leslie IJ, Williams S, Isaac G, et al. High cup angle and microseparation increase the wear of hip surface replacements. Clin Orthop Relat Res. 2009;467(9):2259–65.
22. Callanan MC, Jarrett B, Bragdon CR, et al. The John Charnley Award: risk factors for cup malpositioning: quality improvement through a joint registry at a tertiary hospital. Clin Orthop Relat Res. 2011;469(2):319–29.
23. Tang H, Li Y, Zhou Y, Wang S, Zhao Y, Ma Z. A modeling study of a patient-specific safe zone for THA: calculation, validation, and key factors based on standing and sitting sagittal pelvic tilt. Clin Orthop Relat Res. 2022;480(1):191.
24. Ebramzadeh E. CORR Insights(R): a modeling study of a patient-specific safe zone for THA: calculation, validation, and key factors based on standing and sitting sagittal pelvic tilt. Clin Orthop Relat Res. 2022;480(1):206.
25. Tang H, Zhao Y, Wang S, Ma Z, Li Y, Shi H, Zhou Y. Conversion of the sagittal functional safe zone to the coronal plane using a mathematical algorithm: the reason for failure of the Lewinnek safe zone. J Bone Jt Surg Am Vol. 2022.

7 Robot-Assisted Revision Total Hip Arthroplasty

Yixin Zhou, Hao Tang, Siyuan Wang, and Dejin Yang

7.1 Introduction

Yixin Zhou

Robotic-assisted revision total hip arthroplasty (rTHA) is quite a newly described procedure. The original intention was to improve the precision of implantation in order to reduce the complication rate and improve postoperative outcomes via surgical robots. In view of this, we have preliminarily practiced with more than 100 Mako robotic-assisted rTHAs since mid-2019 with the support of the Mako specialist team. Since revision was not an approved indication of the Mako system, it was not equipped with revision modules in terms of either hardware or software, and little previous work on the Mako system in rTHA was reported in the literature. This work was entirely exploratory.

Nevertheless, the journey we experienced and the results we have observed in robotic-assisted rTHA are pleasing. In addition to improving the precision of implantation, the robotic system enhances surgeons' ability to identify the reasons for failure after THA (dislocation, leg length discrepancy, nerve irritation, etc.), enhance initial and long-term fixation of prosthesis, and improve surgical efficiency.

What is even more exciting is that robotic-assisted rTHA is a process of deconstruction, reorganization, and subversion of the conventional rTHA. With the exploration of robotic-assisted rTHA, our understanding of the principles, goals, and technologies of hip reconstruction, as well as the bone defect itself, has been significantly deepened. It is more beneficial to combine the novel reconstruction theory of "RPC" (rim-point-column theory, proposed by Yixin Zhou) with a robotic system. The whole process of exploration brought alternative feelings of both frustration and excitement, but more of it was the pleasure after an in-depth understanding of the operation, which will be shared here with readers of this book.

7.1.1 Preoperative Simulated Operations: Do Two Times, Win Twice

Image-based robotic systems require preoperative CT scanning and segmentation of the pelvis, bilateral hips, and distal femurs. This allows surgeons to fully evaluate the bone stock and its potentiality for implant fixation before the operation. The robot provides a real-time presentation of the rotating center and the cup version in revision, as well as the contact area of the hemispherical cup and the host bone. Where the bone defect is present, it also shows the gap between the hemispherical cup and the surrounding host bone.

Y. Zhou (✉) · H. Tang · S. Wang · D. Yang
Department of Adult Joint Reconstructive Surgery, Beijing Jishuitan Hospital, Capital Medical University, Beijing, China

Y. Zhou (ed.), *Revision Total Hip Arthroplasty*, https://doi.org/10.1007/978-981-97-9804-9_7

Thanks to the accuracy and precision of robotic surgeries, preoperative planned radiographs always highly predicted the outcomes of postoperative radiographs. The mimicked X-rays generated in the robotic preoperative planning provide surgeons with a possible view of the foreseeable postoperative X-rays, which provides a good insight into controlling the mechanical parameters in hip reconstruction, such as the rotating center, offset, and leg length.

Preoperative 3D images and the measurement of distances between points on various sectional planes also prepare the surgeons well with the selection of various shapes and sizes of metal augments for bone defect reconstruction.

7.1.2 The Intraoperative Role of Robotic Arms

The purpose of the robotic arm is, of course, to constrain the reaming and the position and orientation of the cup implantation. This kind of constraint and guidance is of greater significance for rTHA, especially in complicated cases.

In the presence of a severe bone defect, accurate press-fit, rim fixation or three-point fixation, and a reasonable contact area between the host bone and the hemispheric cup are particularly important. Robotic arm-guided acetabular reaming can shape the bone cavity into a perfect hemisphere without torsion, at the right point of the rotating center, regardless of where the bone defect exists. Even if the residual healthy bone is somewhere only a spot with limited area, it can perfectly contact with the hemisphere cup after robotic reaming and implantation.

Precise reaming assisted by the robotic arm improves the initial stability of the cup and helps form a good contact between the healthy bone and the hemispherical cup which maximizes the potential for osseointegration. In traditional rTHAs, the establishment of initial stability and subsequent biological fixation is often suboptimal when suffering from a severe bone defect, under the circumstance in which mild technical imprecision can lead to the failure of prosthesis fixation. Furthermore, rTHA is still a traumatic surgery for most patients, so it is very important to improve operation efficacy. The robotic system is capable of accurate reaming and facilitating efficient decision-making during surgery, which is critical for damage control in rTHAs.

Another important function of the robotic arms is the precise implantation of the prosthesis. The guiding role of the arms in hemispherical cup implantation will not be further described here; we will focus on the robotic arms functioning in metal augment implantation. The beauty of robotic-assisted revision is that compromise on the rotating center and orientation of the cup is no longer inevitable in revision. In our practice, we usually place the trial cup into the ideal position via a robotic arm, and then we examine the bone contact and support area around the hemispheric trial cup and determine whether and where a metal augment was needed to fill the bone defect and reconstruct the support points based on our RPC theory.

The 3D preoperative planning and robotic arm assistance allow surgeons to only focus on the relationship between the hemispheric cup and the healthy bone left without concerning about the bone defect. This capacity greatly simplifies surgical procedures. One can hardly perceive brevity and simplicity without personal experience with robotic-assisted rTHA. The application of robotic systems, RPC theory, and implants (including cup and augment) coordinate and complement each other. The author once summarized the reconstruction of the cup side as follows: position the cup, find the bone left, and let the augments do the rest. It was well-proved and undoubtedly correct for robotic-assisted rTHA.

7.1.3 Application of the Probe in rTHA

The role of the probe in the initial THA was mainly to capture points or point clouds on the bone surface for registration. Once the registration is completed, the position of the probe relative to the bone structure is established. The function of the probe tip is essentially to indicate spatial coordinates of points, while its body indicates a vector. This function of the probe is of great significance in revision.

The tip of the probe can be used to indicate the specific location of a point (sometimes on the bone surface, sometimes intraosseous) on the entire hemi-pelvis. For example, the distance between a point of interest and the greater sciatic notch helps to determine whether the position of a buttress augment is proper; real-time tracing of the probe can also indicate the real position of the screw hole on the hemi-pelvis and the bone quality along the vector of the screw hole.

The probe generates an approximate geometric shape after collecting points of the bone surface around the augment, such as buttress augment, which is of great help for the accurate placement of the augment under the blockage of visibility by the muscles. The buttress augment is designed to gain bone contact on the outer surface of the ilium which is often required to be placed under the abductors. Any trespassing into the greater sciatic notch would cause irritation or damage to the sciatic nerve and arteriae glataea superior and weaken its mechanical strength of fixation.

Of course, no revision module is equipped in existing systems to date, and the hardware is not specifically designed for revision. This is why we are working on robotic-assisted rTHA with the Mako system, and we will soon develop a new robotic system specific to rTHAs. A specifically designed software and hardware system will greatly improve the efficacy of the rTHA.

7.2 Case 1

Hao Tang, Siyuan Wang, Yixin Zhou and Dejin Yang

7.2.1 Case Summary

Medical History Male, 51 years old, reported "pain accompanied by limited mobility for 6 years after left hip reconstruction 13 years ago." The patient had a pathological fracture on the left femur 13 years ago and underwent left THA using a hip megaprosthesis in another hospital. Malignant histiocytoma was diagnosed after the operation and treated with chemotherapy. The patient recovered smoothly and could walk without obvious discomfort. Six years ago, the patient felt pain and discomfort in the left hip, which was obvious when walking but could be relieved by resting. There was no rest pain or nocturnal pain. Limited mobility was presented, but no special treatment was applied. The symptoms progressed gradually. It was later presented difficulty in squatting and walking up and down stairs. The tolerable walking distance was less than 500 m.

Physical Examination The patient entered the ward on crutches; no pelvis tilting; left lower limb shortening; posterolateral incision scar of the left hip; no obvious swelling around the hip; tenderness in left groin; axial percussion pain (−); obvious limited range of motion; Thomas sign (−) on the left hip; no edema was found in both lower extremities; no hypoesthesia; and the pulse of bilateral dorsal artery was palpable.

Laboratory Examination No abnormality was detected in routine blood tests, including erythrocyte sedimentation rate (ESR) and C-reactive protein (CRP).

Radiographic Data Preoperative X-rays are shown in Fig. 7.1.

CTA examination of both lower extremities: The prosthesis migrated upward into the pelvic cavity in the left hip and pushed the left external iliac artery medially. No definite stenosis or interruption was observed.

Plain CT scan of the hip: left hip prosthesis penetrated into the pelvic cavity after left THA (Fig. 7.2).

7.2.2 Case Analysis

1. Strictly speaking, this was not a case of rTHA, but a conversion THA. According to the Chinese language convention, it could also be considered an rTHA.
2. Difficulties on the acetabular side:

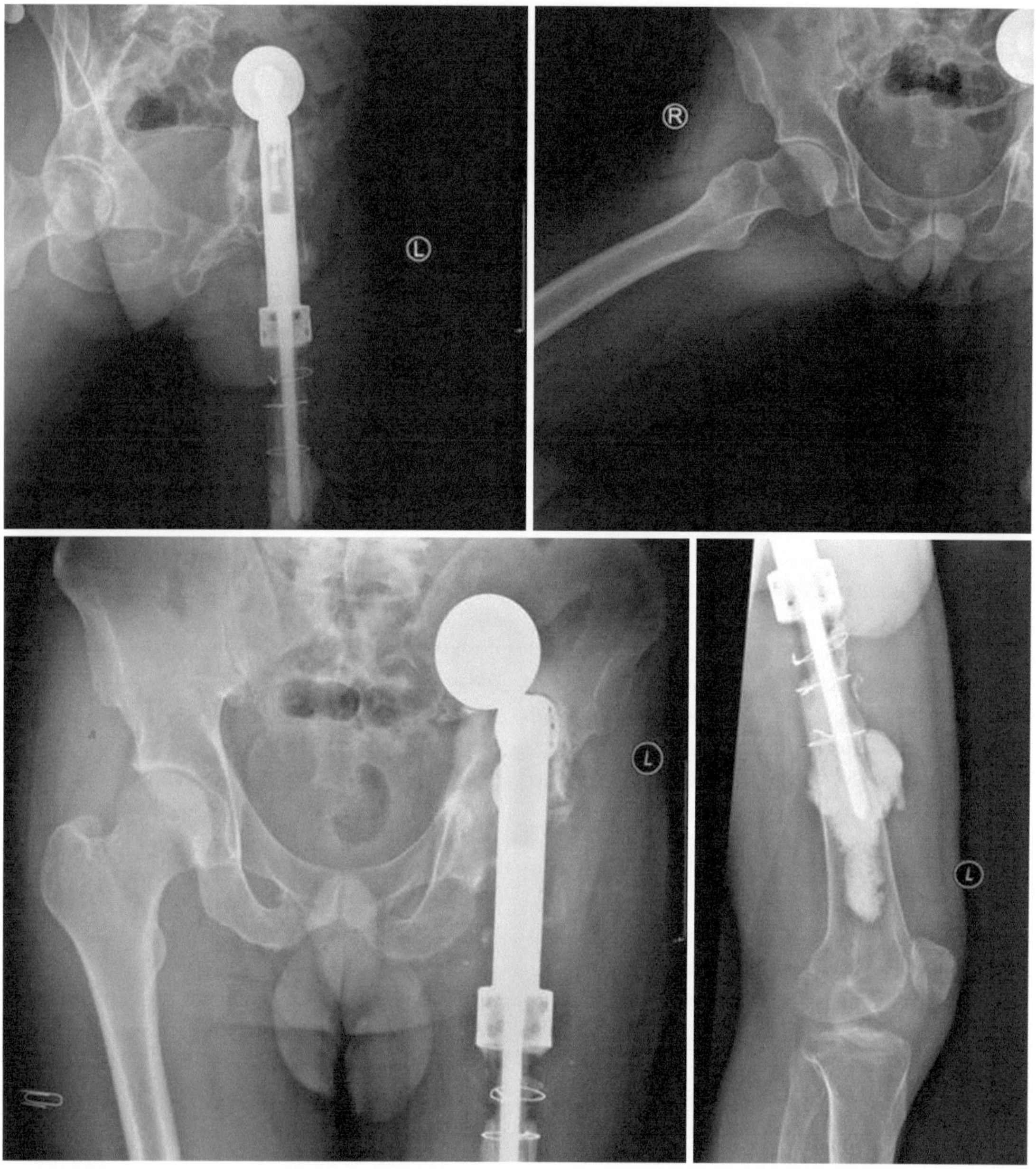

Fig. 7.1 Preoperative X-rays

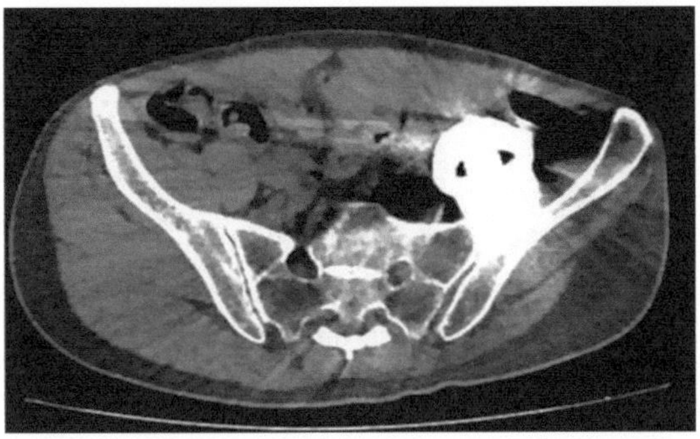

Fig. 7.2 Plain CT scan of the hip

(a) The left acetabulum was possibly discontinued, but teardrop, pubic ramus, and ischial ramus were relatively intact. There were not many points requiring reconstruction, mainly leaving the mediosuperior roof defective, which would be easily dealt with using the robotic system.
(b) The concern of damage to the ureter, major pelvic arteries, and nerves during prosthesis removal should be aware of.
(c) The femoral head might not be easily dislocated and moved out through the acetabular perforation defect, making the exposure and removal process difficult.

3. Difficulties on the femur side: It should not be considered a type IV femur, but rather classified as a femoral remnant. The distal end of the stem was not loose, but well secured in the bone cement. The proximal femur had been absorbed, resulting in more uncertainties on the reconstruction on the femoral side than on the acetabular side.
4. Diagnosis: pelvic penetration after left THA with hip megaprosthesis.

7.2.3 Preoperative Planning

1. Removal of the prosthesis involved great difficulty, as potential damage to the blood vessels or ureters was inevitably concerned. An extensive preoperative investigation and evaluation including CTA and angiography were necessary. The anterior iliac area should be sterilized and draped, and the invaginated prosthetic femoral head could be retrieved through an ilioinguinal incision in case of difficulty via a posterolateral approach. Thorough communication with the vascular surgeons was required before surgery, and a vascular surgeon team standing by was demanded. With a floating supine position, an intravascular balloon could be placed through the catheter in advance of orthopedic surgery. In case of blood vessels rupture during the operation, the balloon could be pumped up to stop bleeding; the patient could be placed in a supine position and the vessels could be exposed through the ilioinguinal approach for repairmen.
2. The bone stock on the femoral side was extremely damaged with weak quality; hence, we determined to recruit the novel technique we developed, endosteal reconstruction. The introduction of endosteal reconstruction not only helped maintain the centralization of the stem and improve the initial stability but was also conducive to maintaining long-term stability. The potential of osseointegration was generated via 3D-printed porous tube-like or ring-like metal augments intubated into the canal of the femoral remnant and scratch-fitted with a refreshed cortical bone bed or cancellous bone (if fortunately) in the femoral canal, which provided a long-term biological fixation for the implant-cement construct. After implantation of the tube-like augments, the stem of a megaprosthesis was cemented into the reconstructed canal. This technique was regarded as a combination of both cemented and cementless techniques. The principle of the endosteal reconstruction is illustrated in detail in Appendix C.
3. How to dislocate the hip during exposure? The limb shortening of the patient was quite significant, and the hip could not be dislocated by intraoperative lower limb traction. The stem possibly needed to be cut off in the middle before being taken out by piece, so a high-speed disc saw and diamond bit specific for metal cutting should be prepared.

4. Thorough informed consent before surgery was needed as there was a higher probability of femoral stem loosening after surgery compared to other cases. Because of the application of modular stem, if the surgery unfortunately failed in the future, only the distal end of the prosthesis would need to be replaced by a component of a total femur prosthesis and the proximal components could be preserved.
5. The risk of postoperative dislocation for this patient was predictably higher due to the uncertainty of abductor continuity and function, as well as the status of the soft tissue sleeve around the hip. To minimize the risk, the location of the acetabular rotating center and the cup orientation should not be compromised. Once compromised on the cup position, together with the aforementioned uncertainty, the risk of postoperative dislocation would dramatically increase. With the help of a robotic system, the acetabulum could be reconstructed perfectly into the desired target to minimize the risk. This is one of the major advantages of robotic rTHA.
6. Preoperative planning in the Mako system: The cup diameter was 62 mm, the diameter of the femoral head was 36 mm, the cup anteversion was 40°, and the cup abduction was 20°, as shown in Fig. 7.3.

7.2.4 Surgical Process

After successful general anesthesia, the floating right lateral decubitus position was adopted. The Mako system was set up and the pelvic tracker was fixed on the iliac crest.

An anterior incision of the left knee and left distal femur was adopted for approaching the distal femur. The quadriceps muscle was bluntly separated to expose the distal femoral stem. The megaprosthesis was well-fixed. We truncated the prosthesis at the beginning of the stem with a high-speed plate saw.

The posterolateral hip approach was adopted through the previous incision. The femoral stem was observed to have migrated upward and protruded into the pelvic cavity. After the surrounding soft tissue scar was released, the stem was pulled out smoothly by hooking the proximal part and holding the cut end distally, but the outer part of the modular head would not get out along with the stem. The first attempt to retrieve the head failed and thus was abandoned, as we were aware of possible vascular injury if we attempted to move out the head more aggressively.

The tissues around the acetabulum were cleaned, and the acetabulum was reamed to 62 mm. The bone defect in the acetabular roof was filled with a metal slope augment (58 mm * 60 mm * 20 mm), and a 62-mm cementless porous cup with multiple screw holes was implanted at 40° inclination and 20° anteversion. Screws were used for auxiliary fixation.

Residual bone cement in the distal femoral remnant was cleaned. A window was opened at the distal femur to remove the residual bone cement. The femur was reamed to 15 mm from the proximal. The distal femoral canal was reamed with a custom-made modular reamer

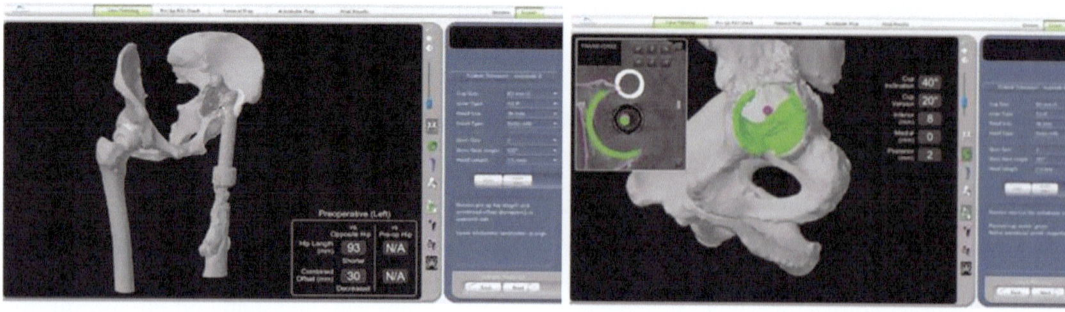

Fig. 7.3 Preoperative planning

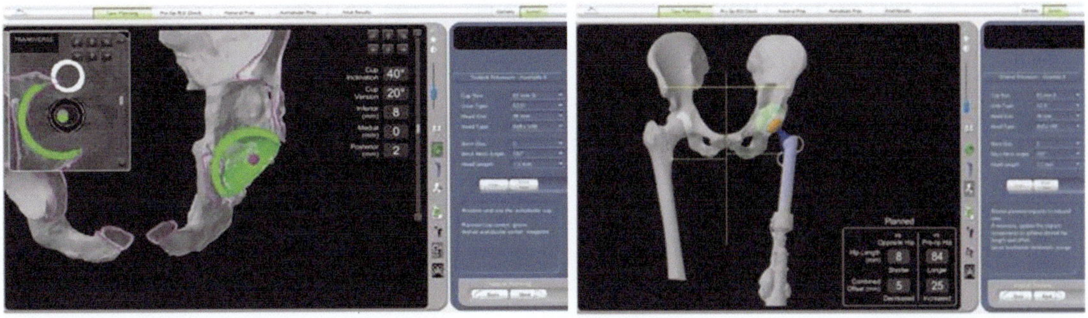

Fig. 7.3 (continued)

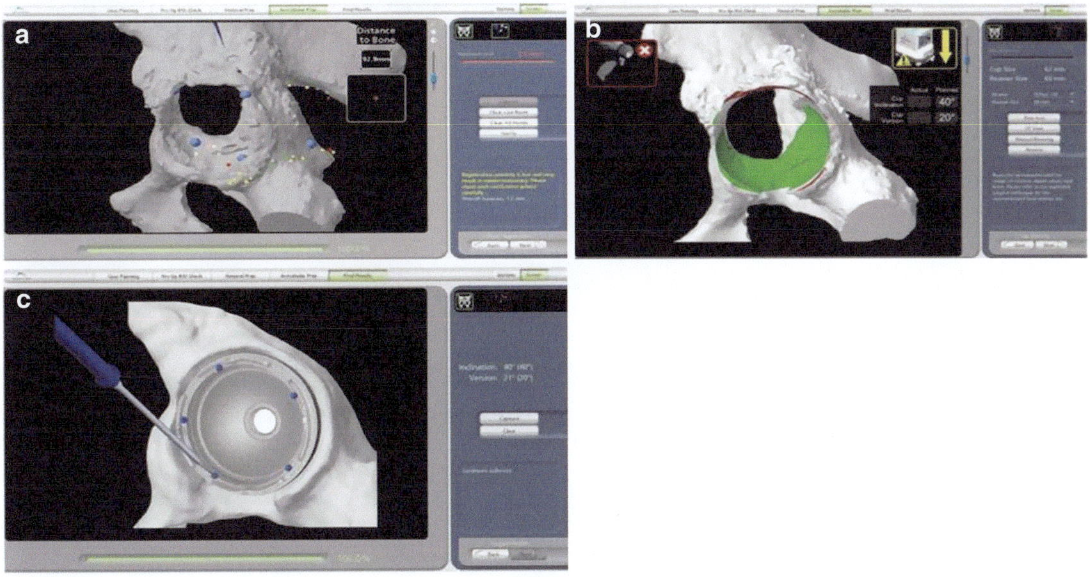

Fig. 7.4 Intraoperative operation interface. (**a**) Intraoperative registration. (**b**) Acetabular reaming. (**c**) Verification

which was put in from the cortical window and driven by a T-shape handle inserted proximally along the canal. A tantalum cone was inserted upside down into the distal canal through the window. The bone block of the window was then placed back and squeezed by a 3D-printed plate and several cerclage cables were placed dispersedly from proximal to distal. Three ring-like metal augments were aligned into the proximal end of the canal with optimal scratch fit. A femoral stem trial with appropriate length was placed in. After hip reduction, the soft-tissue tension and leg length were satisfactory. The final Global Modular Replacement System (GMRS) tumor prosthesis was implanted using cement. A corresponding polythene liner and a 32-mm ceramic femoral head were implanted. After reduction, the wound was thoroughly irrigated and closed.

The operation time was 6 h, with 1300 mL blood loss.

Intraoperative registration results, reaming process, and final cup position are shown in Fig. 7.4.

The intraoperative view is shown in Fig. 7.5.

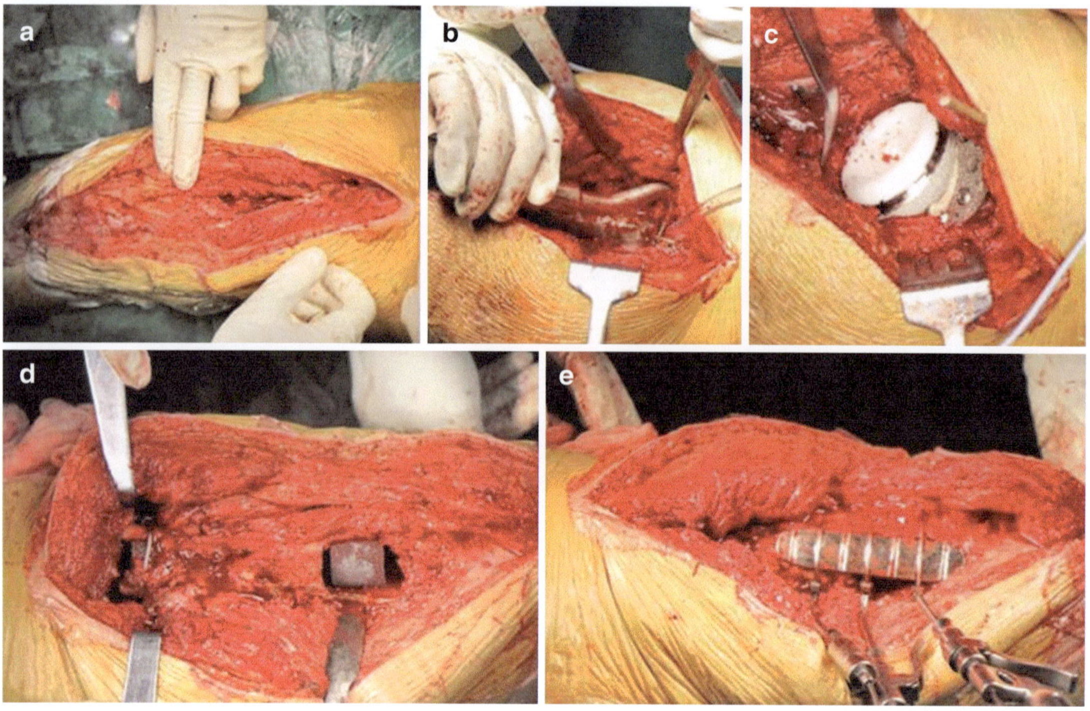

Fig. 7.5 Intraoperative view. (**a**) Exposing the distal femur through an anterior middle incision above the knee. (**b**) Pulling out the stem with a hook holding the proximal part of the stem through the posterolateral hip approach. (**c**) Acetabular reconstruction with 62-mm porous cup and a slope augment. (**d**) A porous tibial cone placed upside-down into the distal canal through the cortical window. (**e**) A 3D-printed plate for fixation and squeezing

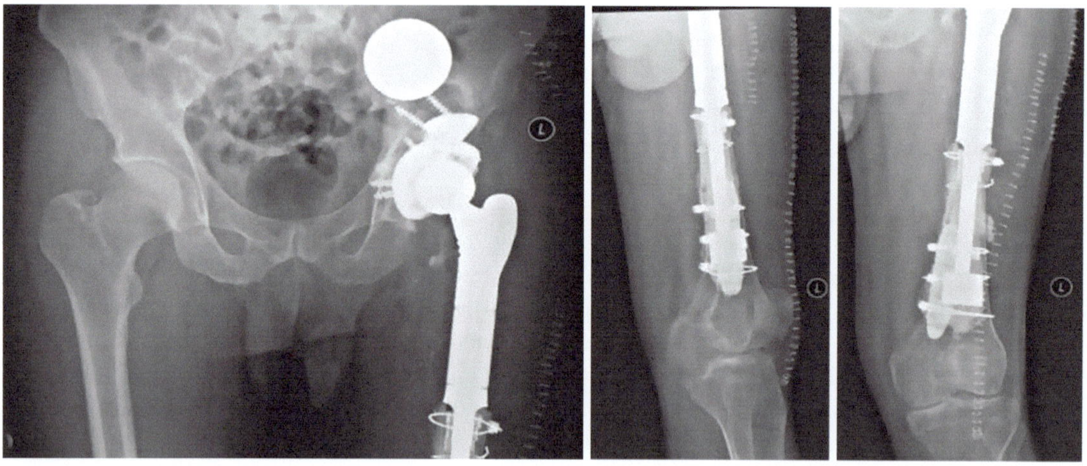

Fig. 7.6 Postoperative X-ray

7.2.5 Postoperative Radiographs

Postoperative X-ray is shown in Fig. 7.6; see Fig. 7.7 for postoperative X-ray in follow-up at 6 months after rTHA.

7.2.6 Conclusion and Reflection

1. How to minimize the risk of damage when retrieving the invaginated prosthesis?

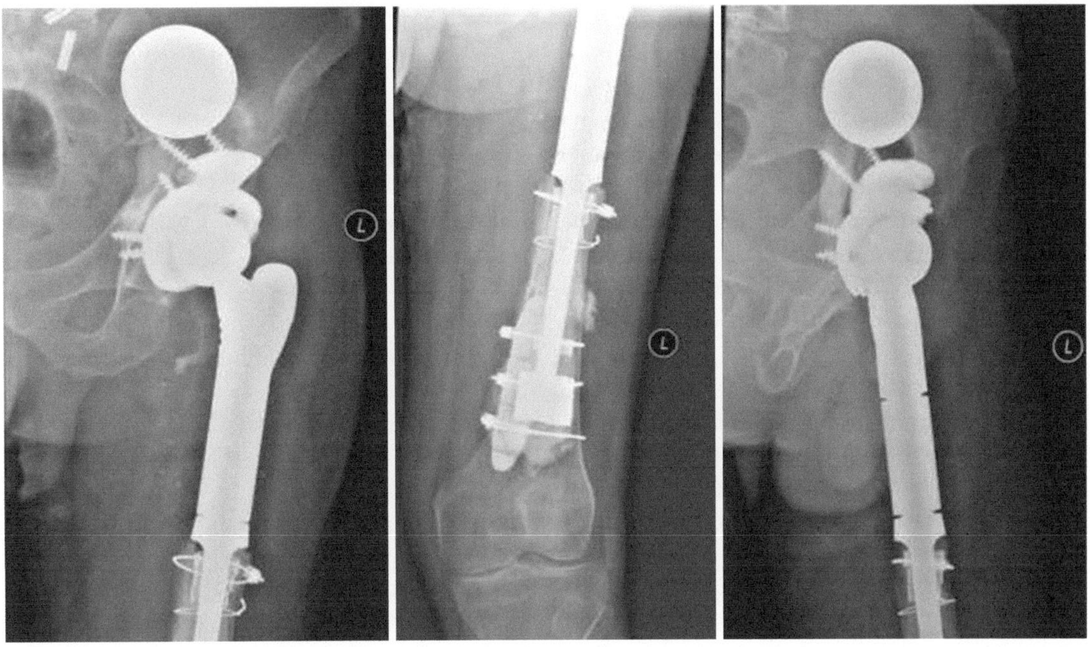

Fig. 7.7 Postoperative X-ray in follow-up at 6 months after rTHA

(a) Retrieval of the invaginated prosthesis was relatively difficult. Possible damage to blood vessels or ureters had to be aware of. Thorough preoperative investigations such as CTA and angiography were necessary.
(b) The anterior iliac inguinal area should be prepared during disinfection. In an unexpected occurrence, the prosthesis could be retrieved via the ilioinguinal incision.
(c) Thorough communication with vascular surgeons before the operation is required. They could provide intraoperative assistance if necessary to prevent unexpected gross bleeding.

2. Why was endosteal reconstruction employed on the femoral side? (See Appendix C for details).

   The bone on the femoral side was quite thin and weak. Cemented fixation of a megaprosthesis in a short femur remnant would have a high possibility of failure in the long term. The introduction of endosteal reconstruction provided not only initial stability but also long-term stability. The ring-like or tube-like 3D-printed porous augment formed the basis for osseointegration, while residual intramedullary cancellous bone and the inner surface of the augment provide a rough interface for cement fixation. It was a combination of cemented and cementless techniques.

3. What are the advantages of robot assistance?
   (a) When facing complex revision cases, preoperative planning in robotic systems can be used to optimize the surgical goals. By adjusting the diameter and position of acetabular reaming, thoughtful planning can be achieved with proper bone retention, prosthesis position, and augment reconstruction. It allows preoperative rehearsals to identify problems and solutions.
   (b) It can accurately execute implantation on the acetabular side, which minimizes the risk of dislocation following rTHA by optimizing the rotating center and cup orientation.
   (c) Find the bone left, well-position the cup, and let augments do the rest. The location and shape of the residual bone beds can be accurately identified through 3D images, and the reconstruction with augments can be planned accordingly.

   (d) Intraoperative use of probes and virtual 3D bone models can accurately evaluate local bone anatomy and reduce surgical risks such as avoiding the great sciatic notch when placing a buttress augment.
   (e) The reaming process can be controlled via the robotic arm, which improves the sphericity of the prepared bone bed and maximizes the contact area of the bone and cup, which will improve the stability of fixation.
   (f) When inserting the metal augment, the robotic arm can firmly hold the cup trial and place it in an accurate position no matter how much bone defect exists. It facilitates the planning and implantation of the porous augment.
4. Surgical difficulties in robotic-assisted revision:
   (a) Preoperative preparation: Metal artifacts brought difficulty in image segmentation and caused larger modeling errors.
   (b) Intraoperative registration: Metal artifacts and bone defects or poor bone quality caused difficulty in registration and commonly a longer registration time than a primary case, which had a certain impact on the patient's overall surgical tolerance. Selection among registration on the prosthesis, registration after prosthesis removal, or registration fully on the extra-acetabular area could be determined depending on the different states of the prosthesis fixation, the material, the degree of metal artifacts, the degree of bone defect, bone quality, and so on.
   (c) Contamination concerns: With the recruitment of new instruments and increased operation time, or even more observation peers, the risk of infection increased.
   (d) Robotic arm positioning: In revision with difficult exposure, the robotic handle of the reamer or cup positioning device could collide with the great trochanter, which may compromise accuracy.

7.3 Case 2

Hao Tang, Siyuan Wang, Yixin Zhou and Dejin Yang

7.3.1 Case Summary

Medical History Female, 82 years old, underwent a THA (right) due to the right femoral neck fracture in another hospital 16 years ago and functioned well after the operation. She developed right hip pain after exercise 1 month ago, which was related to motion and could be relieved by resting and accompanied by limited mobility and difficulty in squatting and walking up and down stairs. There was no nocturnal pain. The tolerable walking distance was less than 100 m. She had hypertension for 20 years and received long-term oral medication treatment. The blood pressure was well controlled. More than 10 years ago, she received a pacemaker implantation in another hospital due to bradycardia. She was diagnosed with "heart failure" in another hospital 2 years ago and did not have an attack after treatment. Gallbladder resection was received 6 years ago. Intake of aspirin was stopped for more than 1 month and low-molecular-weight heparin was continued.

Physical Examination The patient was brought in on a wheelchair; no pelvis tilt; no deformity in the right hip; a 15-cm incision scar on the right hip; no redness or swelling; ilioinguinal area of the right hip and greater trochanter tenderness (+); axial percussion pain (−); mild limited mobility; Patrick's sign (+) on the right; bilateral Thomas sign (−); Trendelenburg sign (+) on the right; Allis sign (+); no edema or hypoesthesia on both lower extremities; and pulse of bilateral dorsal artery palpable. The lower right extremity was about 2 cm shorter than the contralateral side. Abductor force was level 4 in the right hip.

Laboratory Examination No abnormality was detected in a routine blood test, ESR, or CRP.

Radiographic Data Preoperative X-rays (Fig. 7.8): After right THA, the prosthesis was loose.

7.3.2 Case Analysis

1. Osteolysis and subsequent bone defects were found in the ischial ramus, pubic ramus, and ilium. Severe periprosthetic osteolysis was found around the femoral stem.
2. Oblique X-rays showed a thin layer of cortex in the anterior column, while the posterior wall was hollow. Massive osteolysis in the pubic ramus could also be seen in the anterior column.

7.3.3 Preoperative Planning

Defects could be seen through preoperative 3D models. The contact between the prosthesis and host bones could be estimated by preoperative simulation of different sizes and positions of the cup. Preoperative planning is shown in Fig. 7.9.

7.3.4 Surgical Process

After successful general anesthesia, the patient was placed in the left decubitus position and routine sterilization was applied. The Mako robotic-assisted surgery system was set up.

The tracker was fixed on the iliac crest. A previous posterolateral surgical incision of the right hip was adopted for the approach.

The scar tissue around the acetabulum was cleared, and the cup was retrieved without great effort. Registration was performed on the acetabular side with a full extra-acetabular protocol. The acetabulum was reamed to 60 mm sticking to intraoperatively modified planning.

With the robotic arm holding the cup trial to the desired position, two stacked slope augments for superior iliac defect and one slope augment stacked with a disc augment for ischial ramus defect were planned and implanted accordingly. A 60-mm Tritanium multiple screw hole porous cup was implanted with the assistance of the robot, with 43° inclination and 15° anteversion. Screws were applied for additional fixation, and a corresponding polyethylene liner was implanted.

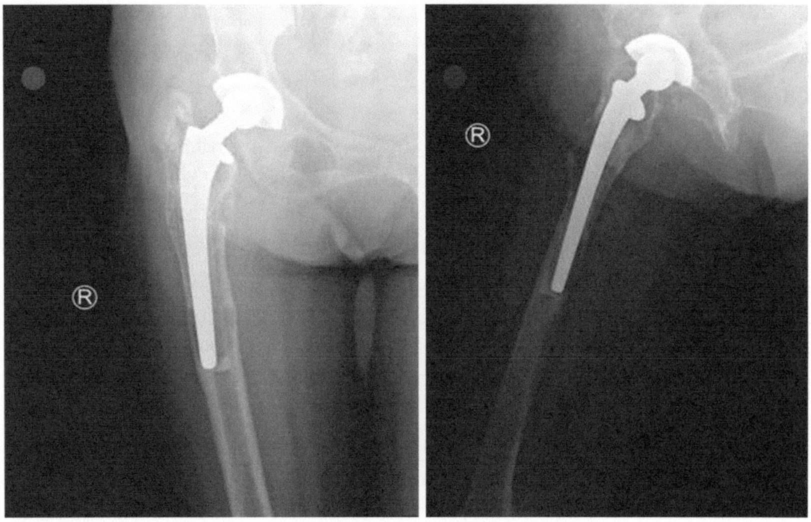

Fig. 7.8 Preoperative X-ray image

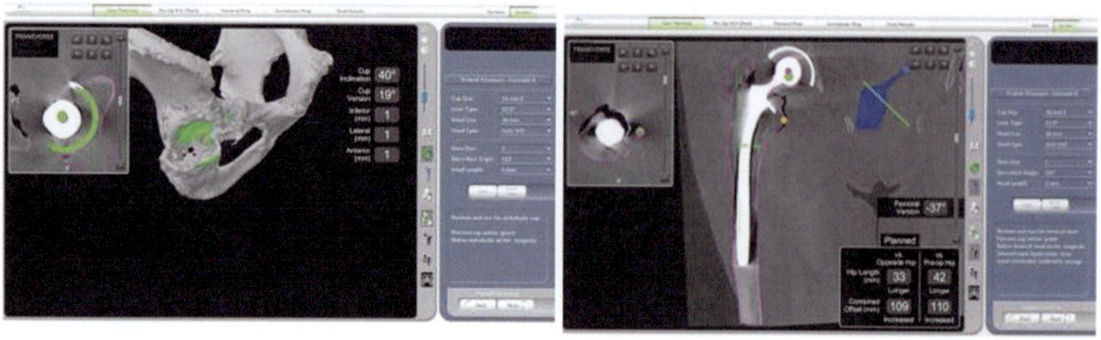

Fig. 7.9 Preoperative planning

ETO was performed with a length of 10 cm. The osteotomy block was subsequently pulled forward together with the abductor. A thin osteotome was employed to open up the gap between the femoral stem and the host bone, and appropriate tools were applied to retrieve the stem and bone cement.

The femoral medullary cavity was reamed to 17 mm, and the press fit was satisfactory. The medullary cavity was rinsed, and a restoration modular system was implanted. A 36-mm ceramic femoral head was inserted.

After hip reduction, the osteotomy block was anatomically reduced. A greater trochanteric claw plate was placed in and fixed with three cables.

Intraoperative considerations:

1. After acetabular reaming, only the bone bed in the dome had a fresh bleeding surface; however, the iliac roof, ischial, and pubic ramus all had significant bone defects. In complex cases of this type, surgeons could still have an accurate registration without much difficulty. The registration could be carried out with or without the original socket. From the robot's point of view, the conditions of the bone defect and its relationship with the hemispherical cup could be presented with good visualization after reaming.
2. Considering that the patient had previous lumbar conditions, it was necessary to calculate an optimal cup orientation for the patient based on the patient-specific safe zone (PSSZ) theory we published before. Subsequently, the appropriately sized cup trial could be placed in the desired position via the robotic arm.
3. A 20-mm slope augment was prepared and tried in the superior roof so that the metal augment was in close contact with the fresh host bone in the anterosuperior area. The gap left between the anterosuperior trial augment and the trial cup is just between a room for another slope augment sized between 20 and 25 mm. A 20-mm augment was too small, but a 25 mm was too big; however, it is impossible to easily enlarge it to a 25-mm gap by reaming as this room was almost between two pieces of trial components. In that circumstance, we changed the cup planning. The rotating center of the cup was moved 1 mm upward and 0.75 mm posteriorly, and its diameter was increased from 58 to 60 mm; thus, the cup's outer face was moved upward by a total of 2 mm. Meanwhile, the second augment was rotated posteriorly by 30–40° and then perfectly sized as 20 mm to ensure a good press fit between the cup and posterosuperior host bone and anterosuperior augment.
4. To accommodate the ischial bone defect shape, the surgeon used a slope augment stacked on a disc augment to support the cup from the distal. In this way, the superior and inferior augments were in close contact with the cancellous bone after being placed in, and with both structural press fit with the cup and further enhancement by cemented fixation, the whole metal construct could be considered an intraoperatively made customized non-spherical cup, which had fantastic initial fixation as well as enlarged bone contact area and promising secondary bone integration.

The intraopesrative process is shown in Fig. 7.10.

Fresh bleeding was observed only in the dome area after reaming, and severe defects were found in the ilium, ischium, and pubis, as shown in Fig. 7.11.

The plan was adjusted accordingly, in which the cup diameter was increased by 2 mm, as shown in Fig. 7.12.

Intraoperative observation is shown in Fig. 7.13.

7.3.5 Postoperative Radiographs

Postoperative immediate radiographs are shown in Fig. 7.14.

7.3.6 Conclusion and Reflection

For patients with severe acetabular bone defects, robotic-assisted revision combined with RPC theory for acetabular reconstruction (Dr. Zhou proposed prior to this book publication) can be mutually beneficial. When the bone defect in intraoperative observation is more severe than expected in some complex cases, an immediate change of preoperative planning is needed. A computer simulation provided by the robotic system helps modify the cup diameter, cup position, augment type, augment size, and position to gain a balance between hip biomechanics, bone contact, and implant fixation. In this way, the surgeons do not have to make a compromise between the hip biomechanics and the implant stability.

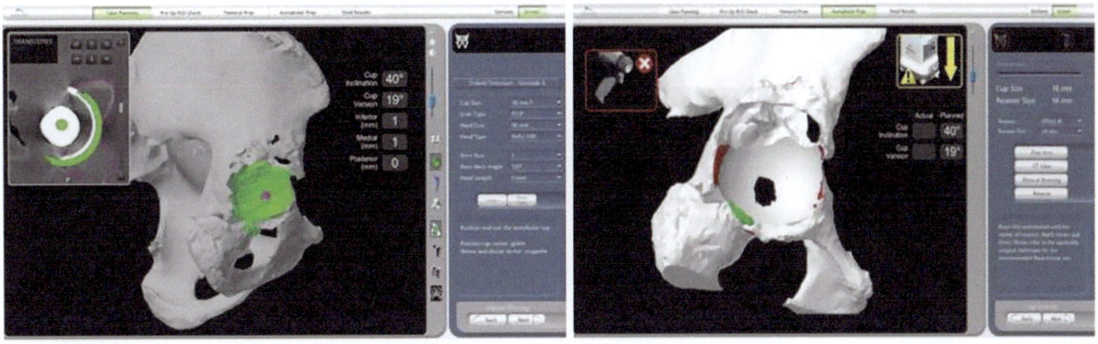

Fig. 7.10 Intraoperative process

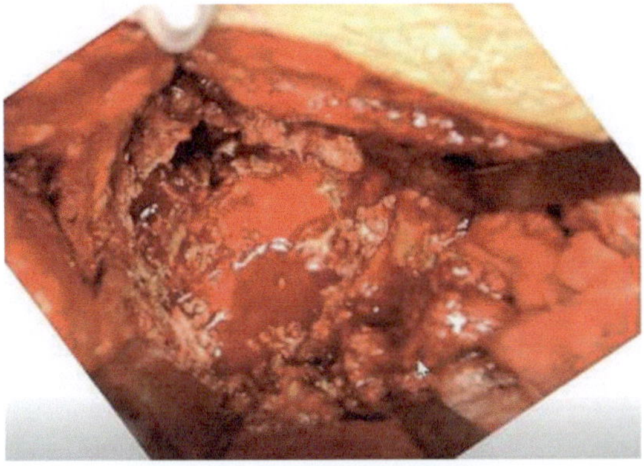

Fig. 7.11 Severe defects in ilium, ischium, and pubis

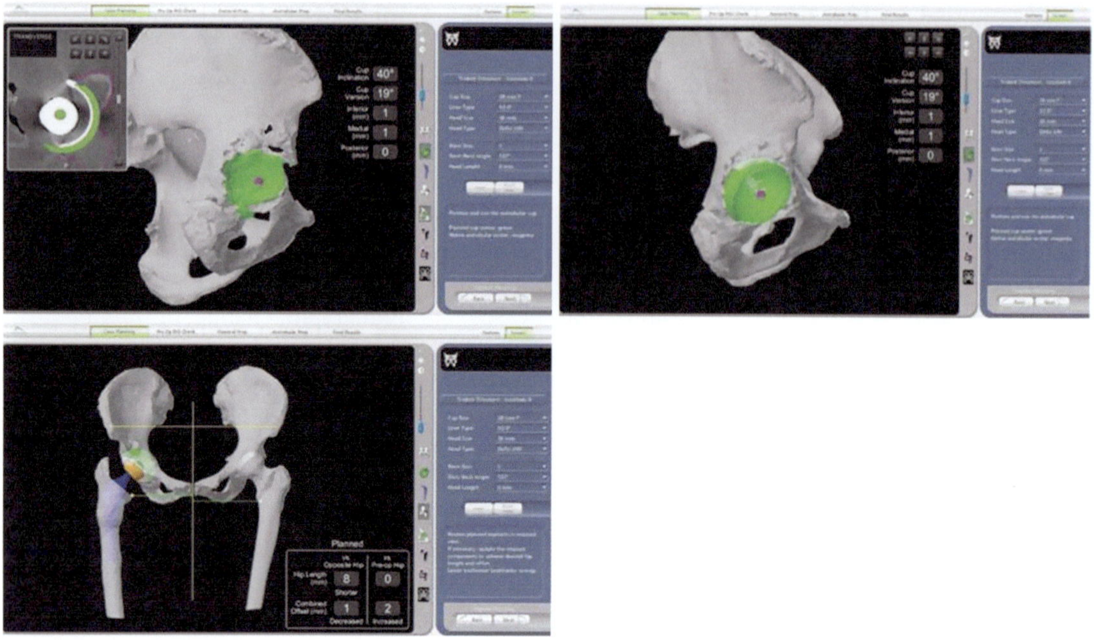

Fig. 7.12 Intraoperative adjustment on the planning

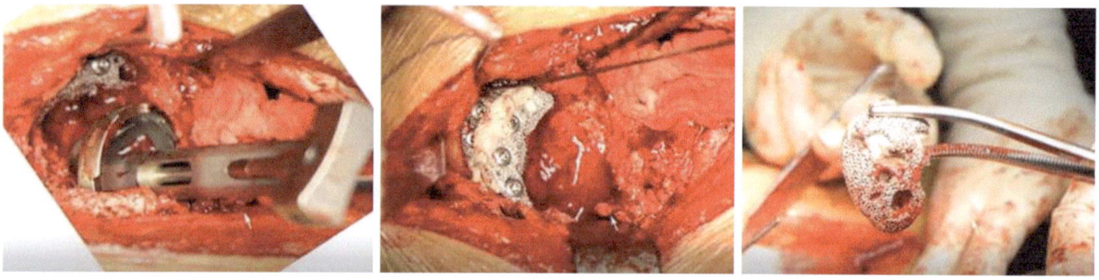

Fig. 7.13 Intraoperative observation

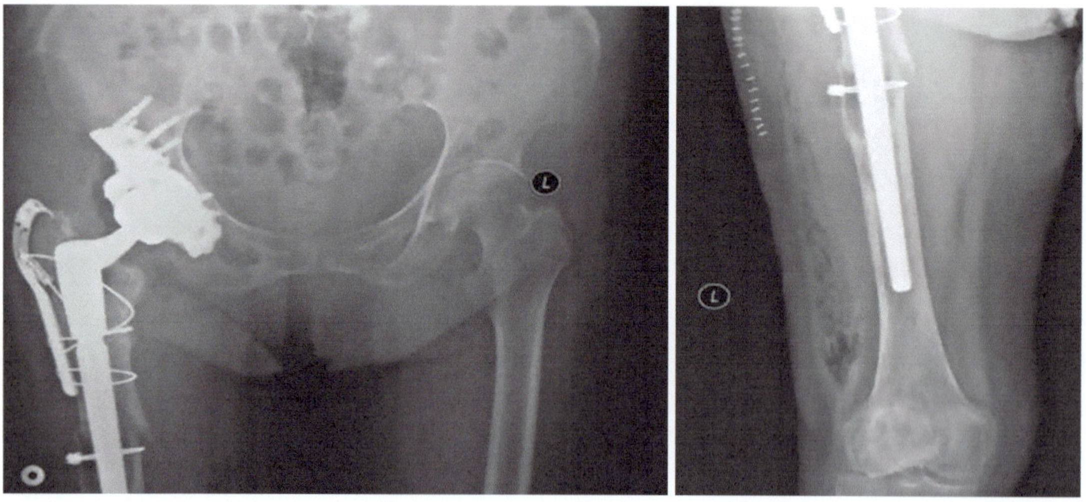

Fig. 7.14 Postoperative immediate radiographs

8 Metallosis Corrosion

Jianming Gu, Xiao Feng, Yixin Zhou, and Hanlong Zheng

8.1 Introduction

Jianming Gu

Metallosis corrosion-related conditions are mainly focused on the hip joint and related to cobalt ions. At present, cobalt has been studied most, while other metal ions such as titanium and aluminum have not been extensively researched due to their benign reactions to humans. Cobalt–chromium–molybdenum prosthesis is a widely used metal material in orthopedics due to its excellent mechanical properties. These prostheses include the femoral head, cementing the femoral stem and knee components. The cobalt–chromium–molybdenum alloy can form a surface layer of oxide after being exposed to air, which reduces exposure and release of the metal. Nevertheless, after implantation, the ions will be released through physical and chemical reactions, resulting in increased serum cobalt concentration. The metal release of hip prosthesis comes not only from the head–socket interface (like in metal-on-metal (MoM) prosthesis) but also from other metal components. These include the femoral head–stem junction as a fretting interface of the metal parts of modular prosthesis, the collision of metal prosthesis and other parts, the motion of prosthesis inside the cement sleeve or bone when loosening, and the direct reaction of the metal prosthesis in body fluids. Cobalt mainly presents as ions in the human body and is excreted through the kidney. The normal concentration of cobalt ions in the human population is 0.19 μg/L, and the upper limit of 95% confidence interval is 0.42 μg/L. A peripheral blood concentration of 1 μg/L is the limit for industrial overexposure, and a concentration over 5 μg/L is considered harmful. The significant adverse reaction of cobalt in the human body has drawn attention due to the extensive implantation of metal-on-metal prosthesis. Our institution conducted relevant studies from January 2016 to December 2018 among revision total hip arthroplasty (THA) patients. Preoperative serum cobalt ion concentration was tested for revision patients with cobalt–chromium–molybdenum prosthesis, among which 27.7% of patients revealed over 0.9 μg/L (38/137). Although higher cobalt concentration alone cannot be considered as an indication of revision THA, understanding the sources of metal ion release and the incidence of abnormal ion concentration is of great significance for the comprehension of THA failure patterns, grasp of surgical indications, surgical decision-making, and the selection of prosthesis for surgeons. Bradberry et al. summarized 18 cases of systemic toxicity related to elevated cobalt ion concentration, which mainly involved heart, thyroid, nervous, and visual systems. There were two main categories: one group used the MoM prosthesis of eight patients with initial THA, of which the ASR pros-

J. Gu (✉) · X. Feng · Y. Zhou · H. Zheng
Department of Adult Joint Reconstructive Surgery, Beijing Jishuitan Hospital, Capital Medical University, Beijing, China

Y. Zhou (ed.), *Revision Total Hip Arthroplasty*, https://doi.org/10.1007/978-981-97-9804-9_8

thesis of Johnson & Johnson was the majority. The cobalt ion concentration of patients was 34.5 (ref range: 13.6–6521) μg/L. For patients with metal-on-metal prosthesis using cobalt–chromium–molybdenum material for the friction interface, the change in serum cobalt concentration is associated with various factors, including prosthesis design, femoral head diameter, and the placement of the prosthesis during operation. DeHaan et al. reported that the serum cobalt ion concentration of patients with well-functioning MoM prosthesis was 2.4 μg/L, while that of patients with prosthesis malposition was 9.8 μg/L. Due to the damage to the bone matrix and soft tissue, revision THA related to adverse reactions to metal has a higher chance of developing complications, associated with a higher rate of infection, prosthesis instability, and loosening. Crawford et al. conducted a follow-up examination of 203 MoM hip revision cases, in which the Harris score improved from 53.6 (preoperative) to 73.5 (postoperative). Notably, 14% of the patients (28 cases) required reoperation, and 16 cases required multiple revisions. Patients with pseudotumors had a significantly increased risk of revision. The survivorship at 4.2 years was 90.5%. Therefore, detailed communication with patients before the operation is necessary. They must be informed of perioperative risks and long-term effects. Fortunately, the revision of adverse reactions to metal related to metal-on-metal friction interface has been undergoing renovation for more than a decade. With the withdrawal of many MoM prostheses and the declined application, serious adverse reactions related to metal ions will not be reported in large amounts. Lainiala et al. reported that of 730 metal-on-metal revision cases in the JOA journal in 2019, the largest number of revision cases appeared between 2011 and 2013, and then the number decreased each year. There are corresponding guidelines on the use of MoM prosthesis and follow-up examinations in countries such as the UK and the US. Due to the late introduction to the domestic market, patient numbers with MoM prosthesis are relatively few. Although there have been no published guidelines for a follow-up examination, it is necessary to conduct a corresponding follow-up examination referring to the experience and data from other countries in order to avoid serious complications. The second category was revision of ceramic component fracture with metal head, ten cases in total. The serum cobalt ion concentration was 506 (353–6521) μg/L. There was an abnormal increase in serum cobalt concentration caused by direct contact between the femoral head and the cup due to PE wearing through, which suggested that follow-up examination should be intensified, especially for patients who underwent an operation before 10 years or more. PE liner wearing through, fracture, and dislocation should be early detected at follow-up.

In addition to these two common conditions, Dahlstrand et al. reported an increase in cobalt concentration in patients with metal-on-polyethylene interfaces, which was mainly caused by micro-friction and corrosion at the femoral head–stem junction. White et al. reported that in the follow-up examination at a mean of 5 years among 60 THA patients with non-cement titanium alloy femoral stem, there were 17 patients (56.7%) out of 30 metal-on-polyethylene patients with increased cobalt ion concentration, with an average of 2.0 μg/L. Peripheral magnetic resonance imaging (MRI) findings of seven patients with cobalt concentration greater than 4.0 μg/L and seven with symptoms showed that four of them exhibited early adverse reactions to metal. Previous studies showed that the combination of cobalt–chromium–molybdenum head and cobalt–chromium–molybdenum stem presents more sources of cobalt ion release. Minor damage at the junction can lead to more cobalt release. The basic process of metal corrosion at the femoral head and femoral stem cone is called mechanically assisted crevice corrosion (MACC). There are various related factors, including the combination of different materials, the diameter of the femoral head, the design of the femoral head and stem cone, and mechanical stress (patient body mass, implantation time, amount of motion). The design of the stem cone includes angle, length, diameter, surface treatment, and so on. Tan et al. have found that 11/13 stem cones have a higher corrosion rate. Triantafyllopouls et al. found that tapered PCA is more corrosion resistant than that of V40 stem cone, and prosthesis with lower stiffness at the stem cone exhibits higher fretting corrosion, the reasons for which are associated with the elastic modulus and cross-sectional area of the material, taper angle, bonding depth of the femoral head, and so on. The general principle is, again, to pay attention to whether there is excessive metal release for prosthesis with metallic femoral heads of large diameters with elongated femoral necks. Bansal et al. systematically recorded 46 revision cases of definitive failure of femoral stem cones, all of which were applied with chromium–molybdenum femoral head. The concentration of cobalt ions was detected in 22 patients of them; the average concentration was 9.36 (0.5–33.6) μg/L. Only three patients had a concentration of <1 μg/L, and the remaining 19 had abnormally elevated figures. This suggests that for patients with MoP prosthesis, once the serum concentration of cobalt ions is found to increase, it is necessary to actively identify the cause and arrange regular follow-ups to closely monitor the progress of metal precipitation and its complications, and to perform revision surgery if necessary. The application of modular stem is also an important source of cobalt ions, and the postoperative complication rate is high after revision. Inoue et al. reported 80 revision cases of patients with adverse local tissue reaction (ALTR) using modular-neck stem, 10% of them developed complications related to prosthesis, and six of them underwent second revision (two for dislocation, two for femur loosening, and two for peripheral fractures), and the 63-month survival rate in this group was 82%. The significance of this chapter is to remind orthopedic surgeons of cobalt-related conditions and to be alert to clinical symptoms, as more than a quarter of revision THA patients who attended our institution exhibited an abnormal increase in the serum cobalt ion concentration, which should arouse alert in physicians.

With the wide use of ceramic heads in China, large-diameter metal ball head is relatively less used. Thus, the problem of cobalt ion release was solved to a certain extent. Ceramic materials contain no cobalt, and electrolysis does not occur to them. As a result, the use of ceramic heads can significantly reduce fretting corrosion. Kocagoz et al. conducted research on retrieved prosthesis from 100 cases of hip revision due to the adverse reaction of the metal, in which the annual metal release of cobalt–chromium–molybdenum femoral head was 0.1 (ref range: 0–8.8) mm^3. The metal release at the stem cone junction occurred primarily on the femoral head side instead of the stem cone side. Metal release of the ceramic head was 0 (ref range: 0–0.4) mm^3. Therefore, they recommended to use ceramic femoral head to reduce abrasion and corrosion at the femoral head–stem cone when a high offset prosthesis was required and the patient had impaired renal function. Wight et al. studied the risk factors of corrosion at the stem cone, suggesting that a high-offset, large-diameter femoral head should be applied with caution, and a large-diameter metal ball head should also be used with special caution for overweight patients with high-level physical activity. In the expert consensus on *The Classification Standard of Metal Ion Corrosion Risk for Metal-on-Polyethene Total Hip Femoral Head–Neck–Stem Cone* jointly published by the American Association of Hip and Knee Surgeons (AAHKS), the American Academy of Orthopaedic Surgeons (AAOS), and the Hip Society in 2021, high-risk factors included high-level activity, cobalt–chromium–molybdenum ball head larger than 40 mm, and high offset femoral stem.

In conclusion, elevated serum cobalt concentration is not rare in revision THA, and patients with MoM friction interface and modular stem should be monitored for serum cobalt concentrations and complications. Follow-up examinations should also be intensified for patients with MoP-bearing hip prosthesis to early detect polyethylene wearout, cobalt ion release, and associated complications. When a femoral head with a large diameter and high offset is applied, the cobalt–chromium–molybdenum femoral head should be carefully decided, especially in patients with renal dysfunction, overweight, and high activity levels. For clinicians, it is necessary to master related knowledge and stretch the ability of preoperative and intraoperative identification, primarily to identify patients who are likely to develop adverse reactions to metal ions and identify sources of the metal ions, including MoM prosthesis, modular prosthesis, and application of metal head joint. Whether the patient developed metal-related systemic and local reactions can be confirmed through medical history and physical examination, and local examination of the hip joint can be performed by ultrasound or peripheral MRI. Meanwhile, blood samples and synovial fluid should be collected for metal concentration determination, and intraoperative samples should be collected and sent for pathological diagnosis.

8.2 Case 1

Xiao Feng, Jianming Gu, and Yixin Zhou

8.2.1 Case Summary

Medical History Male, 64 years old, complaint: left hip pain and limited hip range of motion for 1 year. The patient accidentally injured his left hip 13 years ago, which was diagnosed as "left femoral neck fracture." He underwent left THA. The operation went uneventfully, and postoperative walking was nearly normal. Left hip pain aggravated 1 year ago, which was related to motion and could be relieved by rest. Nocturnal pain and limited mobility were presented. The symptoms gradually progressed. He had difficulty in squatting and walking up and down stairs. The walking distance was less than 200 m once. The patient denied previous chronic disease.

Physical Examination The patient walked with left hip shortening gait; incision cicatrix could be seen without redness or swelling; left inguinal area, greater trochanter area, and proximal thigh tenderness (+); axial percussion pain (+); obviously limited mobility; Patrick's sign on the left (+); Thomas' sign on the left (+); Trendelenburg's sign on the left (+); Allis' sign on the left (+); Ober's sign on the left (−); no edema in either lower extremity; no hypoesthesia; and the pulse of the bilateral dorsal artery of foot was palpable.

Laboratory Examination Preoperative routine blood test: white blood cell (WBC) 5.13×10^9/L, erythrocyte sedimentation rate (ESR): 2 mm/h, C-reactive protein (CRP): 1.10 mg/L.

Metal ion-related results: preoperative serum Cr 3.47 ng/mL, Co 2.38 ng/mL.

Periprosthetic soft tissue Campbell-Aseptic Lymphocytic Vasculitis Associated Lesion (ALVAL) score: 7.

Radiographic Data Preoperative X-rays are shown in Fig. 8.1; preoperative digital tomosynthesis is shown in Fig. 8.2.

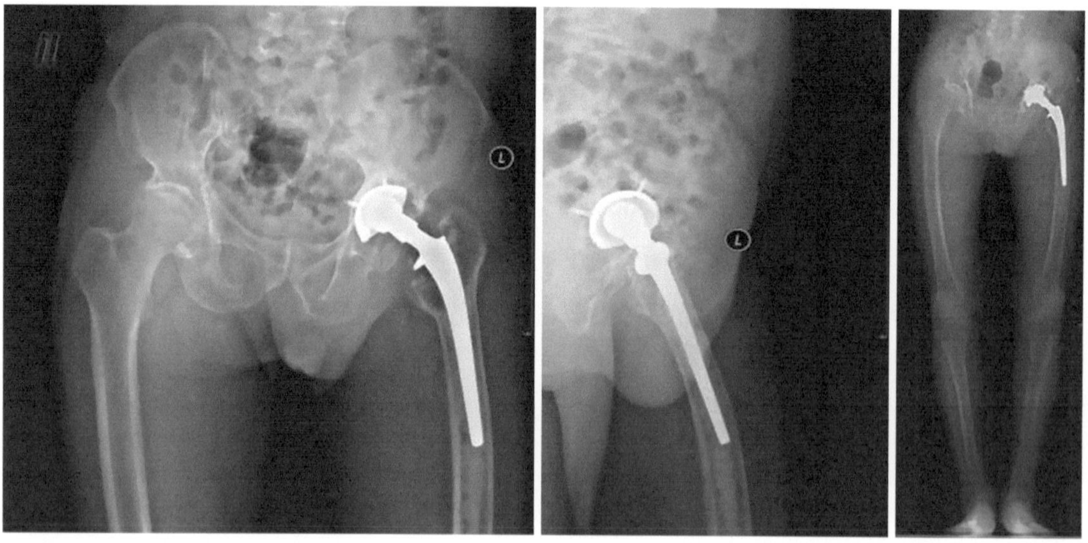

Fig. 8.1 Preoperative X-rays

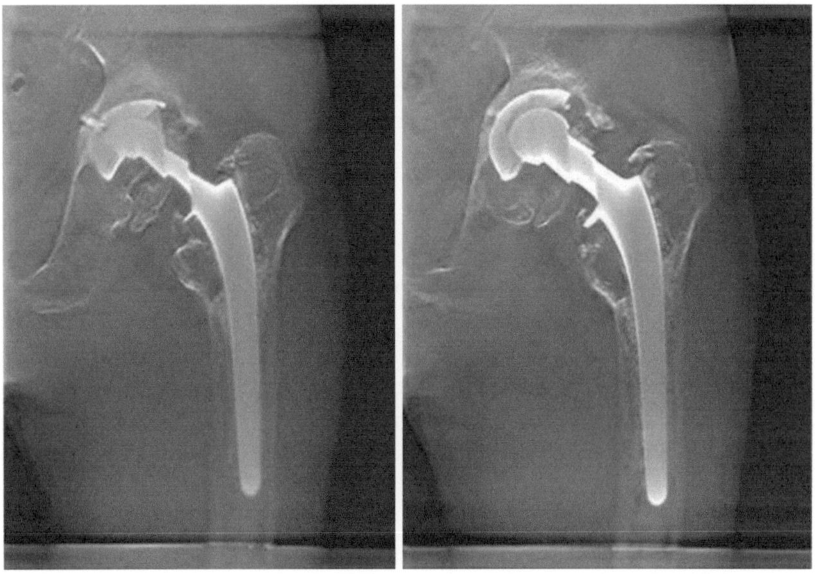

Fig. 8.2 Preoperative digital tomosynthesis

8.2.2 Case Analysis

1. The initial left THA used the MoP-bearing surface with cementing femoral prosthesis. Preoperative WBC, ESR, and CRP were within the normal range. There was no fever, skin ulcer, abscess, swelling, skin redness, or skin warmness. Thus, the possibility of infection was ruled out.
2. The radiographs showed varus migration of the femoral stem and upward migration of the femoral head to the liner. Bone cement could be identified in the periprosthetic area of the femoral stem within the medullary cavity. And a clear periprosthetic radiolucent line could be seen. Osteolysis was observed around the cup and femoral stem in digital tomosynthesis, especially Gruen zones 1 and 7. Aseptic loosening, osteolysis, and polyethylene eccentrically wear were diagnosed.
3. The significantly increased serum Co and Cr ions before the operation were considered a result of corrosion at the metal head–stem taper junction of the left hip prosthesis. In addition, the abrasion between loose cement stem and bone cement could also be one of the sources of metal ions.
4. In conclusion, the reasons for failure in this patient were mainly aseptic loosening due to PE wear, and ALTR should be considered.
5. Diagnosis: aseptic loosening following left THA (MoP prosthesis), ALTR.

8.2.3 Preoperative Planning

1. Radiographs of the patient revealed extensive periprosthetic osteolysis and possible severe bone defect on the acetabular side. If metal reconstruction was planned, preoperative preparation of various types of augments was required. Moreover, a severe bone defect exists in the proximal femur, and a bone substitute could be prepared to restore some bone stock. A longer distal fixation stem should be prepared for the femur side.
2. The osteolysis was mainly due to polyethylene wear; thus, ceramic liner or highly cross-linked polyethylene liner could be employed instead. As the patient had increased metal ion concentration, ALTR should be taken into consideration. The grossly diseased part of the periprosthetic soft tissue should be completely removed during the operation. Prosthesis containing Co and Cr should be

avoided, and the sources of ALTR need to be removed.
3. Cement removal equipment, such as an ultrasonic bone cutter, should be prepared.

8.2.4 Operation Findings

1. The hip joint was exposed and dislocated, and the femoral head was removed.
2. Cicatrix and adverse soft tissue at the proximal femur were removed. We found that femoral stem was loosened and then easily removed. The surrounding adverse soft tissue was removed, as shown in Fig. 8.3.
3. Then the polyethylene liner and acetabular shell were taken out. During the operation, the polyethylene liner had remarkable eccentric wear with impingement marks. Black debris was seen at the junction of the metal ball head and the stem taper. The Goldberg score for corrosion classification was 3 for the taper and 3 for the ball head. The femoral stem was partially polished. The polythene liner and metal prosthesis are shown in Fig. 8.4.
4. After thorough debridement, a serious acetabular bone defect was found. It was subsequently filled and supported with augment, as shown in Fig. 8.5. The acetabulum was reamed to 56 mm with adequate bleeding of the bone bed. The wound was irrigated, and a 58-mm non-cement Trabecular Metal (TM) continuum cup and polyethylene acetabular liner were implanted.
5. Soft tissue with possible ALTR around the femur was carefully debrided and sent for pathological examination for ALVAL grading. Then we started cleaning the femoral cement. Due to the proximal femur deformity, distal bone cement was difficult to remove. Then ETO was performed. Osteotome and ultrasonic bone cutter were used to clean the intra-

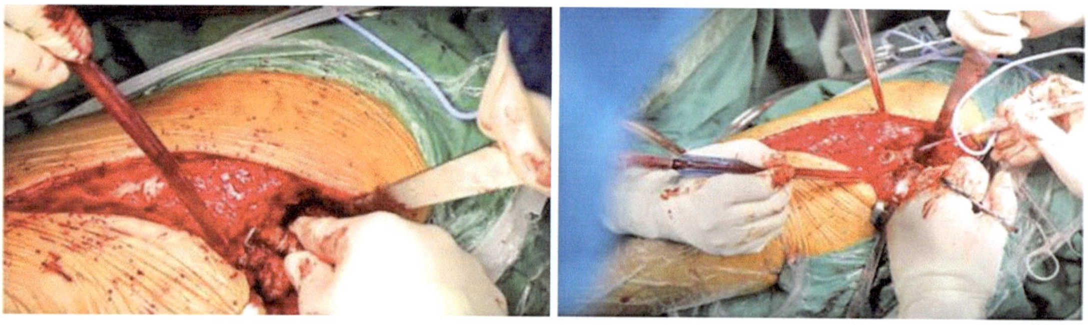

Fig. 8.3 Intraoperative pitures of femoral stem and adverse soft tissue removal

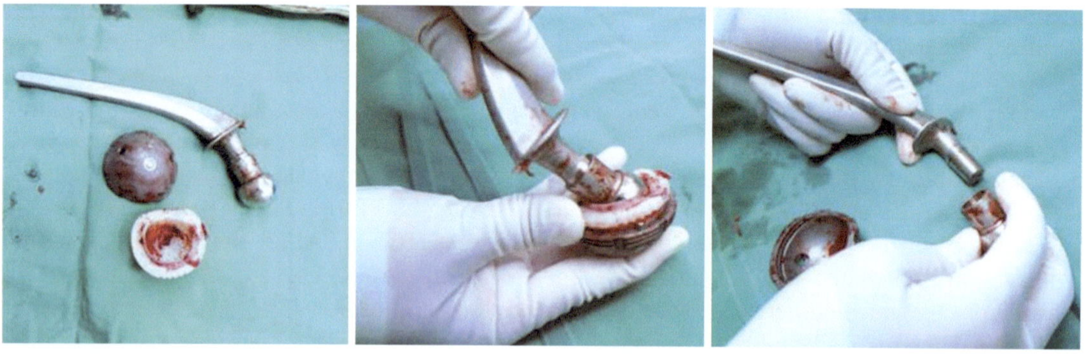

Fig. 8.4 Left: retrieved implants. Middle: polythene liner had impingement with skirt of femoral head. Right: black debris could be found at the junction of metal head and stem taper

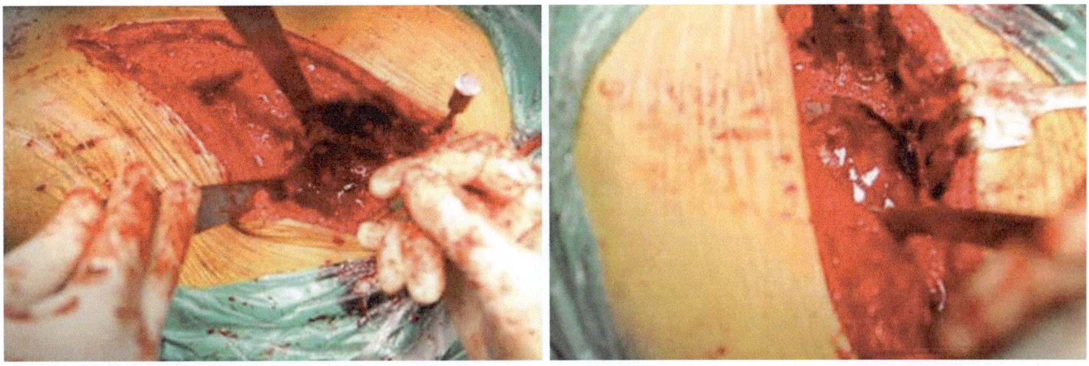

Fig. 8.5 Acetabular bone defect filled with augment

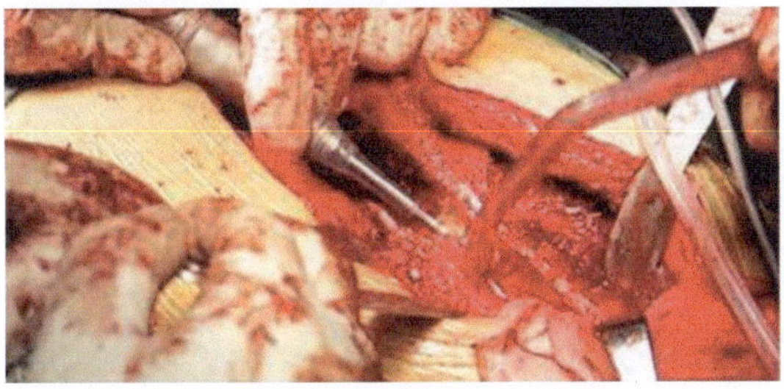

Fig. 8.6 Removing intramedullary bone cement

medullary bone cement, and the distal cement plug was pushed further as it could not be fully removed, as shown in Fig. 8.6.

6. A sequential drill reamer was used for the femoral canal to a satisfactory press fit. A distal 17-mm stem was used. The RM 195-mm femoral stem was implanted. The torsion test was satisfactory. The proximal medullary cavity was then reamed to 23 mm, and a proximal femur 23 + 20 mm stem was implanted and locked tight with the distal end. A 36 + 0 mm ceramic (pink) femoral head was implanted. The great trochanter of the proximal femur was placed back and fixed with cable.

8.2.5 Postoperative Condition and Outcome

1. The serum level of Cr was 2.30 ng/mL and of Co was 1.18 ng/mL. Pathological examination showed a periprosthetic soft tissue Campbell-ALVAL score of 7, confirming ALTR caused by elevated metal ion concentration in the patient. Fortunately, this patient did not have systemic toxicity manifestation for elevated metal ion.
2. The patient recovered well and gradually began to weight bearing normally.
3. At 3 months follow-up, serum Cr and Co levels decreased to 0.93 and 0.70 ng/mL, respectively.
4. Other follow-up results: free of pain; no limitation in walking up and down stairs or on flat ground; and functional recovery was good. The radiographs showed that the prosthesis was in good position and the osteotomy was healing.

Instant postoperative X-rays and postoperative X-rays at the latest follow-up are shown in Fig. 8.7.

8.2.6 Prosthesis Retrieval

The retrieved prosthesis is shown in Fig. 8.8. The femoral stem was polished, by the friction with cement and the femur (see Fig. 8.9). Corrosion and metal deposition could be seen at the head–neck connection, as shown in Fig. 8.10. The taper (light microscope and ultra-depth field microscope views) is shown in Fig. 8.11. The medial view of the femoral head (light microscope and ultra-depth field microscope views) is shown in Fig. 8.12. Polyethylene liner wear and impingement are shown in Fig. 8.13.

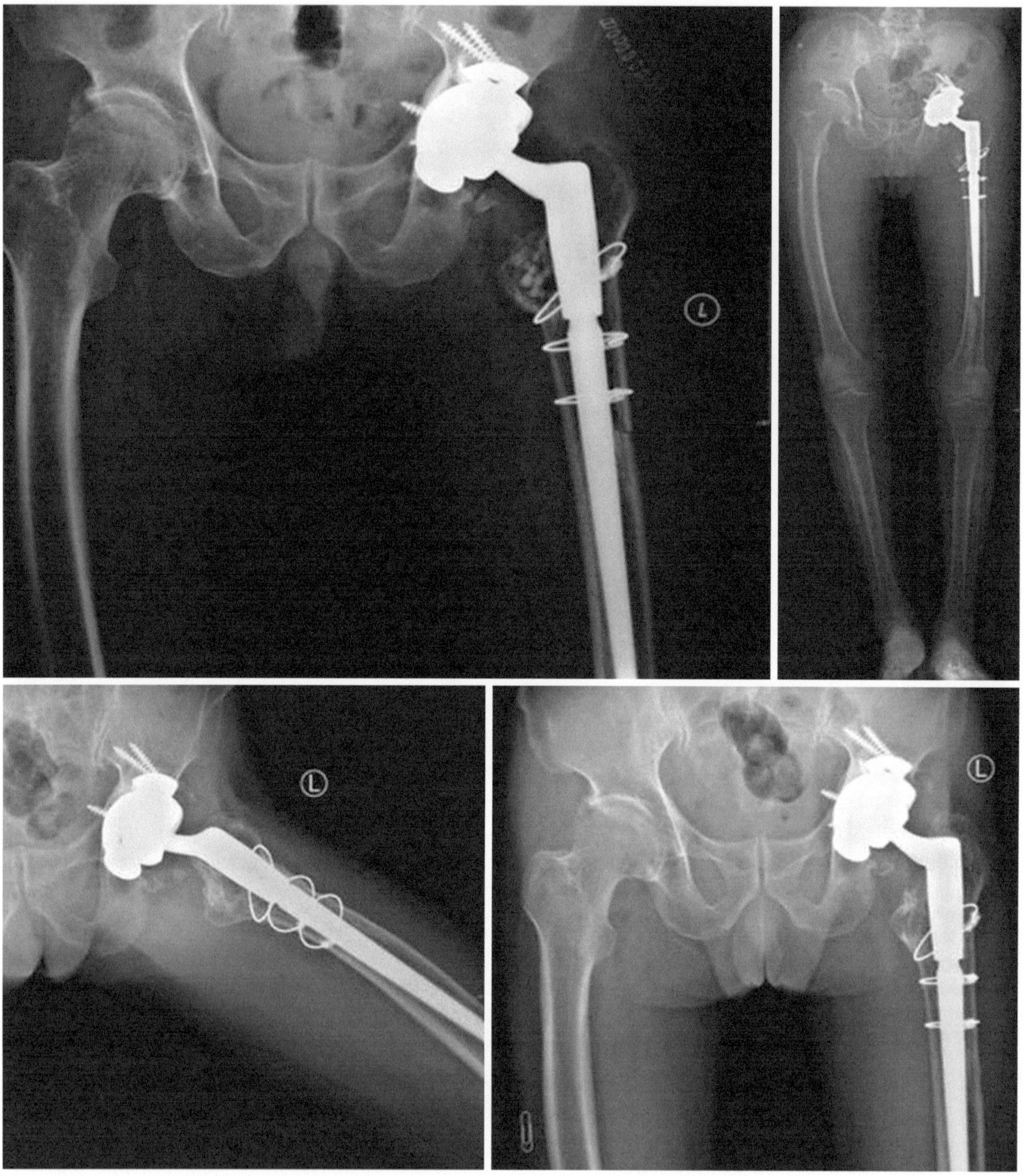

Fig. 8.7 Instant postoperative X-rays and postoperative X-rays at the latest follow-up

8.2.7 Conclusion and Reflection

1. Patients with severe periprosthetic osteolysis may possibly have metallosis as a complication. Patients with elevated metal levels could develop local adverse reactions such as osteolysis, prosthesis loosening, and early failure of the revision surgery. When the osteolysis cannot be fully explained by polyethylene wear, and there are sources of metal ion release, serum metal ion level could be tested to rule out metallosis.
2. CoCrMo is the most common material used for cement stems. CoCrMo heads cannot be combined with stainless steel stems, as it will lead to serious corrosion. The CoCrMo stem

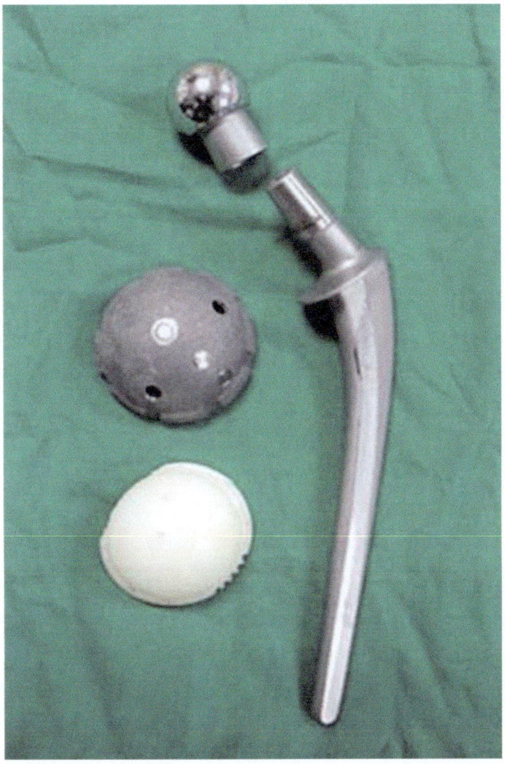

Fig. 8.8 Retrieved prosthesis

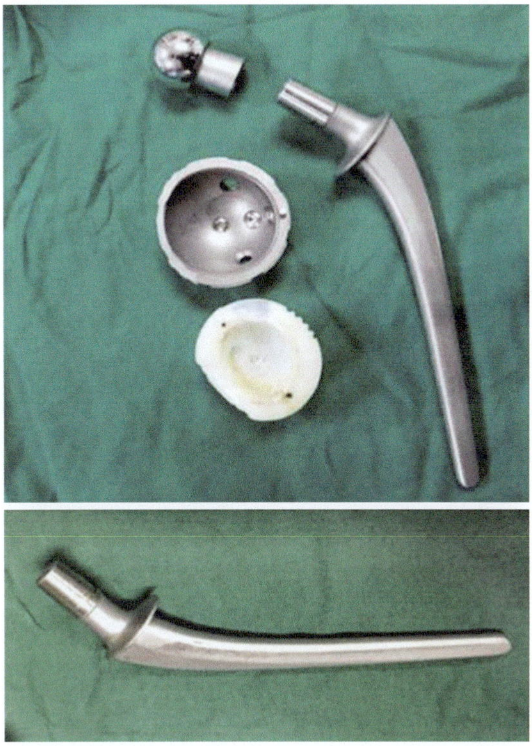

Fig. 8.9 Femoral stem prosthesis

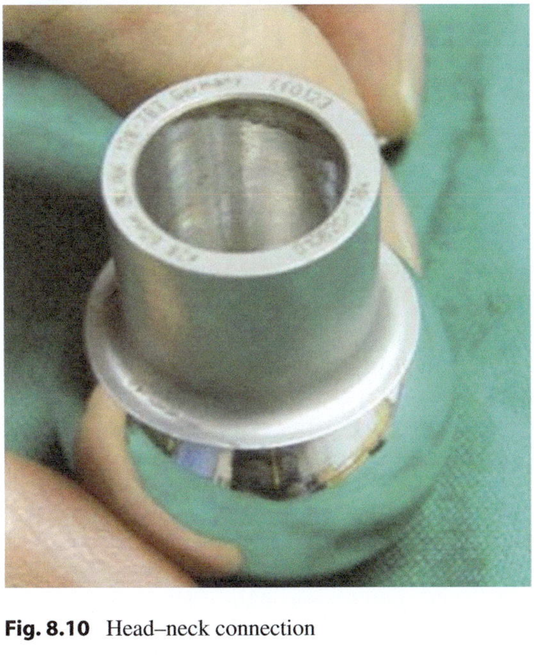

Fig. 8.10 Head–neck connection

usually couples with the CoCrMo head, yet it may develop corrosion. The elongated femoral head of this patient gave increased torsion at the head–neck junction, which was a greater risk of corrosion. When the stem was loosened, there could be motion between the stem and the bone cement. The retrieved stem had shown a loss of metal material at the polished surface. This patient bore more than one metal release source.

3. This patient did not have systemic toxicity manifestation for elevated metal ions. Local reaction to metal ions was confirmed in pathology. Patients with elevated metal ions may develop dislocation or infection after revision. It was due to the soft tissue toxicity of the metal ion. After debridement and prosthesis removal, this patient recovered uneventfully.

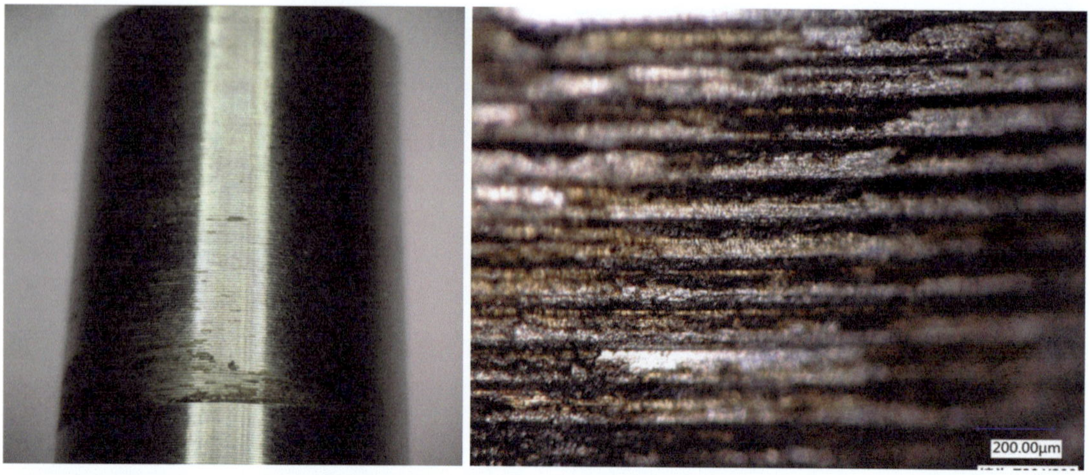

Fig. 8.11 The taper (light microscope and ultra-depth of field microscope views)

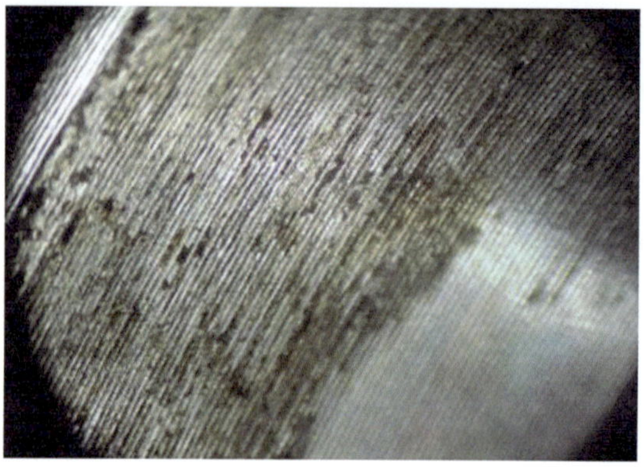

Fig. 8.12 Medial view of the sphere (light microscope and ultra-depth of field microscope views)

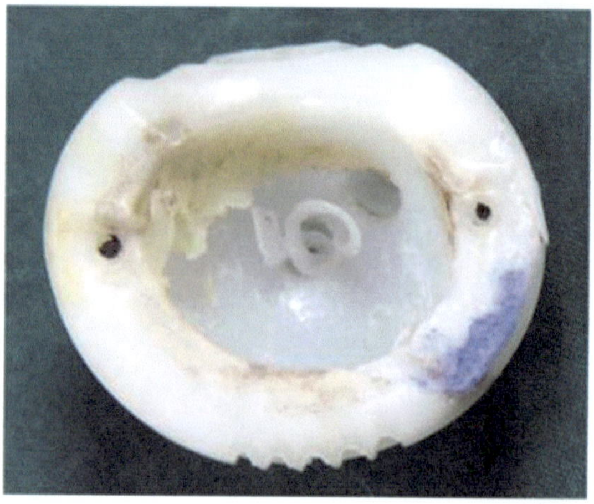

Fig. 8.13 Polyethylene liner

8.3 Case 2

Xiao Feng, Jianming Gu, and Yixin Zhou

8.3.1 Case Summary

Medical History Male, 43 years old, complained of "pain of the right hip for 3 years, after history of right THA for 7 years." This patient underwent right THA 7 years ago in our hospital in 2009 and left THA in 2010 due to ischemic necrosis of the femoral head. Right hip pain occurred 3 years ago, aggravated by movement and relieved by rest. There was no nocturnal pain or obvious restriction in motion. The patient denied a history of hypertension, diabetes, coronary heart disease, hepatitis, tuberculosis, or other infectious diseases. In 2006, he received surgical treatment for craniocerebral trauma.

Physical Examination The patient entered the ward by walking without pelvis tilt; There was an incision cicatrix at the right hip without redness or swelling; There was tenderness at the greater trochanter area and proximal thigh of the right hip, axial percussion pain (+); mild limited mobility; Patrick's sign on the right (+); Thomas's sign on the right (−); Trendelenburg's gait (−); Allis's sign on the right (−); Ober's sign on the right (+); no edema or hypoesthesia in either lower extremity; and the pulsation of bilateral dorsalis pedis was palpable.

Laboratory Examination Preoperative routine blood test: WBC 10.66 × 10^9/L; ESR: 8 mm/h; C-reactive protein: 6.71 mg/L.

Serum metal ion results: Preoperative serum Cr 6.00 ng/mL and Co 9.75 ng/mL.

Radiographic Data See Fig. 8.14 for preoperative X-rays.

8.3.2 Case Analysis

1. This symptomatic patient had MoM prosthesis on the right hip. He had increased WBC before the operation, but the ESR and CRP were normal. No symptoms of fever, skin ulcer, pus formation, local swelling, skin redness, or skin temperature rise were observed; thus, the possibility of infection was low.
2. The preoperative radiographs indicated that the position of the components in the right hip was acceptable. No obvious signs of osteolysis or loosening were observed on the acetabular or femoral side.
3. Preoperative serum Co and Cr ions significantly increased, considering that the main source was at the MoM interface on the right and corrosion at the stem–taper junction. There was a high possibility of ALTR resulting from metal ions.
4. Diagnosis: ALTR at the right hip (MoM).

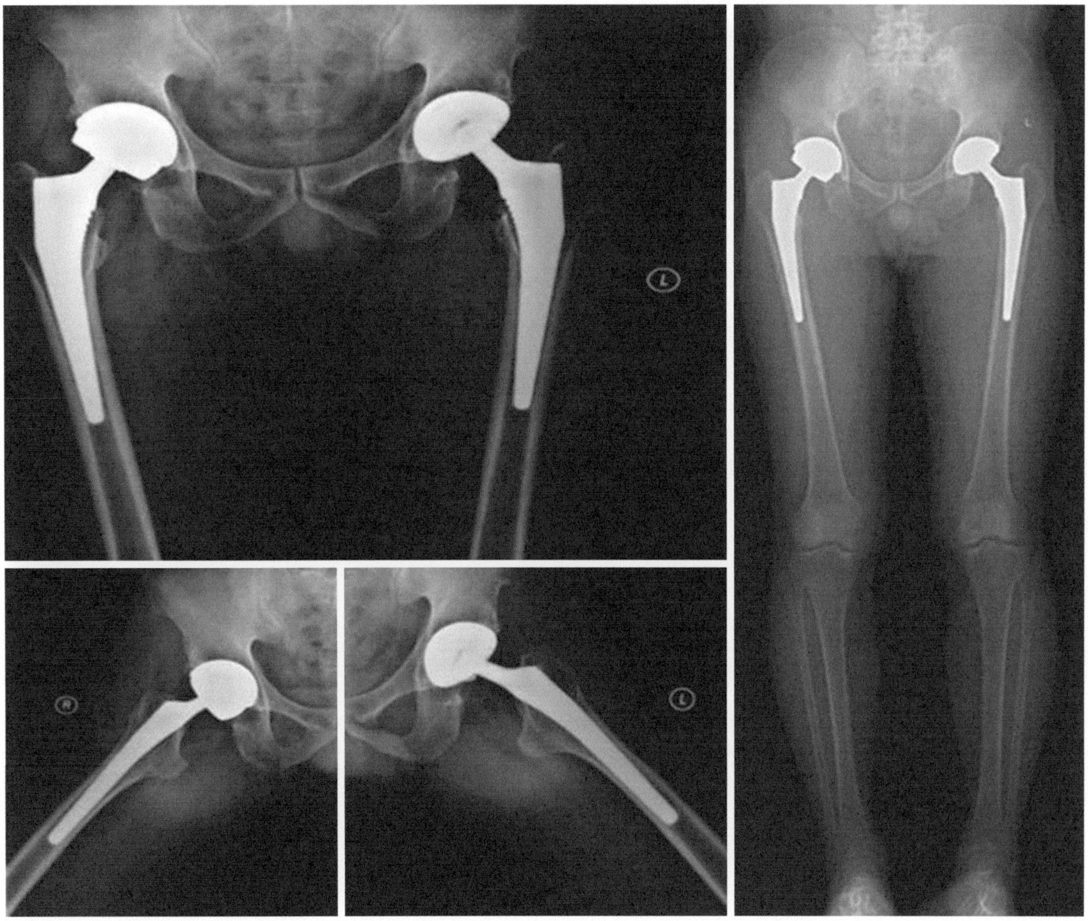

Fig. 8.14 Preoperative X-rays

8.3.3 Preoperative Planning

1. This patient had clinical symptoms and increased Co and Cr serum levels and WBC levels, no sign of loosening or osteolysis could be found in the radiographs, and infection and ALTR should be considered. Intraoperative pathology and culture samples should be collected.
2. For the treatment of ALTR, grossly injured soft tissue needed to be debrided during the operation, and the MoM bearing surface should be changed to eliminate possible sources of ALTR.
3. The non-cement stem on the femoral side was well fixed in a good position, it could be retained, using a metal-sleeved ceramic head for revision.
4. Because ALTR could possibly involve the abductor mechanism, excessive release of soft tissue should be avoided. Appropriate soft tissue tension should be gained to avoid possible hip instability after revision.
5. Implants containing Co and Cr should be carefully chosen in revision.

8.3.4 Operation Situation

1. When the hip was exposed, fluid accumulation and edema of the soft tissue around the joint were observed, as shown in Fig. 8.15.
2. The hip was dislocated and osteotome was used to remove the femoral head from the trunnion. ALTR around the femoral metal head was seen, as shown in Fig. 8.16. Goldberg's score was 3 for the taper and 3 for the ball head.
3. After the acetabular component was removed, soft tissue swelling was identified surrounding the acetabular bone bed. Necrotic tissue and gray pseudomembrane were present, as shown in Fig. 8.17. They were completely debrided and were subsequently sent for pathological examination and ALVAL scoring.
4. After debridement, the acetabular was reamed to 54 mm with good bone bleeding. The incision was thoroughly irrigated, and a 54-mm non-cement Pinnacle acetabular component and ceramic liner were implanted, as shown in Fig. 8.18.
5. The femoral stem was stable; thus, it was preserved. An OPTION femoral head with a metal sleeve and the corresponding ceramic liner was applied, as shown in Fig. 8.19.

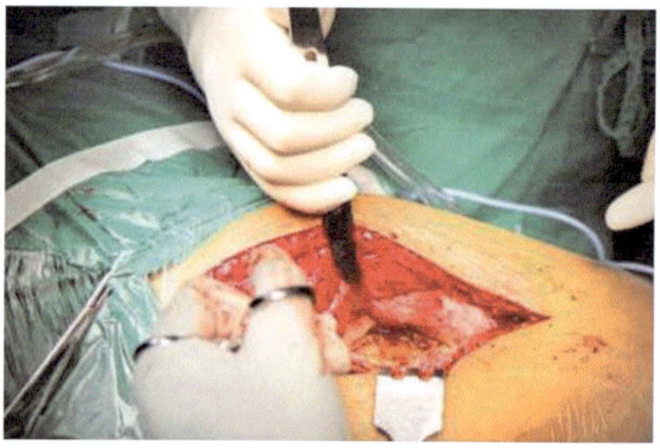

Fig. 8.15 Hip exposure

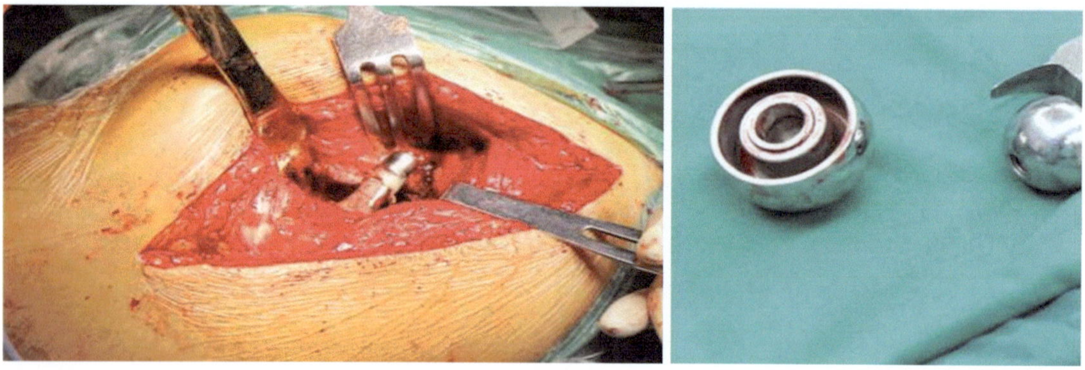

Fig. 8.16 Corrosion at the joint of stem cone and metal ball head

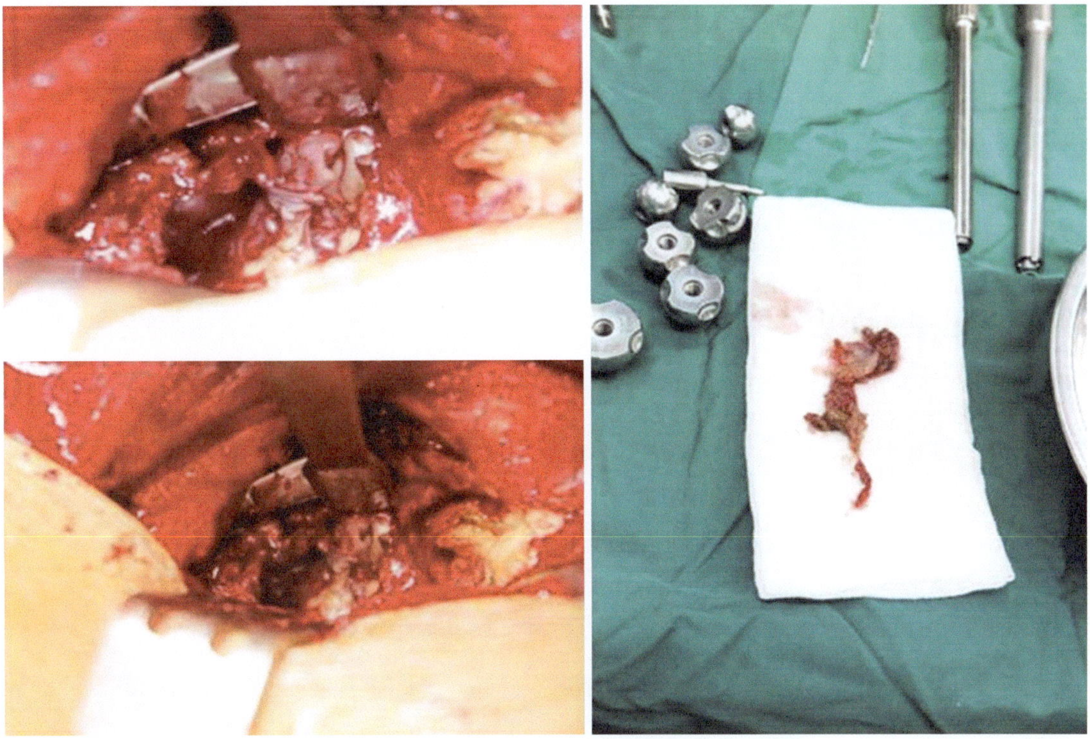

Fig. 8.17 Periprosthetic necrotic tissue and white pseudomembrane

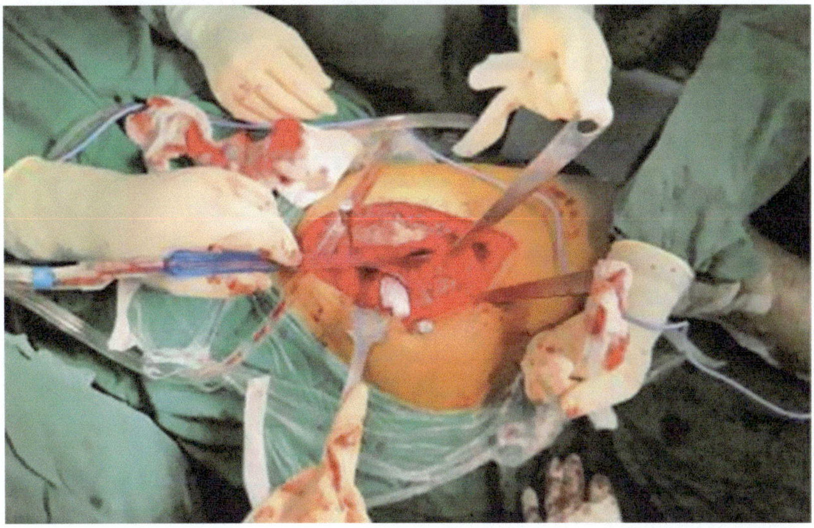

Fig. 8.18 Implanting acetabular component and liner

8.3.5 Postoperative Condition and Outcome

1. Intraoperative synovial fluid Cr level was 841.50 ng/mL, Co level was 331.11 ng/mL, postoperative serum Cr 2.76 ng/mL, and Co 0.87 ng/mL. Campbell-ALVAL score of periprosthetic soft tissue reported by pathological examination was 7.
2. The patients recovered well and walked normally. Serum Cr and Co levels significantly reduced to 0.68 and 0.73 ng/mL, respectively at 3 months follow-up.

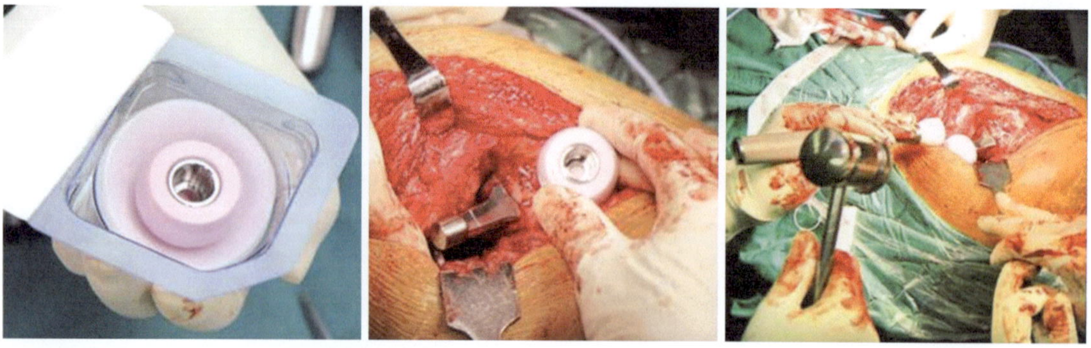

Fig. 8.19 Replacing the femoral head component

Fig. 8.20 Postoperative immediate radiographs

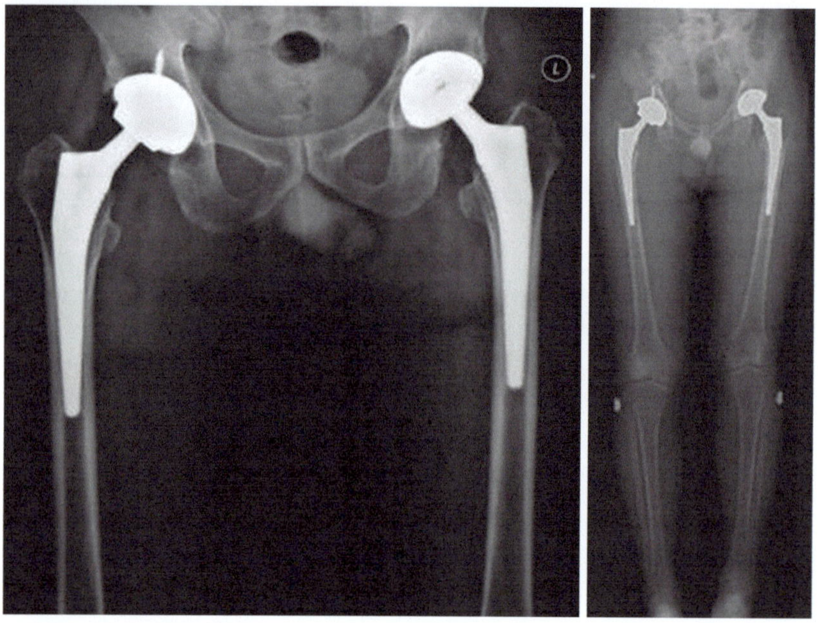

3. Other follow-up examination: Free of pain; walking up and down stairs or on plain ground was not restricted. X-rays showed that the implant was in a good position. Postoperative immediate X-rays are shown in Fig. 8.20. Postoperative radiographs after 3 months are shown in Fig. 8.21. Postoperative radiographs after 6 months are shown in Fig. 8.22.

8.3.6 Prosthesis Retrieval

The acetabular component is shown in Fig. 8.23. Minimal bone loss was achieved when removing the acetabular shell.

See Fig. 8.24 for metal femoral head component.

Corrosion and metal deposition could be seen at the head–neck joint in a microscopic view, as shown in Fig. 8.25.

8.3.7 Conclusion and Reflection

1. Patients with the MOM-bearing surface may develop pain, especially within 3–5 years after the operation. In addition to pain, such patients may experience hip weakness and lower extremity edema. A small number of patients could develop systemic symptoms (e.g., eczema, hearing loss, and heart failure).

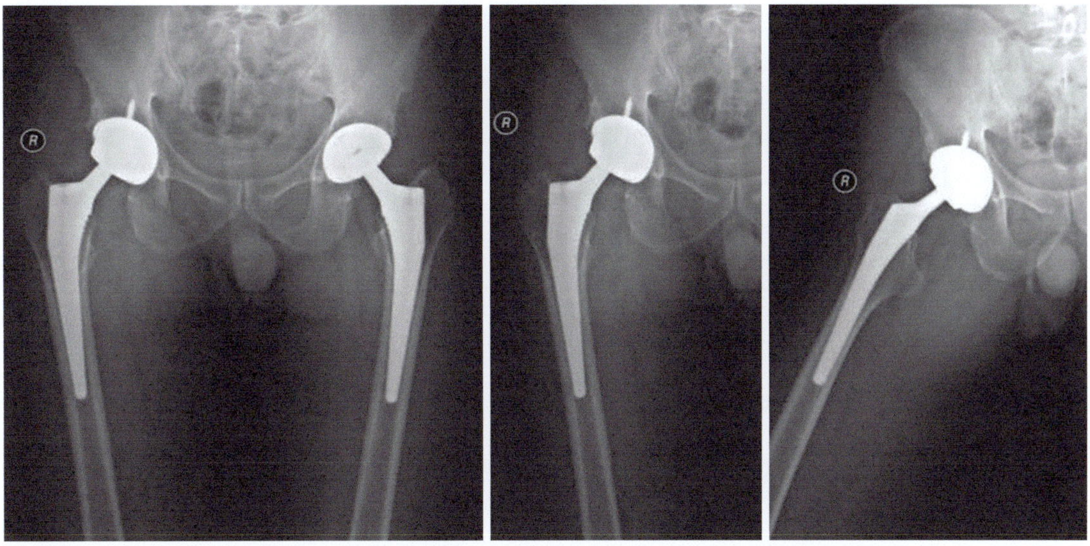

Fig. 8.21 Postoperative radiographs after 3 months

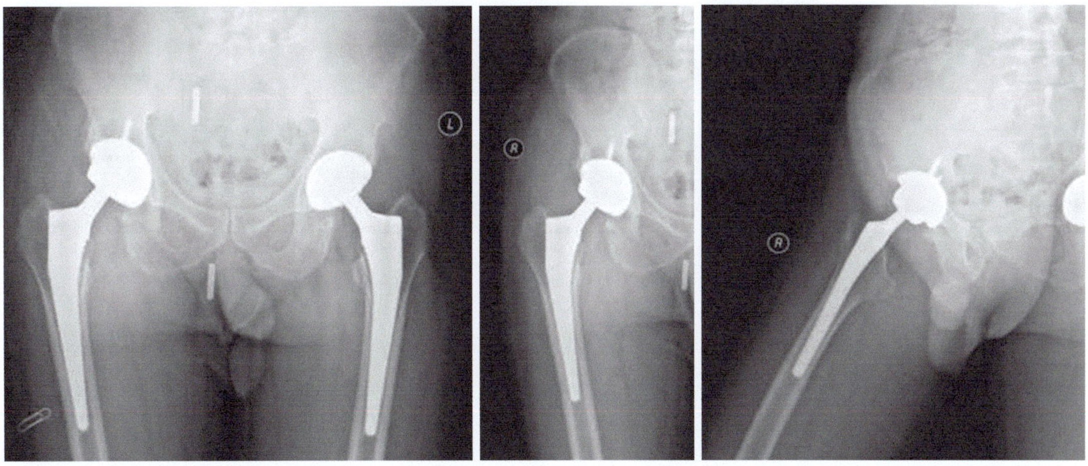

Fig. 8.22 Postoperative radiographs after 6 months

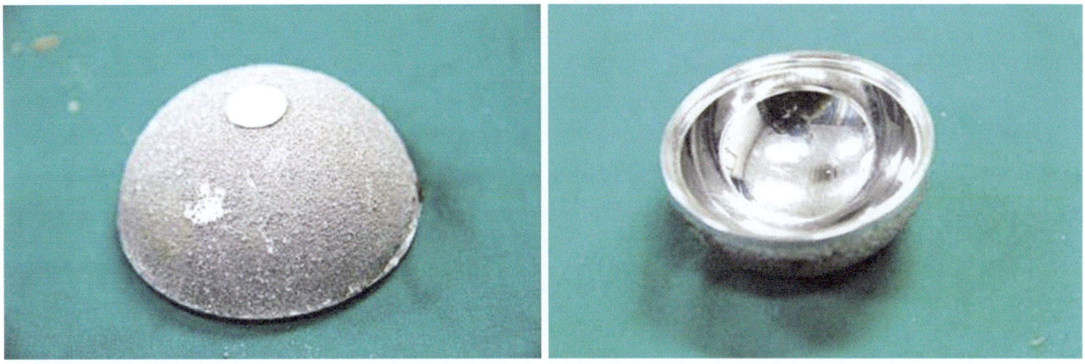

Fig. 8.23 Acetabular component

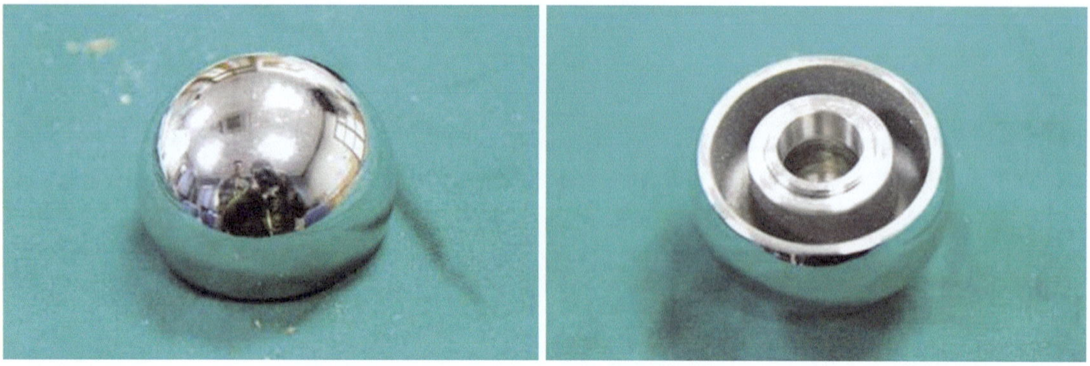

Fig. 8.24 Metal femoral head component

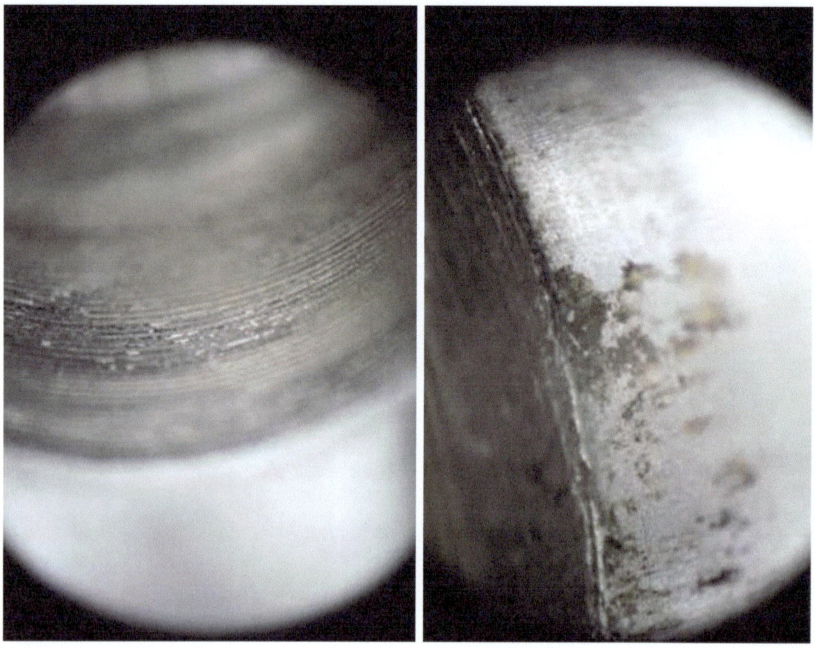

Fig. 8.25 Head–neck joint in microscopic view

2. If no obvious signs of osteolysis and loosening could be found, metal ion-related problems should be taken into consideration. When the patient is symptomatic, preoperative artifact reduction MRI examinations can be considered to detect ALTR surrounding the hip joint, including periprosthetic effusion, pseudotumor, and neuromuscular changes. It could help to determine the diagnosis and area for debridement during surgery. Severe muscle involvement reminds surgeons to prepare for hip instability.
3. By a combination of clinical manifestations and radiographic examination, some clues of metallosis can be found. In some cases, ALTR can be difficult to identify or even coexist with infection. Full preoperative examinations including routine blood test, ESR, and CRP should be performed. In addition, symptoms of fever, skin ulcer, discharge of abscesses, articular swelling, skin redness, and higher skin temperature rise need to be identified. If all the above indicators are normal, then the possibility of infection is minimal. Preoperative diagnosis of metal ion corrosion and ALTR is difficult. Apart from clinical manifestations and radiographic examination (B-ultrasonography, artifact-reducing MRI),

metal ion levels in the blood and synovial fluid are important indicators. Currently, preoperative diagnosis of ALTR should not rely too much on certain individual index; comprehensive evaluation is required.

4. The following aspects should be considered for MoM patients with hip pain:
   (a) If a lucent line around the acetabulum is visible without spot welding, cup loosening should be considered.
   (b) When using a larger femoral head, impingement may occur between the edges of the acetabulum, femoral neck, and the surrounding soft tissue, which can cause irritation.
   (c) Abrasion does not necessarily occur when there is corrosion in MoM, whereas corrosion definitely occurs along with abrasion.
   (d) A larger femoral head comes with greater torque, which may lead to increased motion between mobile parts of the hip and then create motion-associated crevice corrosion. If the stem has a modular neck component, it will also impact the above points.
5. How to distinguish pain caused by soft tissue irritation from that caused by cup loosening?

   If the pain is caused by soft tissue impingement, it may be related to extreme hip movement, such as hyperextension of the hip, Patrick's test, or internal and external rotation during hyperextension.

   If the pain is caused by cup loosening, the patient may experience first-step pain and pain related to standing up from a chair.
6. How to distinguish bearing surface abrasion and corrosion between the stem cone and femoral head?

   It is mainly dependent on ion concentration monitoring. If Cr and Co are disproportionately increased, stem cone corrosion should be considered. If the concentration ratio of Cr and Co is close to 1, it is mainly considered as bearing surface abrasion.

8.4 Case 3

Hanlong Zheng, Jianming Gu, and Yixin Zhou

8.4.1 Case Summary

Medical History Female, 75 years old, complained of "left hip pain for 6 years." The patient had left hip THA more than 20 years ago for ischemic necrosis of the femoral head. She was pain-free after the THA. Six years ago, left groin soreness recurred. The pain aggravated in recent years, she could hardly walk when attending to the hospital. Periprosthetic osteolysis (left) was considered after a physical exam and radiological exam. She had a past medical history of over 20 years of hypertension and over 10 years of Parkinson's disease. She had a left shoulder dislocation and left humeral fracture treated conservatively more than 1 year ago.

Physical Examination Previous posterolateral incision cicatrix healed well without hip redness; left groin tenderness (+); axial percussion pain (−); Patrick's sign (+) on the left; Trendelenburg's sign on the left (+); and Allis's sign (−). A mass was felt in the front of the left thigh without a clear boundary with mild tenderness. Left buttock atrophy.

Laboratory Examination Routine blood test: WBC 6.33×10^9/L, N 75%, eosinophilic WBC percentage 0.8%; CRP 2.4 mg/L; ESR 19 mm/h. Serum metal ion level: preoperative serum Cr was 0.23 ng/mL; Co was 6.69 ng/mL.

Radiographic Data Preoperative X-rays are shown in Fig. 8.26.

MRI plain scan of the left hip after THA; hip joint effusion and synovial hyperplasia in the left hip, multiple hyposignal structures surrounding the prosthesis and bone; and soft tissue edema around the left hip. Cyst in sacral nerve root sleeve. Hyperplasia at the margin of the right

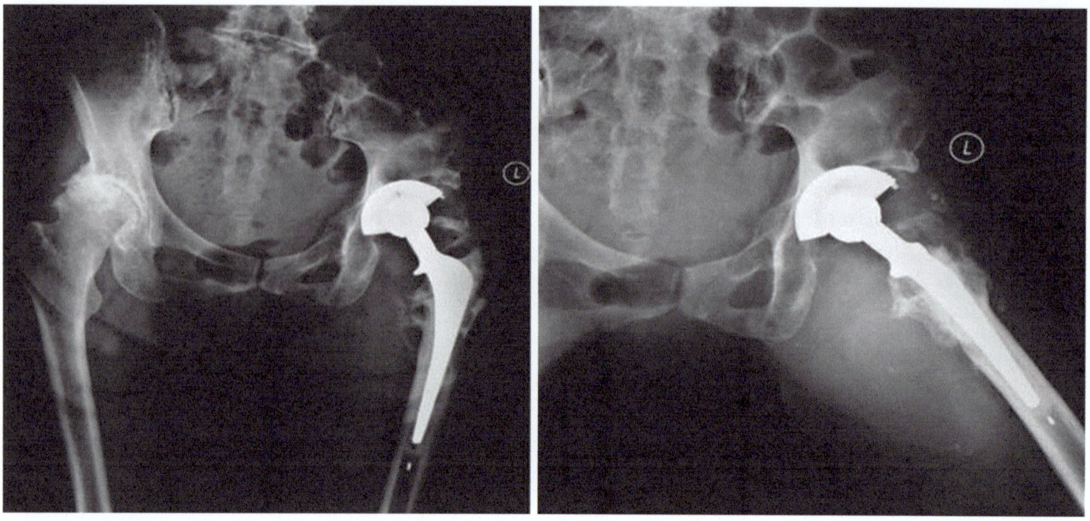

Fig. 8.26 Preoperative X-rays

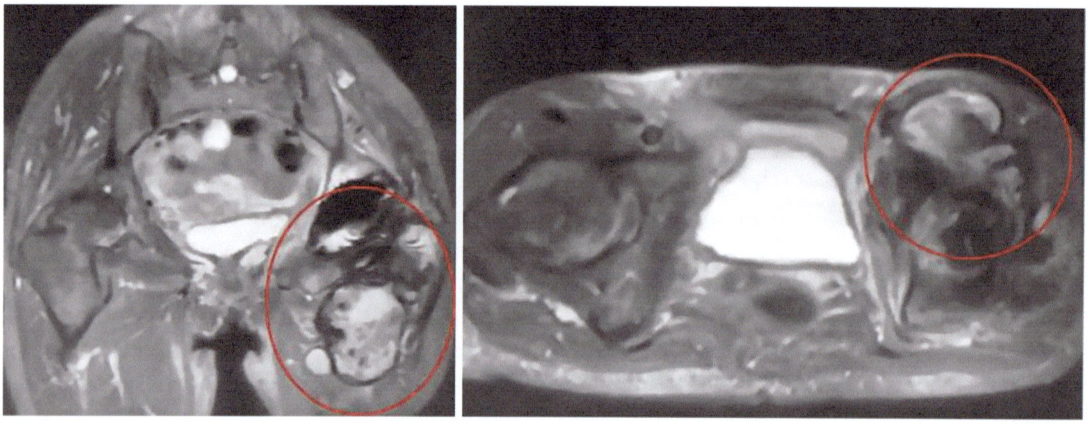

Fig. 8.27 MRI plain scan of the left hip

acetabulum, multiple cysts in the right femoral head and acetabular cartilage, and ischemic necrosis of the right femoral head. MRI plain scan of the left hip is shown in Fig. 8.27.

8.4.2 Preoperative Planning

1. Radiography Illustration: Massive osteolysis was seen in the iliac, ischium, and pubis on the acetabular side, and there was a sign of a previous fracture at the pubic ramus, massive perifemoral osteolysis, and signs of previous trochanteric fracture. No obvious eccentric wear was found in the PE liner. The signs above alerted the surgeons: Why was there massive osteolysis without obvious eccentric wear on X-ray?

   Further analysis combined with clinical manifestations showed that the systemic condition of this patient was poor. She could hardly walk when attending to the hospital. She had renal function damage in the past 2 years. Physical examination and MR revealed a cystic mass around the hip. In combination with the clinical data together, we tested the serum metal ion concentration for this patient and found that the level of cobalt and chromium ions was disproportionately increased.

The treatment strategy: She was senile with a poor general condition and many comorbidities, and the surgical risk was high. The femoral and acetabular components were not significantly loosened. The decision of revision should be carefully made. However, the patient presented with obvious pain, limited mobility, lump in the thigh, severe radiographic osteolysis, and fractures. Without revision, periprosthetic fracture, aseptic loosening, or periprosthetic infection could occur making the treatment more difficult. Inflammatory pseudotumor masses might lead to further impairment of nerve function. Due to the fracture of the greater trochanter and ionotoxic damage to the gluteus muscle, the risk of hip dislocation could increase over time.

In conclusion, the authors decided to perform revision THA for this patient. How to achieve solid fixation with massive bone defects in the superior acetabular, pubic ramus, and ischial ramus? The author planned to use lotus augment at the pubic ramus and ischium separately and a halved buttress augment filling the superior iliac area. Cement was used to link the augments with the hemispherical TM cup. The femoral component was removed by the "hammer-in, hammer-out" strategy. After the stem was retrieved, the Exeter stem could be implanted with the cement-in-cement technique. Cables were used around the trochanteric area preventing fractures. A 40-mm femoral head was placed to increase the jump distance and prevent dislocation following THA.

8.4.3 Surgical Procedure and Intraoperative Observation

Revision THA + inflammatory pseudotumor resection (Continuum + 3 Augment + EXETER, MoP) was performed.

A modified posterolateral Gibson approach along the previous scar was adopted. A cystic mass of 4 cm × 6 cm was found in the deep layer of the gluteus maximus. Dark red fluid was found in it, as shown in Fig. 8.28.

The mass was removed using extracapsular resection technique, and then the implant was exposed. Dark red, paste-like periprosthetic tissue was observed. Debridement was performed for these necrotic and periprosthetic osteolysis tissue. The stem was subsequently removed, as shown in Fig. 8.29.

When the cup was taken out, the bone tissue left was osteoporotic and paste-like. These unhealthy

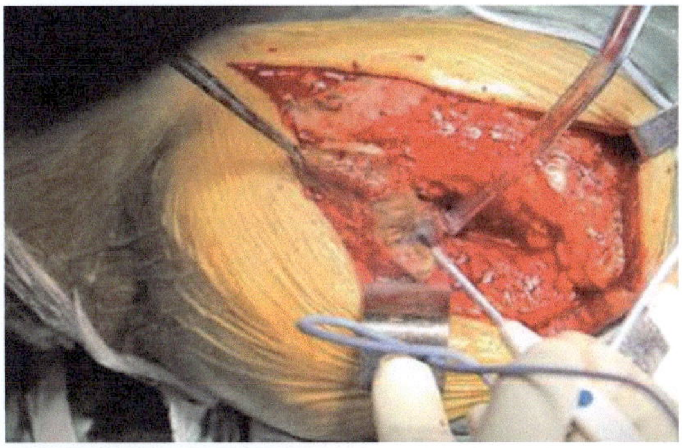

Fig. 8.28 Cystic mass in the deep layer of the left gluteus maximus

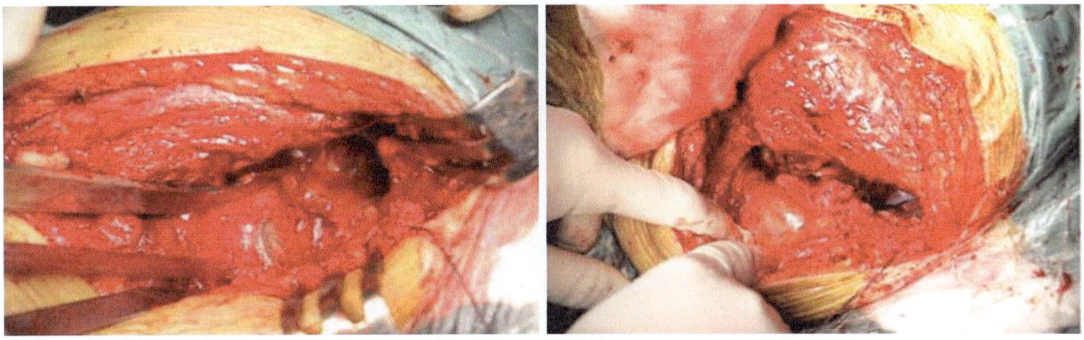

Fig. 8.29 Dark red, paste-like periprosthetic tissue

tissue were curetted till bleeding bone surface. The resected tissue and implants are shown in Fig. 8.30.

Three augments were implanted into healthy bone, and an acetabular reamer was used from small to large to widen the acetabulum. A 62-mm non-cement continuum cup was implanted with a good press fit, and six screws were applied for further fixation. The Exter femoral stem was implanted in cement.

8.4.4 Postoperative Condition and Outcome

The postoperative immediate X-rays are shown in Fig. 8.31.

Postoperative X-rays at 6 months are shown in Fig. 8.32.

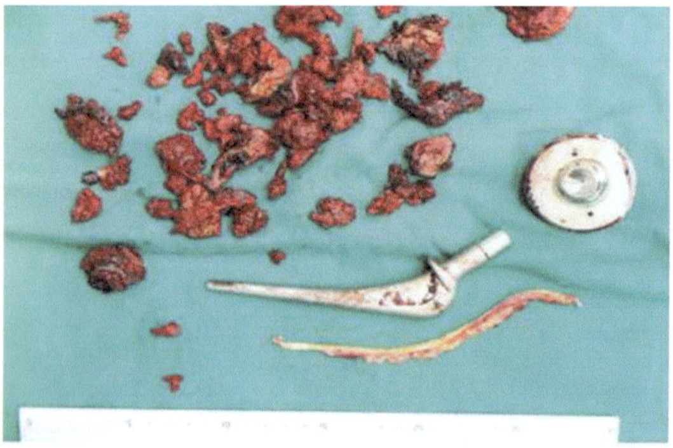

Fig. 8.30 The resected tissue and implants

After 3 months, the Cr was 0.52 ng/mL and Co was 1.19 ng/mL.

8.4.5 Conclusion and Reflection

The patient presented with poor systemic conditions and various comorbidity. After the revision, she had a significant improvement in general condition, walking ability, and hip mobility.

1. How was metallosis corrosion diagnosed in this case?

   In terms of pathogenesis, osteoclast is the cause of radiographic bone resorption. The reasons for the activation of osteoclast could be: (1) bone and joint infection; (2) bone tumor; (3) osteolysis caused by polyethylene particles; and (4) metallosis corrosion. Malignant tumors were excluded by clinical and radiological exams after consulting the oncology department. Infection risk was minimal based on symptoms and serological manifestations. Osteolysis due to PE particles could be considered in consideration of 20 years of PE wear. However, there was no obvious eccentric wear in the X-rays. Where there was soft tissue mass around the hip, metallosis-related osteolysis should be considered.

Fig. 8.31 Postoperative immediate X-rays

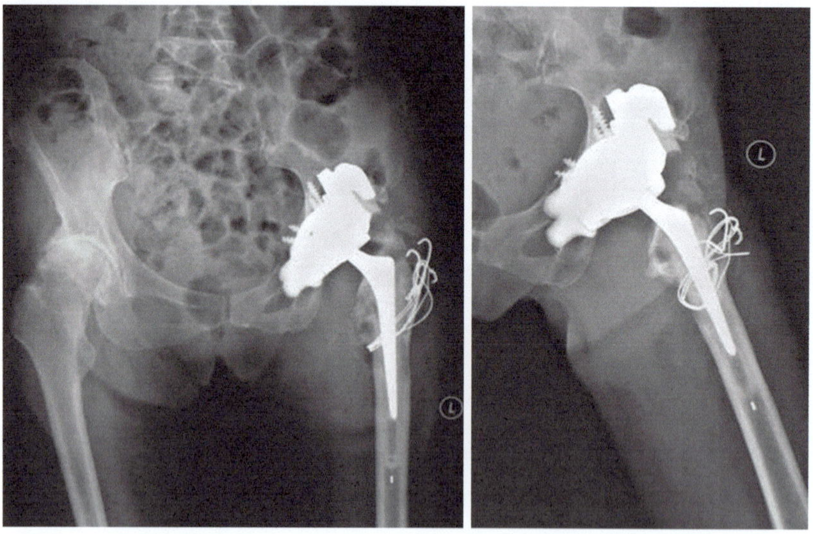

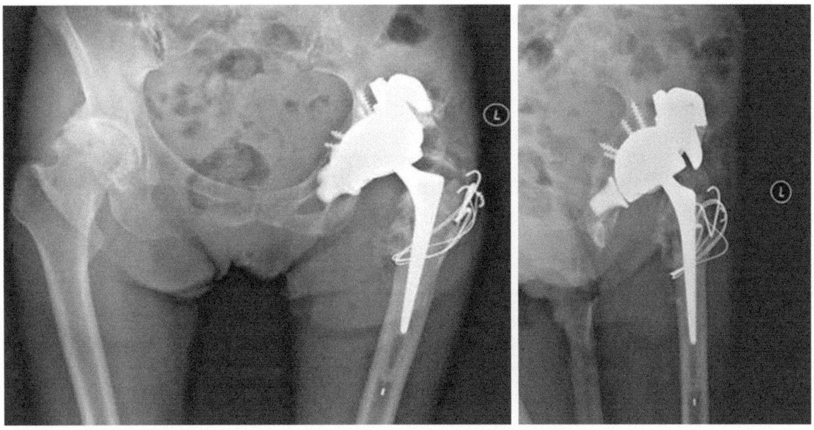

Fig. 8.32 Postoperative X-rays at 6 months

2. Where was the source of the elevated serum concentration of metal ions?

   The following four components typically cause the increase in metal ion concentration following hip surgery: cup, liner, head, and stem. The femoral head and stem were COCrMo. There were no signs of loosening of the femoral stem. When chemical causes were involved, electrochemical etching occurred between the femoral head and the stem cone, and the concentration of cobalt and chromium ions would non-equally increase. The metal release source was considered in the head–stem junction.
3. Was it necessary to debride the intramuscular soft tissue pseudotumor in the proximal femur? How to operate?

   The inflammatory pseudotumor should be removed to decrease the tissue reaction in metallosis. However, the surgeons should avoid overzealous debridement. Complete resection is not required as in periprosthetic infection. Otherwise, over-resection may result in excessive soft tissue damage, subsequently dislocation following THA.
4. Why was the buttress augment "halved" during the operation?

   The superoposterior acetabulum had severe bone loss and was unsupported. It was a large cavity defect, the buttress augment was too large to be put in. It was cut into half. We suggest manufacturers to provide shorter augments so that more complex acetabular defects can be easily treated.
5. Radiographs of the patient showed severe bone damage. How to distinguish it from osteolysis caused by polyethylene particles?

   In this case, the reader may ask: Although the acetabular liner did not show obvious eccentric wear, why can't the osteolysis be caused by polyethylene? According to the clinical experience of the surgeons, metallosis corrosion can cause osteolysis indeed, especially for the MoM interface, it can occur even without polyethylene particles. In terms of radiography, there is no specific difference between the two, as the nature of bone damage is that metal ions or polyethylene particles stimulate cytokines, and further stimulate osteoclasts.

   However, there are still slight differences between the two in X-ray: The fluidity of the lesions in polyethylene-related osteolysis is poor. It will slowly expand in joint space, like the appearance of benign tumors, the area is limited. Osteolysis resulting from metallosis corrosion is often associated with inflammatory pseudotumor. As the metal ion easily goes into fluid, the range of osteolysis is large. In this case, osteolysis spread to the middle and upper femur. However, if the metal ion corrosion is minimal or the tissue reaction is mild, osteolysis is confined to the local releasing area, and it will be difficult to distinguish the osteolysis from that caused by polyethylene particles.

Recommended Reading

1. Semlitsch M, Willert HG. Implant materials for hip endoprostheses: old proofs and new trends. Arch Orthop Trauma Surg. 1995;114(2):61–7.
2. Kocagoz SB, Underwood RJ, Macdonald DW, et al. Ceramic heads decrease metal release caused by headtaper fretting and corrosion. Clin Orthop Relat Res. 2016;474(4):985–94.
3. Kwon YM, MacAuliffe J, Arauz PG, et al. Sensitivity and specificity of metallon level in predicting adverse local tissue reactions due to head-neck taper corrosion in primary metal-on-polyethylene total hip arthroplasty. J Arthroplasty. 2018;33(9):3025–9.
4. Mistry JB, Chughtai M, Elmallah RK, et al. Trunnionosis in total hip arthroplasty: a review. J Orthop Traumatol. 2016;17(1):1–6.
5. Liao Y, Hoffman E, Wimmer M, et al. CoCrMo metal-on-metal hip replacements. Phys Chem Chem Phys. 2013;15(3):746–56.
6. Bijukumar DR, Segu A, Souza JCM, et al. Systemic and local toxicity of metal debris released from hip prostheses: a review of experimental approaches. Nanomedicine. 2018;14(3):951–63.
7. Cheung AC, Banerjee S, Cherian JJ, et al. Systemic cobalt toxicity from total hip arthroplasties: review of a rare condition. Part 1—history, mechanism, measurements, and pathophysiology. Bone Joint J. 2016;98-B(1):6–13.
8. Zywiel MG, Cherian JJ, Banerjee S, et al. Systemic cobalt toxicity from total hip arthroplasties: review of a rare condition. Part 2. Measurement, risk factors, and step-wise approach to treatment. Bone Joint J. 2016;98-B(1):14–20.
9. Liow MHL, Kwon YM. Metal-on-metal total hip arthroplasty: risk factors for pseudotumours and clinical systematic evaluation. Int Orthop. 2017;41(5):885–92.
10. Alimonti A, Bocca B, Mannella E, et al. Assessment of reference values for selected elements in a healthy urban population. Ann first Super Sanita. 2005;41(2):181–7.
11. Sanz Perez MI, Rico Villoras AM, Moreno Velasco A, et al. Heart transplant secondary to cobalt toxicity after hip arthroplasty revision. Hip Int. 2019;29(4):Npl–5.
12. Bradberry SM, Wilkinson JM, Ferner RE. Systemic toxicity related to metal hip prostheses. Clin Toxicol (Phila). 2014;52(8):837–47.
13. De Haan R, Pattyn C, Gill HS, et al. Correlation between inclination of the acetabular component and metal ion levels in metal-on-metal hip resurfacing replacement. J Bone Joint Surg Br. 2008;90(10):1291–7.
14. Crawford DA, Adams JB, Morris MJ, et al. Revision of failed metal-on-metal total hip arthroplasty: midterm outcomes of 203 consecutive cases. J Arthroplasty. 2019;34(8):1755–60.
15. Lainiala OS, Reito AP, Nieminen JJ, et al. Declining revision burden of metal-on-metal hip arthroplasties. J Arthroplasty. 2019;34(9):2058–2064.e2051.
16. Dahlstrand H, Stark A, Anissian L, et al. Elevated serum concentrations of cobalt, chromium, nickel, and manganese after metal-on-metal alloarthroplasty of the hip: a prospective randomized study. J Arthroplasty. 2009;24(6):837–45.
17. White PB, Meftah M, Ranawat AS, et al. A comparison of blood metal ions in total hip arthroplasty using metal and ceramic heads. J Arthroplasty. 2016;31(10):2215–20.
18. Mali S. Mechanically assisted crevice corrosion in metallic biomaterials: a review. Mater Technol. 2016;31:1–9.
19. Tan SC, Teeter MG, Del Balso C, et al. Effect of taper design on trunnionosis in metal on polyethylene total hip arthroplasty. J Arthroplasty. 2015;30(7):1269–72.
20. Triantafyllopoulos GK, Elpers ME, Burket JC, et al. Otto Aufranc Award: large heads do not increase damage at the head-neck taper of metal-on-poly ethylene total hip arthroplasties. Clin Orthop Relat Res. 2016;474(2):330–8.
21. Bansal T, Aggarwal S, Dhillon MS, et al. Gross trunnion failure in metal on polyethylene total hip arthroplasty-a systematic review of literature. Int Orthop. 2020;44(4):609–21.
22. Inoue D, Restrepo C, Nourie B, et al. Clinical results of revision hip arthroplasty for neck-taper corrosion and adverse local tissue reactions around a modular neck stem. J Arthroplasty. 2020;35(6S):S289–93.
23. Wight CM, Lanting B, Schemitsch EH. Evidence based recommendations for reducing head-neck taper connection fretting corrosion in hip replacement prostheses. Hip Int. 2017;27(6):523–31.
24. Kwon YM, Della Valle CJ, Lombardi AV, et al. Risk stratification algorithm for management of head-neck taper tribocorrosion in patients with metal-on-poly ethylene total hip arthroplasty: consensus statement of the American Association of Hip and Knee Surgeons, the American Academy of Orthopaedic Surgeons, and The Hip Society. J Bone Joint Surg Am. 2021;103(5):el8.

9 Ceramic Liner Fracture

Xinghua Yin and Hongyi Shao

9.1 Introduction

Xinghua Yin

The fracture of ceramic parts of hip arthroplasty is one of the serious complications of total hip arthroplasty (THA). The ceramic fragments can not only cause local symptoms but also lead to severe abrasion of metal components, which results in increased serum ion concentration and serious systemic complications such as lower extremity edema, renal dysfunction, and cardiac failure.

In the twenty-first century, Biolox Forte (the third generation of ceramics) and Biolox Delta (the fourth generation of ceramics) have been widely applied in THA. According to the data from the National Joint Registry of the United Kingdom, the fourth-generation ceramics significantly reduced the fracture rate of the femoral head compared to the third-generation ceramics (0.009% vs. 0.119%), but it did not decrease the fracture rate of the liner (0.126% vs. 0.112%).

There are many factors that may be related to ceramic fracture. In general, these factors can be divided into material factors, mechanical factors of prosthesis design, and operation-related factors. Material factors are related to the composition of the ceramics. For example, Biolox Delta contains 17% zirconia, which significantly increases the strength of the alumina ceramics. On top of this, the small plate structure formed by strontium oxide helps to absorb stress, further increasing the strength of the Biolox Delta. More recently, innovative cartilage with higher strength (such as silicon nitride) has paved the way in THA. The design of ceramic components, such as the size and length of the femoral head, thickness of the ceramic liner, and cone lock design, affects the fracture probability when causing different degrees of stress riser. In general, ball heads with a small diameter (e.g., 28 mm femoral head), lengthened or shortened femoral heads, and thinner ceramic liners are relatively easy to fracture. Surgical factors are also directly associated with ceramic component fracture. According to our data, the fracture of the Biolox Delta ceramic liner is often related to the imperfect positioning of the ceramic liner in the metal cup.

The preoperative diagnosis of ceramic fracture mainly relies on radiographic examination. The fracture mainly presents as dense shadows with sharp edges in the X-ray. The density is even or much higher than that of cortical bone, and its location and distribution are highly unpredictable. After the diagnosis of ceramic fracture is confirmed, the possible causes of it should be taken into consideration in the meantime. In addition, the abrasion between the ceramic head and the metal cup after ceramic fracture increases the toxicity of metal ions on the tissue, which

X. Yin (✉) · H. Shao
Department of Adult Joint Reconstructive Surgery, Beijing Jishuitan Hospital, Capital Medical University, Beijing, China

Y. Zhou (ed.), *Revision Total Hip Arthroplasty*, https://doi.org/10.1007/978-981-97-9804-9_9

reduces the anti-infection capability of the tissue and leads to a higher risk of co-infection. Approximately half of patients with high metal ions present with elevated ESR and C-reactive protein. In consequence, an articular cavity aspiration test to exclude infection before ceramic fracture revision is still crucial.

In revision cases of ceramic fracture, residual debris often poses great abrasion risk to the implanted femoral head and liner. Therefore, complete synovium resection is necessary to thoroughly remove all residual debris and particles. Apart from the selection of the articular surface, the treatment of the acetabulum and femoral stem should also be considered. When determining the exchange or retention of the metal cup, possible damage caused by the fragmented ceramic liner should be considered. If the locking mechanism between the metal cup and the ceramic liner is compromised, metal cup retention may increase the risk of future revision. Meanwhile, if the location and angle of the metal cup are inappropriate, it should be replaced and repositioned to prevent future ceramic liner fracture. Retention of the femoral stem should be considered if the stem is well fixed, its cone is not damaged and can be well fastened with the head, and the soft tissue tension can be restored. Otherwise, revision of the femoral stem should be performed to re-establish articular function and ensure better long-term outcomes. If periprosthetic infection is present, subsequent treatment should be followed.

Postoperative long-term prosthesis survival in patients who underwent ceramic fracture revision was relatively poor in earlier studies. Allain et al. published their results of follow-up for revision ceramic head fracture, indicating that the main risk factors for failure were unrevised cup, applying metal femoral head, incomplete synovium resection, and patients under 50 years old. In this study, postoperative dislocation occurred in 8 patients (7.6%). Some studies have reported dislocation rates following THA as high as 33%. The reason for the dislocation is possibly that the debris produced by friction between the metal and ceramic components compromises the soft tissues (articular capsule, glutcus mcdius, ctc.) which maintain the stability of the hip. Meanwhile, excessive intraoperative debridement and exposure may also lead to hip instability. Several factors such as large cup-head difference, inappropriate cup position, or failure to correct the femoral stem angle may also increase the risk of dislocation following THA. Dislocation can be prevented to a certain degree by moving the cup downward (to the location of the original acetabulum) or outward (to improve soft tissue tension), adjusting the angle of the cup, applying dual-mobility articulations, and so on. Good postoperative management is an important part of preventing dislocation and should be highly valued.

Overall, although ceramic fracture is one of the relatively rare postoperative complications of THA and not complicated to diagnose, only by selecting the appropriate bearing surface materials, identifying the causes, and correcting and improving them by revision can ensure good long-term outcomes of revision THA in ceramic fracture patients.

9.2 Case 1

Xinghua Yin and Hongyi Shao

9.2.1 Case Summary

Medical History A 68-year-old female patient presented with "right hip pain accompanied by abnormal sound for 1 month after THA which she received for more than 1 year." The patient underwent right THA in another hospital due to a femoral neck fracture 15 months ago. She was mobilized on the postoperative day 3, was discharged on the fifth day postoperatively, and began rehabilitation. One month ago, sudden pain occurred in the right hip, accompanied by abnormal sound, and slightly limited range of motion (ROM). She rested at home. Three weeks ago, an X-ray examination was performed in another hospital. She was diagnosed with "prosthesis fracture." She came to our hospital for further treatment.

Physical Examination The patient was pushed into thc ward on gurncy; an incision scar was seen in the right hip; no redness or swelling; tenderness (+) in the inguinal region of the right hip; axial percussion pain (+); abductor strength of the right hip was normal; slightly limited ROM in the right hip; and flexion/extension of the right hip was 0–90°.

Laboratory Tests No abnormality detected in complete blood count, erythrocyte sedimentation rate (ESR), or C-reactive protein (CRP).

Imaging Preoperative radiographs are shown in Fig. 9.1.

9.2.2 Case Analysis

1. Infection was basically excluded according to the comprehensive preoperative examination.
2. X-ray films revealed that:
   (a) After right THA, the rotation center and abduction of the cup were acceptable, and the position of the femoral stem was appropriate.
   (b) Dense shadows with sharp edges can be detected around the head and neck junction of the right hip component, with a density far greater than that of the bone cortex.
3. Diagnosis: ceramic liner fracture after right THA.

9.2.3 Preoperative Planning

1. The diagnosis of ceramic liner fracture was confirmed and infection was basically excluded.
2. It was planned to retrieve the broken ceramic liner and debris, retrieve the metal cup, reconstruct the acetabulum, and place a new metal cup and its ceramic liner.
3. After the femoral head component was retrieved, the original femoral stem would be retained and a new ceramic head would be implanted, provided that there was no obvious corrosion or damage in the taper area, the stem was stably combined with the femur, and the anteversion was appropriate.

9.2.4 Intraoperative Findings

1. After exposure through the previous surgical incision, the ceramic liner fracture and scattered ceramic fragments around the acetabulum were observed, some of which revealed sand-like, and some were embedded in soft tissue, as shown in Fig. 9.2.
2. After the ceramic liner was retrieved, the abrasion of the metal cup and black stained tissue around it could be seen, as shown in Fig. 9.3. Excess scar tissue around the ace-

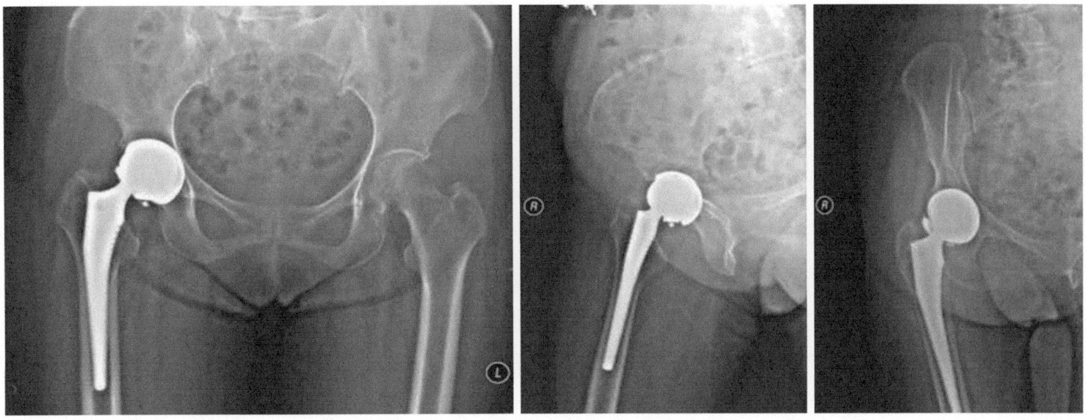

Fig. 9.1 Preoperative radiographs

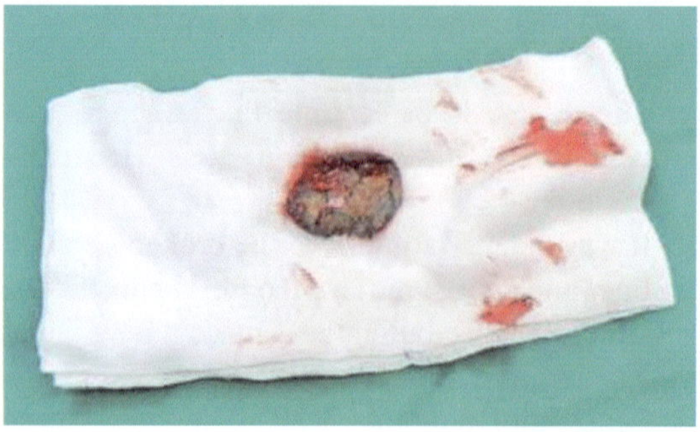

Fig. 9.2 Broken ceramic liner

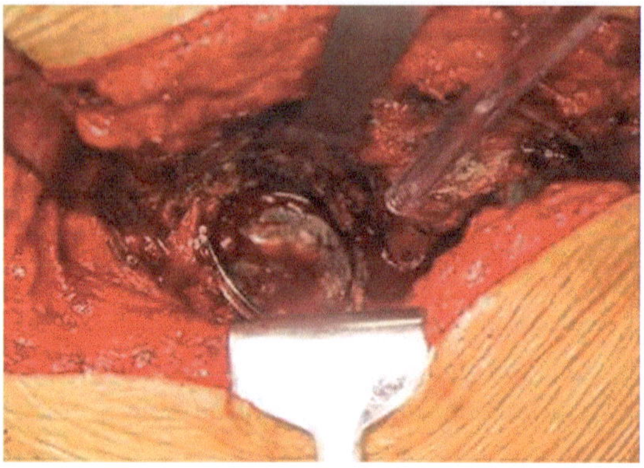

Fig. 9.3 Black stained tissue

tabulum was resected, then the acetabular component was retrieved, the osseous acetabulum was refreshed and reamed, and a new metal cup and ceramic liner were implanted.

3. Fibrous scar tissue and some osseous tissue in the proximal femur were resected. It could be seen that the femoral stem was stable, its taper area was in good condition, and thus the stem was reserved. The ceramic head was replaced with a new one.

9.2.5 Postoperative Rehabilitation and Outcome

1. The patient was encouraged to get off the bed, walk with crutches, and perform rehabilitation exercises.
2. The postoperative immediate antero-posterior (AP) view is shown in Fig. 9.4.

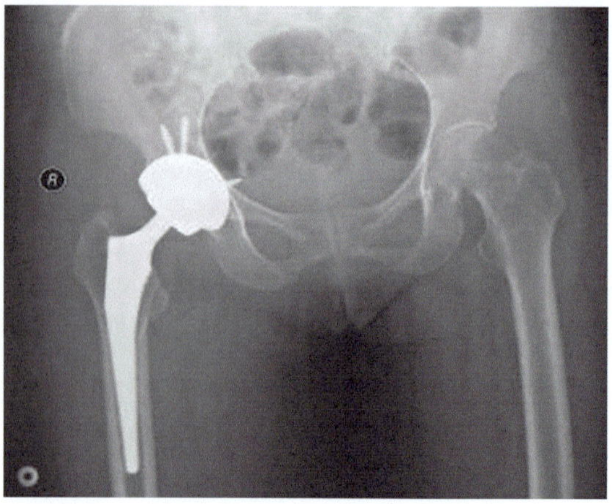

Fig. 9.4 Postoperative immediate AP view

9.2.6 Conclusion and Reflection

1. How to diagnose the ceramic fracture?

   When the ceramic fracture occurs, it accelerates the abrasion of the metal, like a scrub. In some ceramic fracture cases, the fracture can be insidious and may not be visible in X-ray. However, some of them may present with abnormal sounds and further computed tomography (CT) scans can be performed to confirm the ceramic fracture. Meanwhile, a serum ion concentration examination can also be performed to support the diagnosis. From the perspective of ceramic materials, compared with third-generation ceramics (FORTE), the density of fourth-generation ceramics (DELTA) is significantly higher. Thus, the high-density periprosthetic shadow can be seen in X-ray if the fourth-generation ceramic fracture occurs (as in this case).

   In addition, after the introduction of fourth-generation ceramics (DELTA), the fracture rate of the ceramic head decreased significantly, whereas the fracture rate of the ceramic liner did not. This provides a reference for the diagnosis of ceramic fracture.
2. How to minimize the occurrence of ceramic fracture?
   (a) About the liner: After reaming the acetabulum, if a thin ceramic liner and its metal cup are determined, proper over-reaming of the acetabulum can be further per-

formed to increase the diameter of the outer cup and to increase the liner thickness in the setting of the same diameter of the femoral head. However, it should be noted that in some commercially available hip systems, as the cup diameter increases, the thickness of the metal cup increases with the thickness of the ceramic liner remaining unchanged in the setting of the same femoral head diameter. Therefore, preoperative awareness of the components employed for the surgery is required.

After placing the ceramic liner, make sure with your fingers the feeling of "lined up" with the edge of the cup. It should not be rushed to knock the ceramic liner in until the ceramic is appropriately "lined up."

(b) About the ceramic head: When an extremely lengthened or shortened head is expected to be employed during operation, other methods should be used to best align the femoral head length to the standard one. Because lengthened or shortened head is easier to concentrate stress in the cone region, making it easier to fracture.

3. What is the cause of the ceramic liner fracture in this case?

   In postoperative immediate radiographs, it could be seen that the ceramic liner did not "sit" well into the metal cup (see Fig. 9.5, the edge of the ceramic liner did not line up with the metal cup). It is worth mentioning that the impingement between the ceramic liner and the femoral neck is a very important cause of fracture.

4. In revision surgery of ceramic liner fracture, is it possible to only replace ceramic liner?

   Generally, the fractured ceramic liner damages the metal cup as well. If the locking mechanism of the metal cup and ceramic liner is damaged, it is easy to cause problems if the metal cup is not replaced. Also, there is usually a cause for ceramic liner fracture, such as the positioning of the cup, in which case the metal cup needs to be replaced to improve the rotation center and angle. Finally, merely replacing the bearing surface cannot eliminate the influence of fracture on soft tissue, and it may lead to hip instability.

5. How to select the bearing surface if there are lots of fragments (metal or ceramic, etc.) in the joint during revision? Ceramic on ceramic, ceramic on polyethylene, or metal on polyethylene?

   As the third body, metal or ceramic fragments in the joint will increase the abrasion of the bearing surface. As a result, wear-resistant materials should be applied as much as possible, ceramic on ceramic being preferred. If the ceramic-on-ceramic coupling cannot be applied due to other considerations or constraints, then ceramic on polyethylene can be considered. Metal on polyethylene should never be used (including metal heads with zirconia surface on polyethylene). When a ceramic on polyethylene coupling is applied, fragmented ceramics can be pushed into the polyethylene, resulting in no catastrophic problem. But with a metal head, once the fragments wear out the bearing ceramic surface and expose the rough metal, abrasion will increase rapidly.

9.3 Case 2

Xinghua Yin and Hongyi Shao

9.3.1 Case Summary

Medical History A 61-year-old male patient presented with "right hip pain, limited mobility and repeated dislocation after THA for 6 years." The patient suffered a right acetabular fracture in a car accident and received open reduction and internal fixation in another hospital 16 years ago. Six years ago, he received THA for the right hip in another hospital for avascular necrosis of the femoral head. Pain and limited mobility of the right hip were not obviously improved after THA, and recurrent dislocation began to occur.

Fig. 9.5 Postoperative immediate radiographs

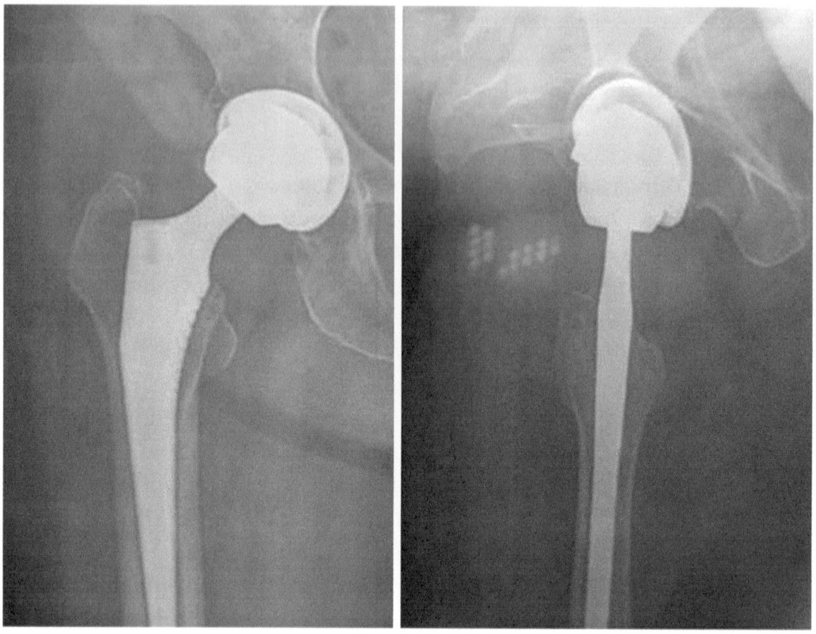

Physical Examination He presented with claudication and was on crutches; no pelvic tilt; no deformity in the right hip; no redness or swelling; right greater trochanter tenderness (+); axial percussion pain (−); mildly limited range of motion; rightside Patrick's sign (+); rightside Thomas test (+); rightside Trendelenburg sign (+); no edema or hypoesthesia in lower extremity; and pulses of bilateral dorsalis pedis arteries were palpable.

Laboratory Tests Blood tests: ESR 48 mm/h, CRP: 34.5 mg/L; WBC: 5.60×10^9/L; Neutrophil %: 59.5%.

Imaging The preoperative AP view of both hips is shown in Fig. 9.6. A preoperative hip CT examination is presented in Fig. 9.7.

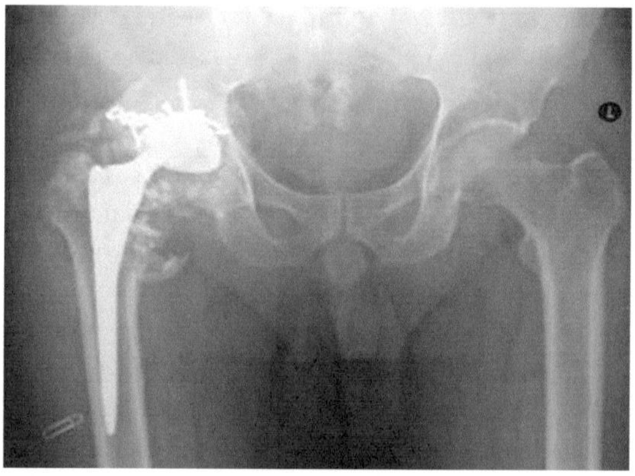

Fig. 9.6 Preoperative AP X-ray of bilateral hip joints

Hip Aspiration Test

1. Aspiration fluid routine: turbid fluid with blood, white blood cell count: 2624/mm3, leukocyte mononuclear ratio: 8%, multinuclear leukocyte ratio: 92%. Characterized by the Rivalta test.
2. Aspiration fluid culture: no bacterial (aerobic or anaerobic) or fungal growth for 5 days.
3. Aspiration fluid biopsy: collagen-rich fibrocystic parietal tissue in the right hip joint. Crushed collagen fibers with numerous pigmentations around the hip prosthesis. The biopsy pathological section is shown in Fig. 9.8.

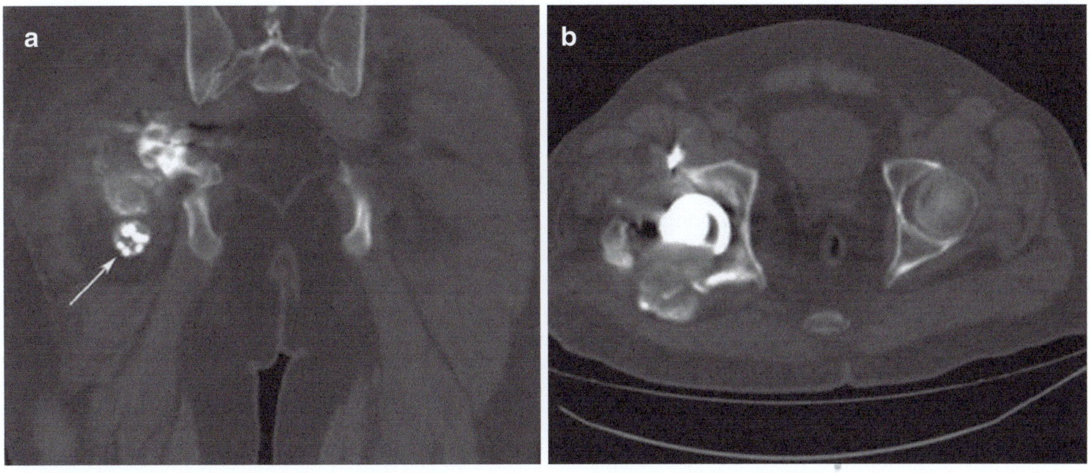

Fig. 9.7 Preoperative hip CT examination. (**a**) In the coronal plane, scattered high-density shadows can be seen where the arrow points, which are surrounded by soft tissue shadows. (**b**) In the transverse plane, the head directly contacted with the metal cup, and the cup was tilted backward

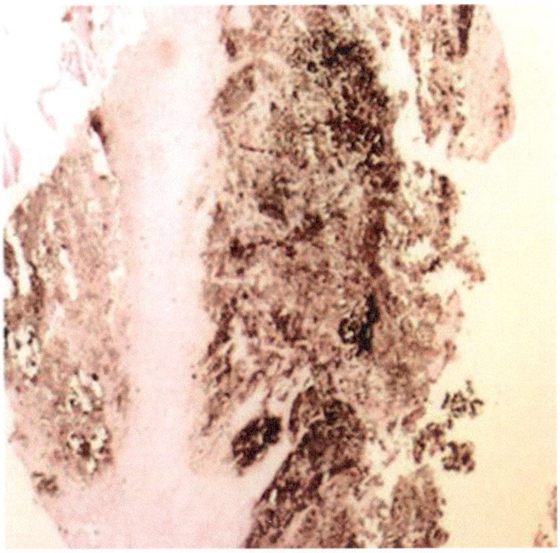

Fig. 9.8 Biopsy pathological sections

9.3.2 Case Analysis

1. Although the positioning and angle of the prosthesis in this patient are not perfect, the possibility of infection should be considered when problems occur within a few years after THA, combined with laboratory examination and aspiration test results.
2. The multiple soft tissue dense shadows scattered around the acetabulum were originally considered to be heterotopic ossification (HO) as the patient underwent internal fixation after the acetabular fracture and subsequent THA. However, CT showed that the femoral head was in contact with the metal cup, and there was a very high density of particles wrapped with soft tissue around the hip, which were considered to come from the prosthesis.
3. X-rays and CT scans suggested that:
   (a) X-rays showed postoperative changes following right THA. Superior-lateral migration of the rotation center of the femoral head and multiple scattered dense shadows around the hip could be seen.
   (b) CT showed that the granular high-density shadows were surrounded by soft tissue shadow, and the femoral stem was not in the same rotation center as the cup.
4. Diagnosis: ceramic liner fracture of the hip implant, hip instability, and periprosthetic infection not excluded.

9.3.3 Preoperative Planning

As the possibility of infection cannot be excluded, it was planned to conduct a two-stage revision.

9.3.4 Intraoperative Finding

1. The incision was made, and as the subcutaneous tissue and deep tissue were exposed, massive black stained tissue was encountered. The stained tissue and suspicious necrotic tissue were removed, and all components were retrieved. Plenty of black stained tissue was contained in the suction fluid, as shown in Fig. 9.9.
2. The articular surface was exposed, the fractured liner was retrieved, and the metal cup was exposed. It could be seen that the femoral head had completely worn through the metal cup, confirming ceramic fracture, as shown in Fig. 9.10.
3. The spacer was implanted after retrieval of the implants. A postoperative immediate radiograph is shown in Fig. 9.11.

9.3.5 Subsequent Treatment and Outcome After Components Retrieval and Spacer Implanting

A postoperative blood sample was taken and sent for metal ion examination. It was found that the concentration of titanium ions increased, which was caused by metal cup abrasion by the ceramic head after ceramic fracture.

The second-stage revision was conducted 6 weeks later, and the postoperative AP X-ray is shown in Fig. 9.12.

Dislocation occurred within 2 months. Closed reduction was performed in the emergency department, followed by the application of an anti-rotation boot and immobilizing at the overcorrection position for 6 weeks. No further dislocation occurred.

9.3.6 Conclusion and Reflection

1. Is aspiration necessary for patients with hip revision?

   We believe that aspiration should be routinely performed for all hip revision patients, as there is often no clear boundary between infection and no infection. In our clinical practice, some patients with normal ESR and CRP were found to be infected (tuberculosis) according to the postoperative pathology examination. There were also cases without suspicion of infection preoperatively, whereas intraoperative culture revealed positive, suggesting common strains of periprosthetic infection. In the meantime, some patients have susceptibility factors such as metal corrosion. It is due to the toxicity of metal ions on the tissue, which reduces infection resistance of the tissue, resulting in a higher risk of co-infection than ordinary patients. Therefore, we believe that even if a patient shows a clear failure mechanism, such as metal corrosion or ceramic fracture, it should not be taken for

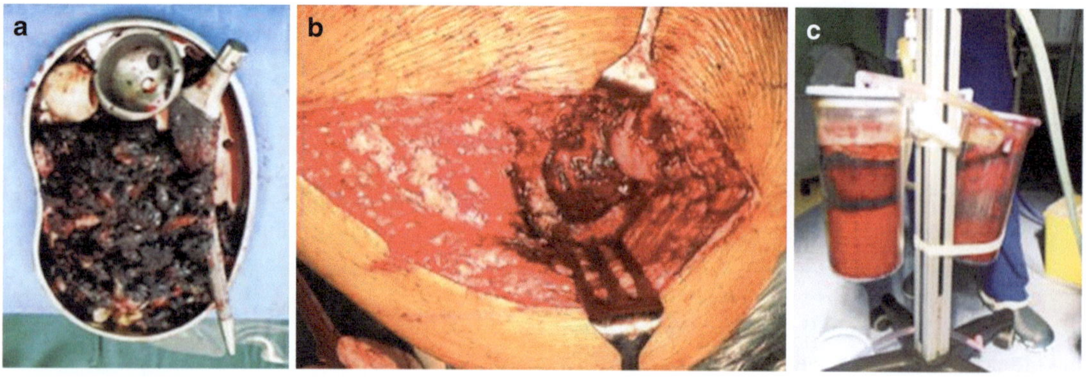

Fig. 9.9 Massive black stained tissue observed during operation. (**a**) The massive black stained tissues and the retrieved components including metal cup, metal stem, ceramic head, and fractured ceramic liner. (**b**) Black-stained tissue can be seen in the operative field. (**c**) The suction fluid was black stained

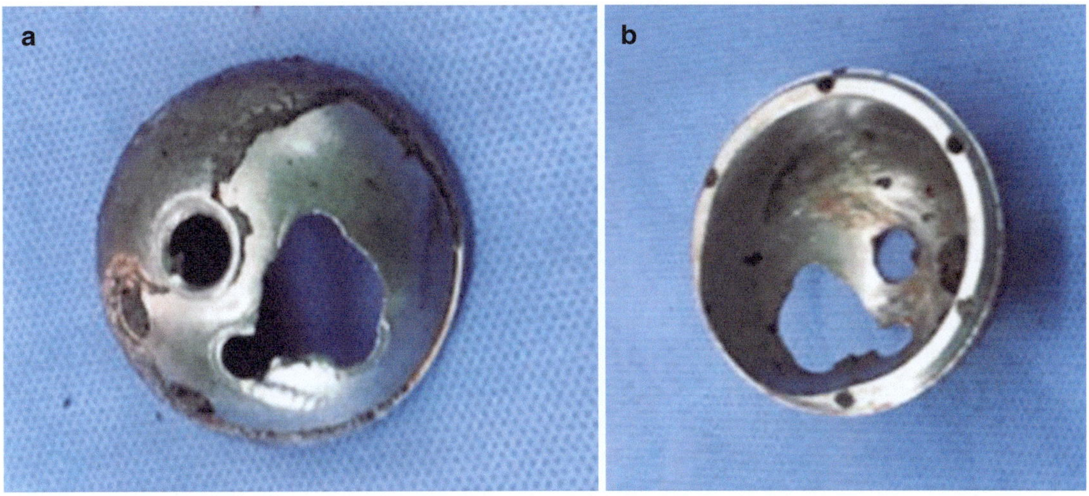

Fig. 9.10 Metal cup worn. (**a**) External view of the metal cup. (**b**) Internal view

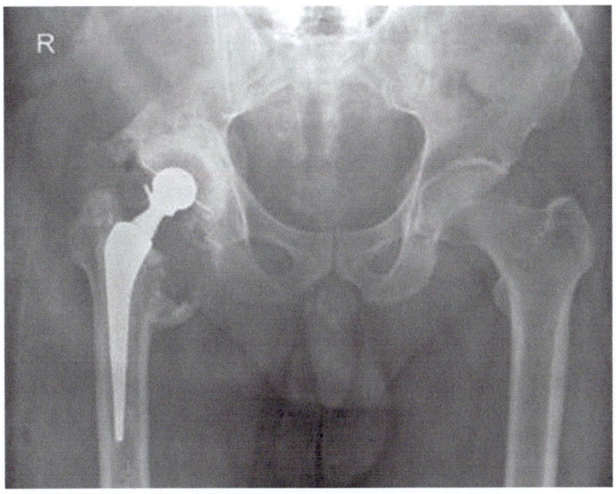

Fig. 9.11 Postoperative immediate radiograph

granted. Further infection exclusion should also be considered.

An aspiration for articular cavity should be routinely performed at least in patients with early failure or suspected infection (even if ESR and CRP are normal) if the clinical situation does not afford for all revision patients.

In addition, pathological examination is of great guiding significance for revision cases. It reports tissue damage score to the clinicians and indicates the presence of metal debris, cement debris, polyethylene debris, etc., as well as the presence of bacteria and even tuberculosis.

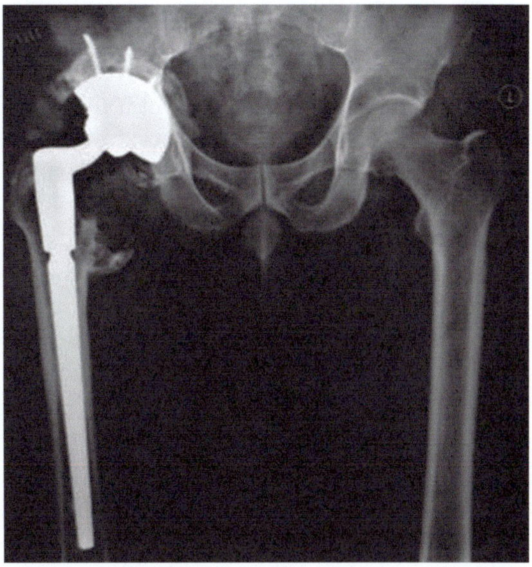

Fig. 9.12 Postoperative AP X-ray

2. How to differentiate heterotopic ossification (HO) and ceramic fracture?

   HO develops in a process, and its distribution around the hip has a certain pattern. Generally, HO is connected to the host bone, the edge is round and blunt, and the density is uneven. HO differs from calcification in that the former has a bone structure and the latter does not.

   On the contrary, ceramic fracture usually occurs immediately, with great uncertainty in location and distribution, and it reveals sharp edges in radiographs. As for the ceramic itself, the radiographic density of fourth-generation ceramics (DELTA) is higher than that of third-generation ceramics (FORTE). In consequence, if high density is observed around the joint and the ceramics is the fourth generation, it further indicates ceramic fracture.

3. What was the cause of ceramic fracture and metal cup abrasion in this case?

   Traces of impingement were seen in the femoral neck of this patient by the acetabular component. In terms of the position and angle in this case, the rotation center of the cup was lifted, the abduction of the cup was small, and the stem was in varus increasing the offset, thus, the ceramic fracture caused by impingement was highly suspected.

4. Abrasion occurred between the cup and the femoral head of this patient, but if there was no abrasion between the femoral head and the femoral cone, was revision required for the stem?

   If the stem had good fixation, soft tissue tension was fine, the stem would not loosen in the short term, the stem cone was fine, and a ceramic head matching the stem cone was available, the femoral stem could be considered reserved.

5. How can infection or non-infection be distinguished in patients with high ESR and CRP?

   Radiography showed a ceramic fracture and an abnormal relationship between the femoral head and the cup. Besides, aspiration fluid was black with relatively moderate levels of neutrophils and white blood cells. Along with the fact that about half of the patients with high concentrations of metal ions reveal high ESR and CRP, it could be summarized that the increase in ESR and CRP was caused by a series of lesions caused by ceramic fracture.

6. Why did dislocation occur following the second stage revision?

   Debris from the metal abrasion affected the soft tissue (joint capsule, gluteus medius, etc.) that maintains the stability of the joint, eventually causing hip instability. Other possible factors of hip instability include intraoperative debridement on soft tissue (overzealous debridement of soft tissue that is considered adverse, including black stained tissue, etc.). When there is a large cup-head difference, dislocation can occur easily. In this case, the anteversion of the cup was not large enough, which may contribute to dislocation.

   The patient presented no dislocation after 6 weeks of restriction in an over-correction position with anti-rotation boots after closed reduction. Therefore, for this type of patient with high dislocation risk, good postoperative management plays an important role in preventing the occurrence of dislocation, which should be paid more attention to.

   For those at risk of dislocation, the cup can be moved down (to the location of the original acetabulum), laterally (to improve soft tissue tension), or its orientation angle be improved. Dual-mobility articulations can also be considered.

7. How to read postoperative hip radiographs?

   We can follow the order of A-B-C to read. Take this case for example:

   A: Alignment, the position of the rotation center of the cup was not ideal in this case. The cup orientation (such as abduction) was not ideal, and the stem was in varus.

   B: Bone, periprosthetic bone was compromised in this case (e.g., the lesser trochanter).

   C: Cartilage (the bearing surface), the center of the cup and the head were staggered in this case, which indicated that the articular surface was seriously faulty. In addition, high-density shadows could be seen scattered around the joint. The density was higher than the bone cortex.

Recommended Reading

1. Toni A, Traina F, Stea S, et al. Early diagnosis of ceramic liner fracture. Guidelines based on a twelve-year clinical experience. J Bone Joint Surg Am. 2006;88(Suppl 4):55–63.
2. Hallan G, Fenstad AM, Furnes O. What is the frequency of fracture of ceramic components in

THA? Results from the Norwegian Arthroplasty Register from 1997 to 2017. Clin Orthop Relat Res. 2020;478(6):1254–61.
3. Zywiel MG, Brandt JM, Overgaard CB, et al. Fatal cardiomyopathy after revision total hip replacement for fracture of a ceramic liner. Bone Joint J. 2013;95-B(1):31–7.
4. Chen YW, Moussi J, Drury JL, et al. Zirconia in biomedical applications. Expert Rev Med Devices. 2016;13(10):945–63.
5. Hamilton WG, McAuley JP, Dennis DA, et al. THA with Delta ceramic on ceramic: results of a multicenter investigational device exemption trial. Clin Orthop Relat Res. 2010;468(2):358–66.
6. Chang JD. Future bearing surfaces in total hip arthroplasty. Clin Orthop Surg. 2014;6(1):110–6.
7. Howard DP, Wall PDH, Fernandez MA, et al. Ceramic-on-ceramic bearing fractures in total hip arthroplasty: an analysis of data from the National Joint Registry. Bone Joint J. 2017;99-B(8):1012–9.
8. Traina F, Tassinari E, De Fine M, et al. Revision of ceramic hip replacements for fracture of a ceramic component: AAOS exhibit selection. J Bone Joint Surg Am. 2011;93(24):el47.
9. Yi PH, Cross MB, Moric M, et al. Do serologic and synovial tests help diagnose infection in revision hip arthroplasty with metal-on-metal bearings or corrosion? Clin Orthop Relat Res. 2015;473(2):498–505.
10. Rambani R, Kepecs DM, Makinen TJ, et al. Revision total hip arthroplasty for fractured ceramic bearings: a review of best practices for revision cases. J Arthroplasty. 2017;32(6):1959–64.
11. Allain J, Roudot-Thoraval F, Delecrin J, et al. Revision total hip arthroplasty performed after fracture of a ceramic femoral head. A multicenter survivorship study. J Bone Joint Surg Am. 2003;85(5):825–30.
12. Zagra L, Bianchi L, Giacometti CR. Revision of ceramic fracture with ceramic-on-polyethylene in total hip arthroplasty: medium-term results. Injury. 2016;47(Suppl 4):S116–20.
13. Lee SJ, Kwak HS, Yoo JJ, et al. Bearing change to metal-on-polyethylene for ceramic bearing fracture in total hip arthroplasty; does it work? J Arthroplasty. 2016;31(1):204–8.

10 Revision Total Hip Arthroplasty in Patients with Ankylosing Spondylitis

Yixin Zhou, Lang Chen, Tao Bian, and Liang Zhang

10.1 Introduction

Lang Chen

Ankylosing spondylitis (AS) is the most common spondyloarthrosis (SpA) that involves the hip. Hip involvement is common in young AS patients, mostly bilateral. Total hip arthroplasty (THA) is by far the most effective treatment for severe hip involvement. With the gradual popularization of THA treatment in AS patients, revision THA has become increasingly common in AS patients. However, there is still a lack of follow-up studies and a systematic classification of revision THA in AS patients.

10.1.1 Epidemiology

About 24–50% of AS patients present some degree of hip involvement, and about 5% require THA. The patients who require THA usually present at a relatively young age, with a male-to-female ratio of 2:1. Most patients have satisfactory outcomes after primary THA [1]. Due to characteristics involving systemic inflammation, spinal fusion, and sagittal disequilibrium in AS patients, the incidence of complications such as dislocation following AS THA and heterotopic ossification (HO) is possibly higher than that of routine revision surgery. However, a cohort study conducted by our institution suggested that there were more AS patients who presented joint stiffness [2], whereas fewer patients had dislocations after THA. The incidence of other complications such as infection and aseptic loosening was not significantly higher.

The 10-, 15-, and 20-year prosthesis survival rates of patients with initial THA reported in the literature are 90%, 78%, and 64%, respectively [3]. Only a few studies focused on the outcome of revision THA in AS patients. It was also reported that the 5-, 10-, and 15-year prosthesis survival rates are 95%, 89%, and 89%, respectively [4]. In our follow-up study, the 5- and 10-year prosthesis survival rates of revision THA in AS patients were 95% and 91%, respectively.

10.1.2 Treatment Plan

Highlights of the perioperative treatment plan of revision THA in AS patients include

1. Conducting bath ankylosing spondylitis disease activity index (BASDAI) and bath ankylosing spondylitis functional index (BASFI) scoring to evaluate the degree of AS motion and articular function of perioperative patients.
2. Developing a perioperative AS medication regimen.

Y. Zhou (✉) · L. Chen · T. Bian · L. Zhang
Department of Adult Joint Reconstructive Surgery, Beijing Jishuitan Hospital, Capital Medical University, Beijing, China

Y. Zhou (ed.), *Revision Total Hip Arthroplasty*, https://doi.org/10.1007/978-981-97-9804-9_10

3. Evaluating the severity of bone defect on the acetabular side and femur side, and developing a reconstruction plan.
4. A full-length spinal X-ray or EOS examination is required for patients with spinal involvement to assess the severity of sagittal imbalance.
5. When necessary, pelvic-hip CT examinations should be performed to identify the best cup and augment positions. Preoperative planning can be achieved with the assistance of intraoperative navigation or surgical robots.
6. Preoperative grading and postoperative treatment/prevention of HO.

10.1.3 Surgical Outcomes and Complications

According to the follow-up examination of our institution, the postoperative HHS and BASFI scores were significantly improved in the AS THA revision. In consistency with AS patients undergoing initial revision, the postoperative flexion and extension range of motion (ROM) after THA are lower in AS patients than that in regular THA patients, whereas the dislocation rate had no significant increase. Despite the postoperative stiffness of hip motion, most patients with AS were still satisfied with the results of the revision. The possible reason is that the spine and pelvis are completely fused in most AS patients undergoing revision THA, while the torso motion mainly relies on hip and knee compensations. Revision THA can significantly improve the motion of the hip compared with the preoperative condition. The incidence of HO in AS patients was also significantly higher than that of regular revision THA patients, but most HO lesions following revision THA were Brooker Class I or II, which had no effect on postoperative range of motion. Other complications include infection, periprosthetic fracture, aseptic loosening, delayed wound healing, deep vein thrombosis (DVT), unequal length of double lower extremities, limb pain, or numbness. No spine-related complications were reported in our follow-up examination.

10.1.4 Summary

The main differences between revision THA for AS patients and regular revision THA include preoperative AS motion evaluation, adjustment of perioperative drug regimen, and the prevention of postoperative HO. In terms of surgical principles, cases with severe spinal involvement require careful preoperative designs to reach sagittal balance and the most ideal placement of the cup. For cases of preoperative hip stiffness, it is necessary to perform appropriate intraoperative release in order to improve postoperative motion.

10.2 Case 1

Lang Chen, Tao Bian, and Liang Zhang

10.2.1 Case Summary

Medical History Male, 65 years old, complained of "pain in both hips and limited mobility for 1 year after bilateral THA 18 years ago". The patient underwent bilateral THA in another hospital for AS involving both hips in 1996. Postoperative recovery was uneventful. In 2013, there was a bilateral increase in hip pain with decreased ROM. The pain was aggregated upon movement and gradually worsened.

Physical Examination The patient entered in a wheelchair; posterolateral incision scar was seen in both hips, no redness or swelling or sinuses were seen; greater trochanter tenderness (+); axial percussion pain (+); and severely limited hip mobility. ROM: right hip flexion 50°, extension 0°, abduction 5°, adduction 0°, internal rotation 10°, external rotation 10°; left hip flexion 80°, extension 5°, abduction 15°, adduction 10°, internal rotation 15°, and external rotation 15°. Stiffness in the spine. Neurovascular examination had no abnormal findings.

Laboratory Examination Routine blood test, erythrocyte sedimentation rate (ESR), and

C-reactive protein (CRP) were all in the normal range.

Radiographic Data See Fig. 10.1 for preoperative radiographs.

10.2.2 Case Analysis

1. Infection was basically excluded according to comprehensive preoperative examination.
2. Plain radiographs and CT radiographs showed that:
   (a) Alignment: posterior pelvis tilt; sacroiliac and spinal fusion; the Shenton's line was disrupted and the center of rotation migrated proximally.
   (b) Bone: The iliac crest, trochanter, and ischial tubercle had signs of calcification; expansive osteolysis was seen around the greater trochanter. The bone defect was noticed around the acetabulum; only bone mass around the acetabular floor was left, whereas the projection of the anterior and posterior acetabulum margins could not be seen. It was speculated that the anterior and posterior column defects of the acetabulum occurred, more obviously in the lateral area. The Kohler line of the right hip was interrupted and the boundary was not clear. Partial defects of a teardrop, pubic ramus, and ischial ramus were observed. The orientation of the "flared" pelvic defect: In this case, the "flared" opening of the right pelvic defect was outward-facing, resulting in better stability than one with an inward-facing opening after reconstruction.
   (c) Cartilage: Eccentric wear presented at the articular interface. No definitive signs of metal cup wear.
   (d) Others: As an intraoperative prediction of the functional position of the cup was not realistic, even if the intraoperative placement of the cup is ideal based on anatomical markers, functional positioning of the cup might not be satisfactory in postoperative loading, resulting in abrasion and osteolysis from edge loading and impingement.
3. Diagnosis: AS; prosthesis loosening following double THA; and osteolysis.

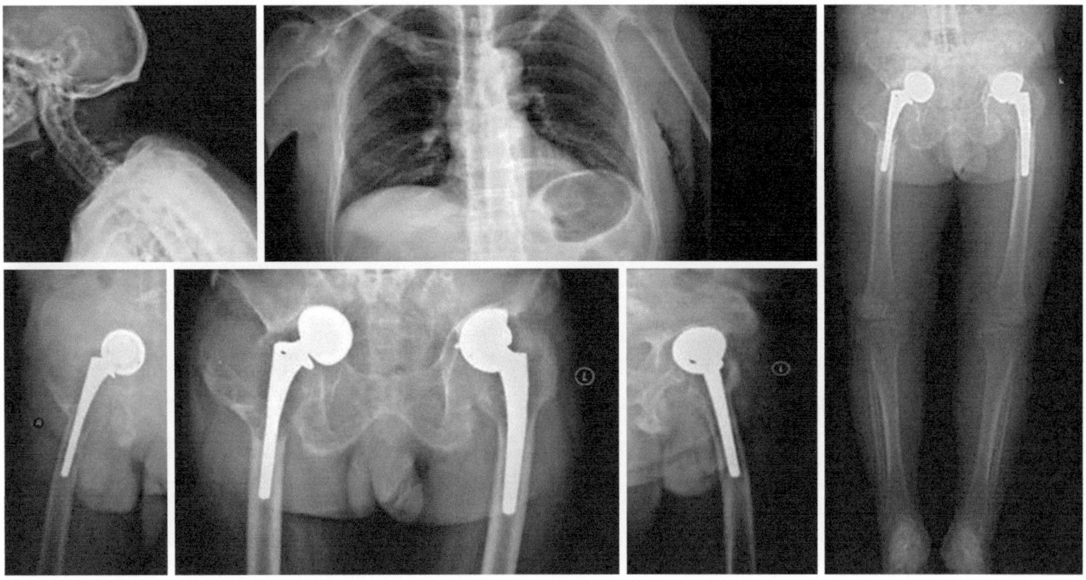

Fig. 10.1 Preoperative radiographs

10.2.3 Preoperative Planning

Previous history of AS.

1. BASFI and BASDAI scoring for disease activity and functional assessment.
2. Drug therapy for perioperative-active AS:
   (a) Diagnosis and treatment by Systematic and Rheumatology Department: Non-steroidal anti-inflammatory drugs (NSAIDs), Disease-modifying antirheumatic drugs (DMARDs), and monoclonal antibody therapy.
   (b) The principle of suspending NSAIDs was the same as previously.
   (c) DMARDs: such as MTX, leflunomide, and salazine sulfamethazine. Continued with normal dosage, no addition, no reduction, no suspending, and not expected to increase the risk of complications.
   (d) Monoclonal antibody therapy: It is very commonly applied in treating AS; patients with a high degree of motion tend to take 2~3 months before indicators return to normal. Afterward, normally 1 drug cycle of suspension is enough, such as a dose of etanercept every 2 weeks, in which the 2 weeks is a cycle. In a conservative treatment period, it can be suspended for 2 cycles.
   (e) Monoclonal antibodies should not be started until 1–2 months after surgery.
   (f) Hormone therapy/Chinese medicines containing hormones: Hormone therapy is of no value for AS. AS patients using hormones should be paid special attention to, as it suggests, previous diagnosis and treatment tissue and/or poor compliance. In this situation, hormone application should be suspended following the hormone reduction and suspension strategy before the surgery.
3. Effect of spinal sagittal balance on revision THA:
   (a) Posterior pelvic tilt, the ratio of vertical to transverse diameters of obturator foramen exceeds 2:1.
   (b) Whether to have spinal orthopedic surgery first should be considered.
   (c) The angle of anteversion and abduction should be adjusted according to the position of the pelvis.
   (d) If the posterior pelvic tilt exceeds 45°, both anteversion and abduction should be adjusted by 15°. The angle of the cup is better smaller than larger.
4. Prevention of HO:
   (a) HO is one of the relatively severe postoperative complications for AS patients, with a high incidence. However, Brooker 3 and 4 are not common. It mainly affects ROM flexion and rotation.
   (b) Postoperative NSAIDs and radiotherapy are two common prevention methods.
   (c) NSAIDs: Any inhibitor. Indomethacin is not necessary. The effects are the same.
   (d) Radiotherapy should be performed 0.5–1 day before the operation.
5. Infection is not a major problem for AS and there is no definite postoperative increase in infection risk.
6. HLA-B27 gene covers locus 01-04, in which 04 is more commonly found in the Chinese population. However, this is a double-edged sword: It is likely to develop AS with HLA-B27, whereas the risk of infection is reduced.
7. In 2013, 220 AS patients receiving THA were taken into statistics in our institution, two of them were presented dislocation. The low dislocation incidence might be related to low postoperative range of motion.
8. Risk factors of low postoperative ROM: (1) preoperative contracture; (2) high preoperative CRP; (3) postoperative HO; and (4) small diameter of femoral head.
9. THA should not be attempted to address deformity and imbalance in the spine. Consulting the Department of Spine is required. If necessary, the spinal deformity can be treated with corrective spinal osteotomy.

The surgical plan and design of the left hip corresponding to the specific characteristics of this case were as follows:

(a) Acetabular side: In terms of the three-point fixation theory, the anterosuperior point might exist, and the bone mass was relatively adequate for the posteroinferior ramus point. The weight-bearing area as well as the posterior column required reconstruction. Thus, augment should be prepared before the operation.

(b) Femoral side: Bone mass in the middle femur was good. The proximal end, presenting with massive inflated osteolysis, needed to be fixed with a femoral stem with proximal osseointegration.

10.2.4 Operation Situation

1. Right hip:
   (a) A large segmental and inclusive bone defect with a diameter of 4 cm was seen in the upper margin and medial wall of the acetabulum. The scar tissue was removed. The acetabulum was reamed to a diameter of 62 mm. A curved augment was fixed with a screw in the medial superior acetabulum. A 62-mm porous TM cup was placed in, with anteversion 30° and abduction 40°, and bone cement was filled in between the cup and the augment. Multiple screws were used to fix the cup.
   (b) A massive inflammatory pseudotumor lay in the medial greater trochanter. When the cyst wall was incised, a large amount of gelatinoid inflammatory tissue was revealed. The pseudotumor content was removed and the cyst wall tissue was scraped off with curette. The severe contained bone defect was seen in the greater trochanter. The abductor attachment point was intact, and the middle and distal femur was good. The femoral stem was loose. The distal medullary cavity mobilization of the femoral stem was attempted with difficulty. The femoral cortex was longitudinally sectioned at 2 cm. After traction, the femoral stem was successfully retrieved from the distal medullary cavity.
   (c) Restoration Modular (RM) No. 14 distal femoral stem was applied. The torsion test was negative. A 27 mm +10 mm proximal RM stem sleeve was implanted, with anteversion 10°; a claw cable-plate system was applied to anchor the greater trochanter and the middle femur cortex.
   (d) Polyethylene liner was applied, and a 32-mm standard ceramic head (pink) was implanted.
2. Left hip:
   (a) A large segmental and inclusive bone defect was seen in the upper margin and medial wall of the acetabulum. The upper margin of the acetabulum was reconstructed with two curved TM augments. A 68-mm porous TM cup was subsequently applied.
   (b) The RM 14 distal femoral stem was implanted. The torsion test was negative. A 36-mm RM 21 sleeve with 4 mm proximal eccentricity was applied, with anteversion 10°.
   (c) Polyethylene liner and 36 mm ceramic femoral head were implanted.

10.2.5 Postoperative Condition and Outcome

1. The patient was instructed to walk on crutches 2 weeks after the operation, partial weight bearing at 6 weeks and complete weight bearing at 3 months.
2. Clinical follow-up: Harris score 87; free of pain; and no limitation walking up and down stairs or on flat ground. Functional exercises of hip flexion and abduction were gradually intensified within 3 months after the operation. The walking distance was 2 km.

The postoperative immediate anteroposterior (AP) view is shown in Fig. 10.2.

10.2.6 Conclusion and Reflection

1. In revision in AS patients, the possible influence of spinal and pelvic imbalance on the hip should be carefully considered.

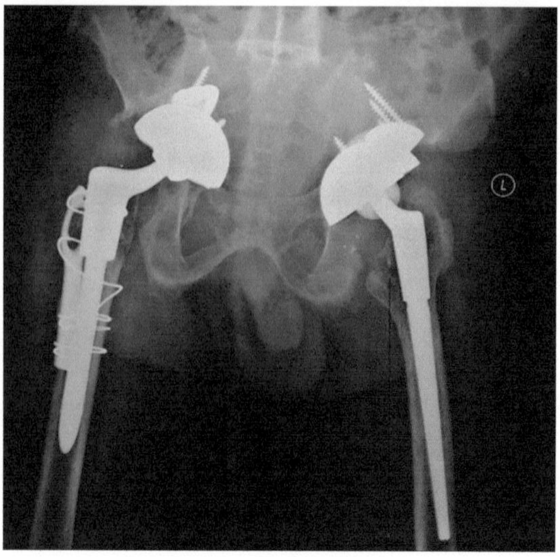

Fig. 10.2 Postoperative immediate AP view

2. If there is a severe deformity of the spine, the hip condition should be treated after corrective spinal osteotomy. In addition, THA should not be applied to overcompensate for functional disorders caused by severe spinal deformity and sagittal disequilibrium.
3. Perioperative AS medication strategies should be carefully formulated, including the treatment of AS in the motion stage and the prevention of AS-related complications.
4. Robotic surgery can be helpful in optimal positioning of the acetabular cup and controlling leg length.

Recommended Reading

1. Vander Cruyssen B, Munoz-Gomariz E, Font P, et al. Hip involvement in ankylosing spondylitis: epidemiology and risk factors associated with hip replacement surgery. Rheumatology (Oxford). 2010;49(1):73–81.
2. Tang WM, Chiu K. Primary Total Hip Arthroplasty in Patients With Ankylosing Spondylitis. J Arthoplasty. 2000;15(1):25–8.
3. Sweeney S, Gupta R, Taylor G, Calin A. Total hip arthroplasty in ankylosing spondylitis: outcome in 340 patients. J Rheumatol. 2001;28(8):1862–6.
4. Bukowski BR, Clark NJ, Taunton MJ, et al. Revision Total Hip Arthroplasty in Patients with Ankylosing Spondylitis: Long-Term Results. J Arthroplasy. 2020;35(9):2573–80.

Appendixes

1.1 Appendix A: Paprosky Classification of Acetabular and Femoral Bone Defect

1.1.1 Paprosky Classification of Femoral Bone Defect (Table A.1, see Fig. A.1)

1.1.1.1 Paprosky Classification of Acetabular Bone Defect (Table A.2)

Type IIIA is also called up and out. Type IIIB is also called up and in.

Table A.1 Paprosky classification of femoral bone defect

Classification	Definition	Metaphysis	Diaphysis	Proximal remodeling	Reconstruction method
I	Minor cancellous defect in metaphysis	Intact	Intact	None	Proximal press fit non-cement fixation
II	Extensive cancellous defect in metaphysis, with intact cortex in diaphysis	None	Intact	Minor	Non-cement stem with extensive coating
IIIA	Severely damaged metaphysis, no support, but more than 4 cm intact cortical bone in diaphysis	None	Femoral isthmus longer than 4 cm	Notable	Non-cement stem with extensive coating is suitable for medullary cavity less than 19 mm, and modular or non-modular ridged tapered titanium stem for medullary cavity less than 19 mm
IIIB	Severely damaged metaphysis, no support, less than 4 cm intact cortical bone left in diaphysis	None	Femoral isthmus less than 4 cm	Notable	Taper Modular Fluted Titanium stems (TMFT)
IV	Both the metaphysis and diaphysis are severely damaged, and the femoral medullary cavity expanded, no support from isthmus	None	None	Minor	Allograft prosthesis composite, compression bone grafting combined with cement stem, or proximal femoral arthroplasty

Y. Zhou (ed.), *Revision Total Hip Arthroplasty*, https://doi.org/10.1007/978-981-97-9804-9

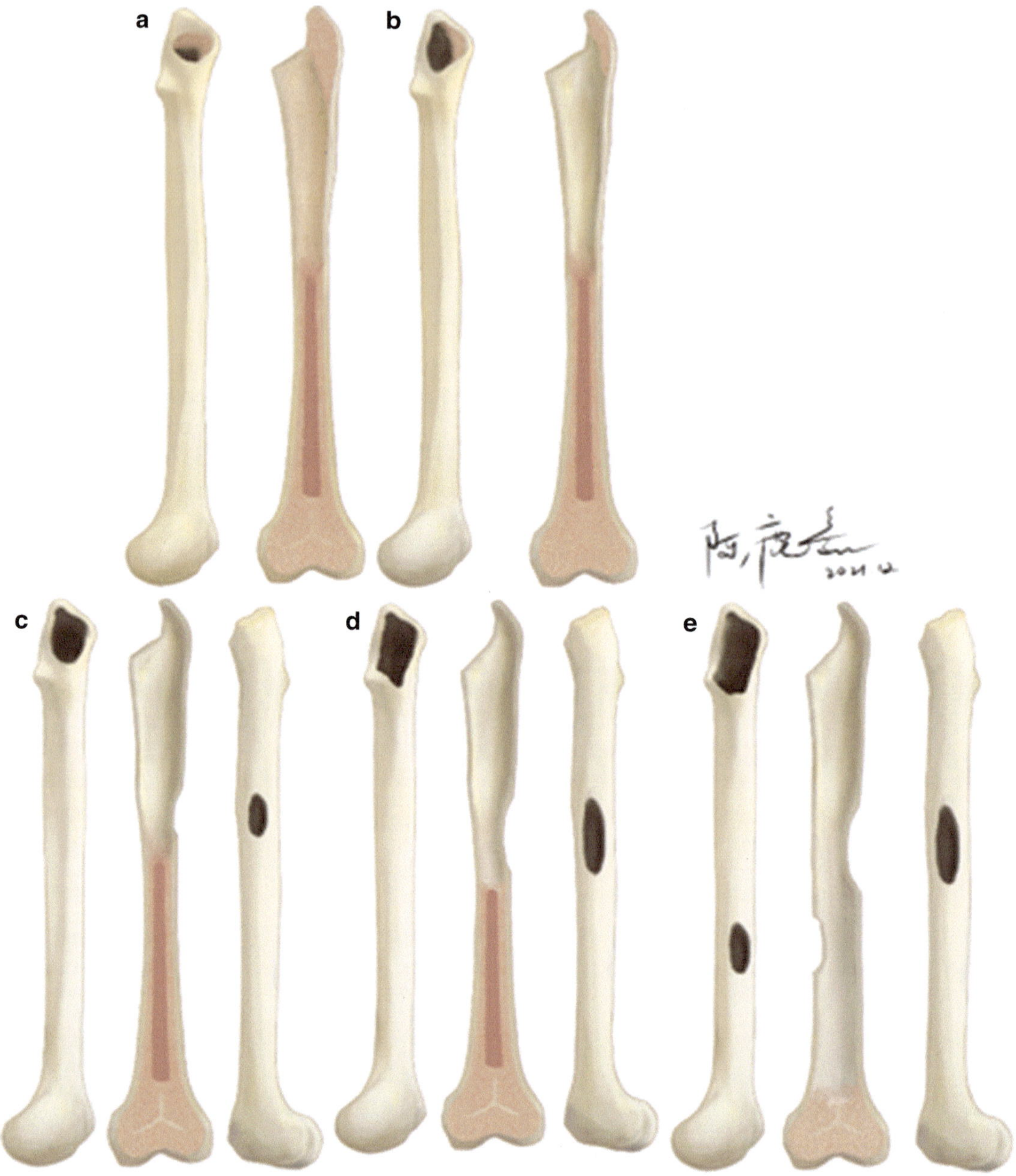

Fig. A.1 Diagram of Paprosky classification of femoral bone defect. (**a**) Type I; (**b**) Type II; (**c**) Type IIIA; (**d**) Type IIIB; and (**e**) Type IV

Table A.2 Paprosky classification of acetabular bone defect

I	No significant defect in acetabular rim or migration
II	Acetabular defect with an intact supporting column; less than 2 cm of up and in or up and out migration of the implant A. Up and in B. Up and out (acetabular roof missing) C. Medial defect only
III	Superior migration greater than 2 cm, severe ischiatic and medial wall defects A. Kohler line intact, bone defect position: 10 to 2 o'clock B. Kohler line is disrupted, and bone defect location is more extensive: 9 to 5 o'clock
IV	Pelvic discontinuity (PD)

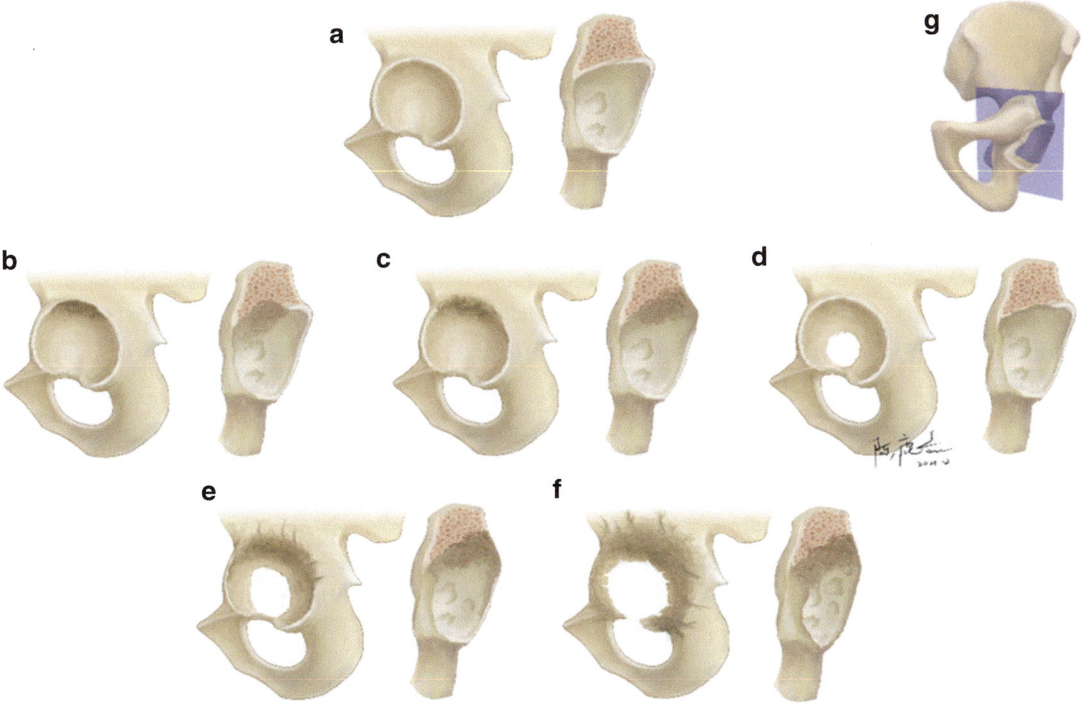

Fig. A.2 Diagram of Paprosky classification of acetabular bone defect. (**a**) Type I; (**b**) Type IIA; (**c**) Type IIB; (**d**) Type IIC; (**e**) Type IIIA; and (**f**) Type IIIB. (**g**) Type IV

Recommended Reading

1. Paprosky WG, Perona PG, Lawrence JM. Acetabular defect classification and surgical reconstruction in revision arthroplasty. A 6-year follow-up evaluation. J Arthroplasty. 1994, 9(1):33–44.
2. Paprosky WG, Aribindi R. Hip replacement: treatment of femoral bone loss using distal bypass fixation. Instr Course Lect. 2000,49:119–30.

1.2 Appendix B: Vancouver-UCS Classification of Periprosthetic Fracture Following THA

Duncan et al. proposed the Vancouver Classification, which is the most widely used classification of periprosthetic femoral fracture following THA.

Vancouver A fracture occurs in the trochanter region of the proximal femur. It is further categorized into the greater trochanter fracture (Vancouver AG) and the lesser trochanter fracture (Vancouver AL).

Vancouver B occurs around or slightly lower than the distal femur stem, which is the most common type clinically. It is further categorized into B1 (well-fixed prosthesis), B2 (loose stem with good bone stock), and B3 (loose stem with severe bone loss) according to the degree of fixation and bone mass.

Vancouver C occurs in the distal femur, in which the stem is usually stable without significant bone loss.

Subsequently, the creator of this classification proposed a Unified Classified System (UCS Classification) in 2014, which was almost exactly consistent with the Vancouver Classification principle, with the addition of fracture between hip and knee prostheses as type D (Table B.1 and Fig. B.1).

Table B.1 Vancouver-UCS Classification

Vancouver classification	UCS classification	Definition	Treatment
A		Fracture occurs between trochanters	
AG	A1	Greater trochanter fracture	Conservative treatment; surgical treatment if the migration is major
AL	A2	Lesser trochanter fracture	Conservative or surgical treatment
B		Fracture occurs around or at the tip of the stem	
B1	B1	Prosthesis is well fixed	Open reduction and internal fixation; revision is occasionally required
B2	B2	The stem is loose and has good bone stock	Long stem revision
B3	B3	The stem is loose with severe bone loss	Long stem revision and reconstruction of bone mass
C	C	Fracture occurs beyond the tip of the stem	ORIF
None	D	Fracture occurs between the hip and knee	Personalized treatment, special prosthesis needs to be customized for complex cases.

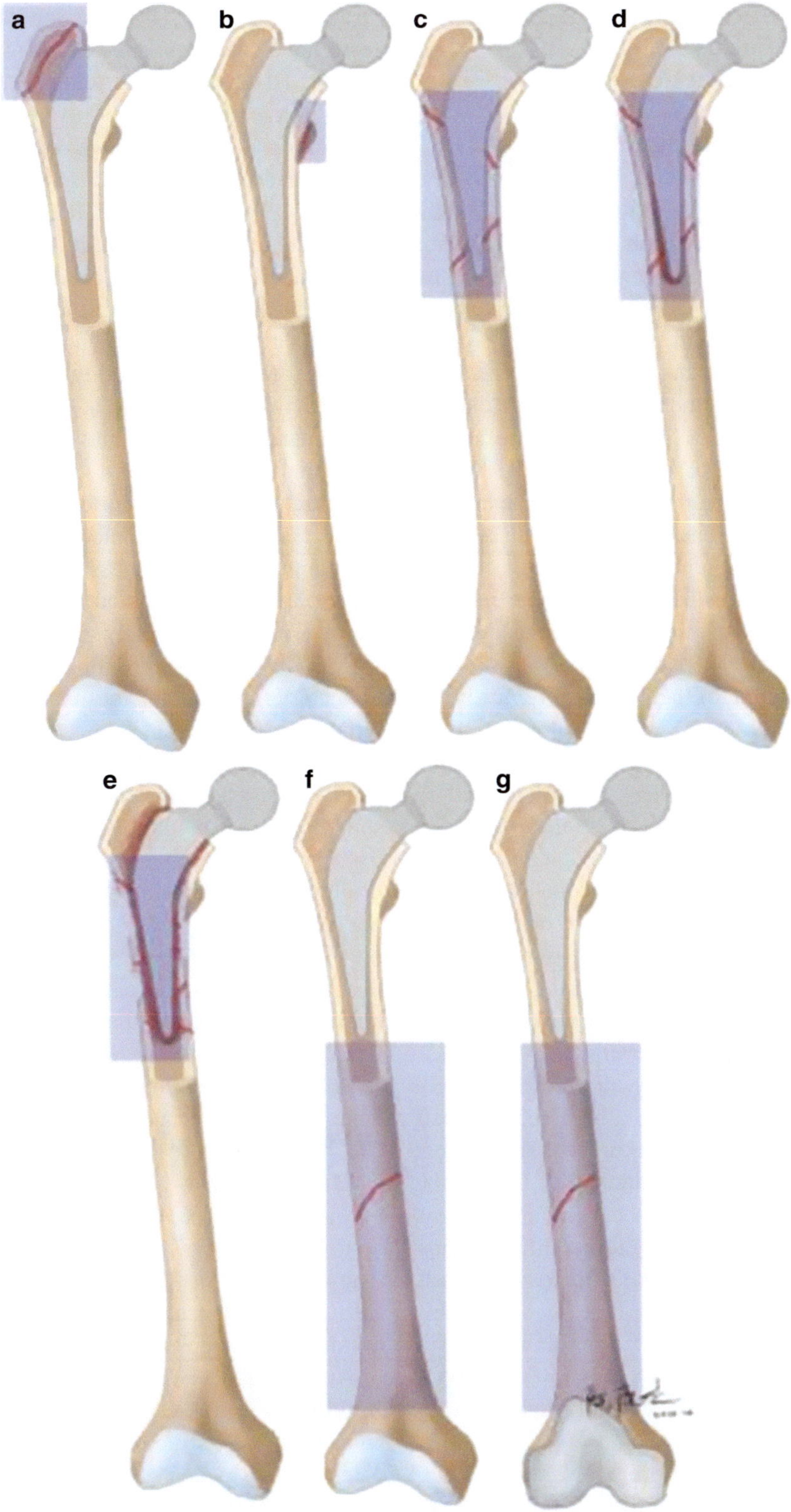

Fig. B.1 Vancouver-UCS Classification diagram. (**a**) Type AG (A1); (**b**) Type AL (A2); (**c**) Type B1; (**d**) Type B2; (**e**) Type B3; (**f**) Type C; and (**g**) Type D

1.3 Appendix C: Isthmusplasty and Endosteal Reconstruction

1.3.1 Isthmusplasty

At present, the main trend of Paprosky IV femoral defect reconstruction is distal fixation TMFT. However, it has been reported that complications such as intraoperative fracture, prosthesis subsidence, and stress shielding occur more frequently. Huang Yong et al. from the Orthopaedics Department of Jishuitan Hospital, Beijing, conducted a retrospective follow-up examination on 182 cases of revision THA with TMFT in our hospital. A follow-up examination of femoral reconstruction over an average of 6 years revealed a high incidence of complications such as prosthetic subsidence, intraoperative fracture, postoperative stress shielding, and postoperative poor new bone formation in the osteolysis area of the proximal femur in the Type N femoral defect, which is close to previous literature. These complications were found to be related to the wider femoral medullary cavity in Paprosky Type N femoral defect patients, with no obvious femoral stem isthmus larger at the top and smaller at the bottom for fixation of TMFT. During the operation, a thicker and longer femoral stem is required to achieve initial stability by sticking at one or more points (usually anterior) with the weak distal cortical bone. However, such fixation is usually not stable and the valid fixation length is insufficient, resulting in a high risk of postoperative stem subsidence or even loosening. The thicker the femoral stem, the higher the stiffness, the less strain of the stem, and the less contact area with the femoral medullary cavity, consequently the more likely to have a stress riser and higher intraoperative fracture incidence. In addition, stress riser caused by a thicker femoral stem also tends to cause postoperative periprosthetic femoral fracture, leading to stress shielding, and subsequently results in a weaker femur and more severe bone defect, which also creates difficulties in future reconstruction surgery. The research results of our team have been published in the top orthopedic journal JBJS Am and articular surgery journal JOA (Appendix E).

Aiming at the insufficient distal valid fixation length caused by lack of femoral isthmus in Paprosky Type N femoral defect patients with tapered stem, Zhou Yixin et al. from the Orthopaedics Department of Jishuitan Hospital creatively proposed isthmusplasty to increase the valid fixation length of femoral stem, so as to enhance the initial stability of stem fixation. Isthmusplasty is to create an isthmus in a femur without an original isthmus. The practice is to create a 4–7 cm long and 1–1.5 cm wide ligulate osteotomy in the lateral cortex of the distal femur. A 3D-printed wedged plate is bound with multiple titanium cables to press the ligulate block in the distal lateral cortical bone into the medullary cavity. Thus, an artificial isthmus with a medullary cavity of large proximal and small distal diameter is created for the fixation of TMFT to reduce the risk of subsidence or even loosening. Meanwhile, thicker femoral stem implantation can be avoided to prevent stress riser and stress shielding, so that intraoperative and postoperative fracture risks are reduced. When the augment is relatively longer, with the proximal end exceeding the position of the greenstick fracture and the distal end exceeding the lateral osteotomy position, the titanium cable can bridge the stress after binding and reduce the risk of iatrogenic fracture.

A model of isthmusplasty reconstruction of Paprosky Type IV bone defect is shown in Fig. C.1.

The long-term 3D-printed long, wedged, porous augment was expected to obtain lateral cortical bone ingrowth (Fig. C.2), thus achieving long-term fixation. The femoral stem was stable with no subsidence and functioned well in the 6-month follow-up examination.

At present, the Orthopaedics Department of Jishuitan Hospital, Beijing, has performed isthmusplasty reconstruction of Type IV femoral defect in six patients. All implants have been stable, and patient functioning is good.

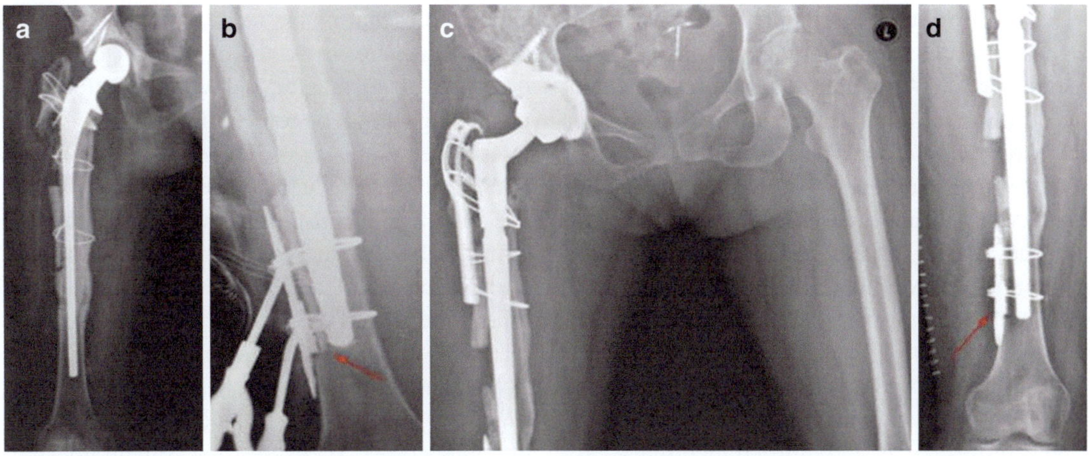

Fig. C.1 A model of isthmusplasty reconstruction of Paprosky Type IV bone defect. (**a**) Female, 51 years old, preoperative right hip AP radiograph showed that no isthmus could be used for femoral stem fixation following second-stage revision Spacer of infection. (**b**) During the operation, isthmusplasty was performed, where titanium cables were applied to tie the 3D-printed wedged plate to squeeze the distal ligulate osteotomy block of the lateral cortical bone into the medullary cavity, forming an artificial femoral isthmus, so that the valid fixation length of the femoral stem increased. (**c**, **d**) Postoperative immediate left hip AP radiographs of the patient showed that the femoral stem was fixed on the distal artificial isthmus

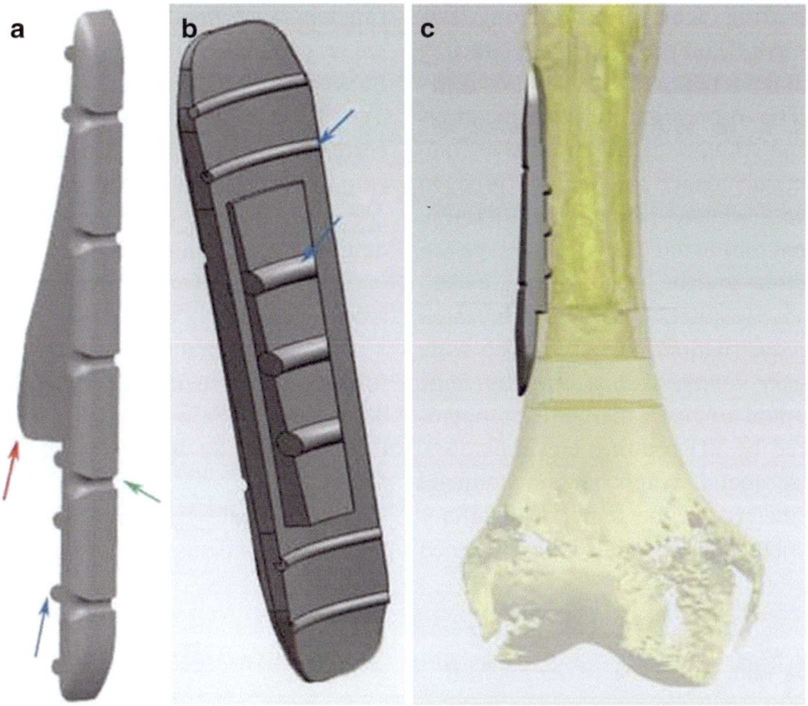

Fig. C.2 The long-term 3D-printed long, wedged, porous augment. (**a**) Titanium cable bound 3D-printed wedged plate, side view. (**b**) The 3D-printed wedged plate, medial side view. (**c**) Ligulate osteotomy is performed in the lateral cortex of the distal femur; the 3D-printed wedged plate was bound with multiple titanium cables to force the ligulate block of distal lateral cortical bone into the medullary cavity, forming artificial isthmus with large proximal and small distal diameter of its medullary cavity, in order to fix the modular TMFT

1.3.1.1 Endosteal Reconstruction

Bone cement fixation remains an effective method for THA, which relies on bone cement penetrating into the trabeculae of cancellous bone to form micro-entanglement. However, the femoral medullary cavity sclerosis of Type N bone defect means it lacks cancellous bone trabeculae; thus, cement entanglement fixation cannot be achieved in revision THA. Therefore, some surgeons proposed impaction bone grafting, in which the allogeneic cancellous bone is driven into the wide medullary cavity to cover the original sclerotic and smooth bone, creating a new, more coarse, and mottled medullary cavity. Subsequently, a modern bone cement technique is employed to implant a highly polished collarless double-tapered stem into the newly compressed allogeneic bone bed. Fixation is realized through the entanglement between bone cement and cancellous bone. Many follow-up examination results showed that compression bone grafting achieves good long-term efficacy. However, compression bone grafting has high technical requirements and is time-consuming. The proportion of complications caused by bone resorption, intraoperative fracture, and stem subsidence is relatively high. In order to obtain the micro-entanglement fixation of bone cement and avoid the disadvantages of compression bone grafting, the orthopedic team at Jishuitan Hospital, Beijing, invented Endosteal Reconstruction. Namely, in the wide femur medullary cavity, porous titanium rings with the potential of bone ingrowth preoperatively produced by 3D printing are implanted. These porous metal rings are customized according to the size of the femoral medullary cavity. The metal ring can also be designed expandable, that is, the teeth on one side of the metal ring are interlocking. After hydraulic pressure or expansion screw distraction, the metal ring cannot be retracted after the teeth are interlocked, so as to realize good press fit fixation in the intramedullary. The porous surface of the metal ring can form micro-entanglement with the bone cement, which plays a role like the trabeculae of cancellous bone. Cement penetrates the porous metal to form micro-entanglement, fixing the femoral stem in the medullary cavity. The middle layer of the porous metal functions as a seal and has a close press fit with the bone cortex. It ensures that cement does not reach the interface between porous metal and bone so that bone ingrowth is not affected. The high-hat-shaped metal ring is inserted in the broken end of the proximal femur, with the brim sitting at the broken end of the femoral cortex, as it helps prevent femoral subsidence. In the long term, the high-hat-shaped porous metal ring can reach bone ingrowth. Besides avoiding the lack of micro-entanglement fixation between trabeculae of cancellous bone and cement in Type IV bone defect due to the smooth sclerotic cortex of the medullary cavity, the porous metal ring can also enhance the strength of the bone cortex and avoid bone resorption and time demanding in compression bone grafting.

See Fig. C.3 for an illustration of endosteal reconstruction.

In clinical practice, we have already performed reconstruction of Type IV femur bone defect using this method in six patients. All of them currently show good stability and functioning.

The clinical application of endosteal reconstruction in patients is shown in Fig. C.4.

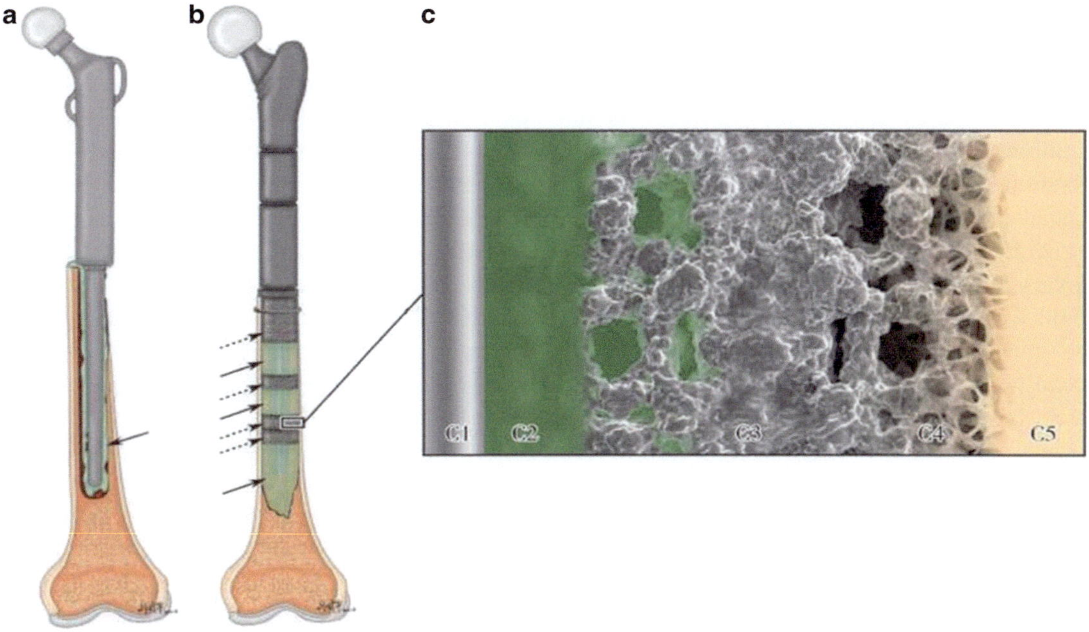

Fig. C.3 Illustration of endosteal reconstruction. (**a**) In Type IV bone defect, due to the sclerotic femoral medullary cavity, there is a lack of trabeculae of cancellous bone; thus, micro-entanglement fixation of bone cement cannot be obtained. (**b**) 3D-printed porous titanium metal ring with bone ingrowth potential. (**c**) Interface of Endosteal Reconstruction. (**c1**) Femoral stem. (**c2**) Bone cement. (**c3**) Porous metal ring. (**c4**) Interface between metal ring and cortical bone. (**c5**) Cortical bone

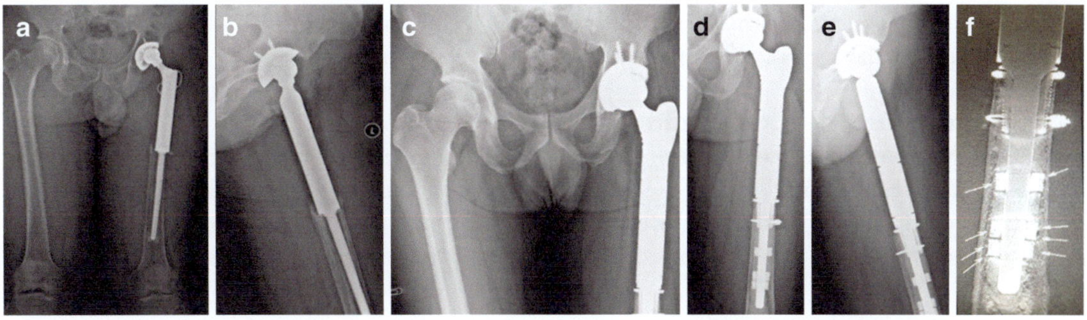

Fig. C.4 Endosteal reconstruction in clinical practice. (**a**, **b**) Preoperative AP X-rays. The patient presented bone tumor and had proximal femoral stem loosening following arthroplasty. This patient had only distal part of the femur left, lack of femoral isthmus and with wide, horn-shaped medullary cavity. (**c–e**) The femur was revised with a mega prothesis with endosteal reconstruction at the distal part. (**f**) At 1-year follow-up, bone ingrowth was found on the 3D printed metal rings

1.4 Appendix D: Non-cement Acetabular Reconstruction Based on RPC Theory

In triangles we trust.

The initial stability of non-cement acetabular reconstruction comes from "rim fixation" or "three-point fixation"; thus, the anterior and posterior columns of the acetabulum, especially the integrity of the posterior column, play a crucial role in determining the supporting capacity of the fixing point. "Three-point fixation" refers to when presented with bone defect, there are three stable points in the bone close to the acetabular rim, but it can still provide sufficient initial stability for the cup. "Rim fixation" can also be considered a mechanical fixation combined with several "three-point fixations." The reconstruction of the acetabular floor was designed to form several triangles inward and outward via the combination of "rim fixation" and "three-point fixation" from the acetabular rim, consequently enhancing the stability of the reconstruction structure. The concept above is named the ring-point-column theory of acetabular reconstruction (see Fig. D.1). Indeed, the rings, points, and columns mentioned here are not sheer geometric definitions, in which ring and point possess no area. In what we have presented, the rings and points are abstract of a relatively small area of bone or metal structure. RPC theory can be comprehended from the following aspects.

1.4.1.1 Rim Fixation

When the acetabular rim is intact, the hemispherical cup protrudes and forms a constriction hooping grip on the acetabular periphery at the equator. This hooping grip provides the initial stability of the hemispherical cup. When presented with defects at the acetabular rim, its integrity can be reconstructed with augment, or the loose rim (ring) can be tightened up with slope augment. This reconstruction strategy to stabilize the cup is called rim fixation.

1.4.1.2 Jumbo Cup: The Cornerstone of Non-cement Acetabular Reconstruction

Jumbo cup can resolve most of the acetabular reconstruction problems that surgeons face in revision THA. The ratio of jumbo cup reconstruction certainly depends on the severity and complexity of the acetabular defect as well. The basic idea of the jumbo cup application is simple, namely, reaming the acetabulum into a larger diameter to increase the area of contact between the outer cup and the bone matrix, under the premise of not causing further significant loss. More importantly, three stable points are established within the area of the remaining acetabulum, and then the hemispherical cup is wedged within the three points, forming a stable three-point fixation.

In clinical practice, the surgeon may also move the rotation center upwards and ream the superior bone to form a high-center acetabulum, so as to reach initial stability and good contact between the cup and the bone matrix. Although the high-center acetabulum remains partially acceptable in clinical practice as a means of compromise and damage control, it should never be routinely applied, much less the target of intraoperative reconstruction efforts. The harm of high rotation centers has been documented in many literatures, which will not be discussed here. It is worth emphasizing that avoiding high-center acetabulum is a technical key that the surgeons should be alarmed about in the initial and revision THA.

The application of the jumbo cup is apparently dependent on the increase of acetabular reaming. The decision between reaming or retaining bone mass thereby arises. In general, the bone mass to

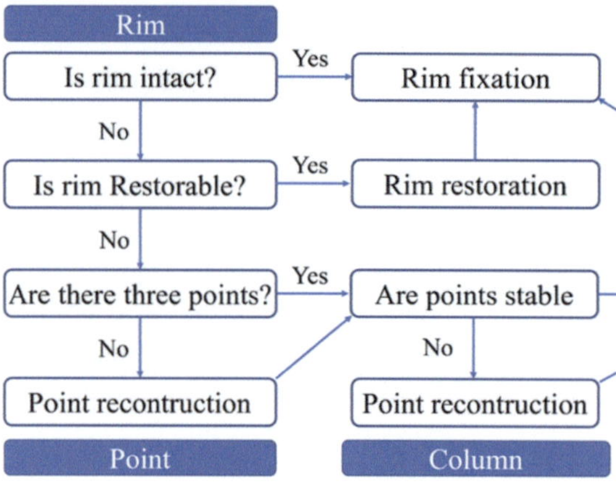

Fig. D.1 Flow chart of RPC theory in acetabular reconstruction

be reamed and sacrificed first is the anterior bone. Nevertheless, the continuity of the anterior bone should be maintained as much as possible. Even if the anterior bone is thin, its continuity can significantly increase the stability of three-point fixation. Another benefit of preserving anterior bone is to avoid impingement between the porous surface and anterior soft tissue, which can cause pain. Even if the anterior column is completely interrupted, the surgeon can still make use of the anteriosuperior, posterosuperior, and inferoposterior bone and create an effective three-point fixation.

1.4.1.3 Three-Point Fixation and Point Reconstruction of the Cup

The three-point fixation of acetabular reconstruction refers to the strategy of establishing three relatively small and stable areas (points) and subsequently wedging the hemispherical cup within the three points to form stable cup fixation (Fig. D.2) in the hemipelvic region (it has been previously expressed as "in the range of the acetabular residual bone," but the emergence of extending-fixation technique allows fixation based on bone mass outside of the acetabulum; consequently, the reconstruction of the non-cement acetabulum expanded beyond the acetabular boundary, involving the entire hemipelvis) in non-cement reconstruction of the acetabulum. These three points can be either bone-based or porous metal-based in reconstruction.

The major pattern of three-point fixation is to select and establish each fixation point in anteriosuperior, posterosuperior, and inferoposterior acetabulum, respectively. In certain cases, for example, when the anterior column of the acetabulum is broken, the surgeon can still make use of the anteriosuperior, posterosuperior, and inferoposterior acetabulum to provide three-point fixation. However, with a limited volume of the pubis and thin pubic rami, the support from the anteroinferior point is limited. Therefore, the anteroinferior, inferoposterior, and posterosuperior points should not be considered the priority for three-point fixation in this situation. Of course, the support of the anteroinferior point can also be enhanced by augments (such as lotus-shaped augment).

The three-point fixation of the cup relies on the support of the three points. Supportiveness is a term often used here. Supportiveness of point has two meanings: (1) Whether the bone mass at this point can provide sufficient and tight attach-

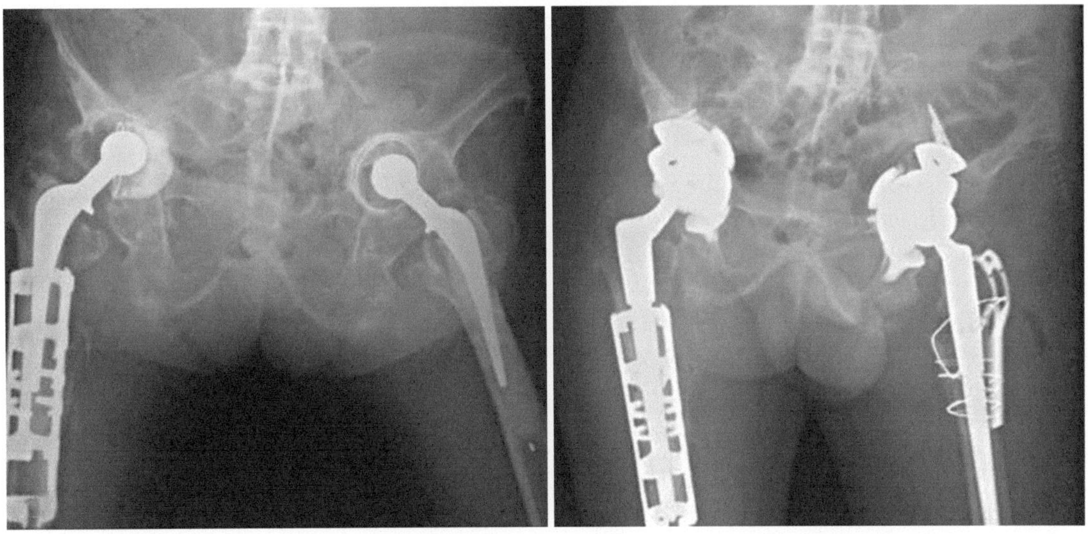

Fig. D.2 Case of three-point fixation. (**a**) Preoperative AP view of both hips. (**b**) Postoperative AP view of both hips (slope augment was applied to reconstruct the superior fixation point and lotus-shaped augment was applied to reconstruct the inferior fixation point. The medial wall of the acetabulum was reconstructed with disk augment)

ment between active bone and the surface of the cup, as well as whether the bone mass at this point can provide enough mechanical strength (it is not difficult to perceive that the point here is not a geometric point, but a relatively small surface area). (2) Whether it is static and stable between two points. If there is relative migration and fluctuation in between points, that is, they are shaking points, they are not supporting points, and stable three-point fixation cannot be obtained.

1.4.1.4 Significance of the Anterior and Posterior Columns

In any case, the three points of the three-point fixation are distributed on the acetabulum, or between the upper and lower hemipelvis, or the iliac segment and the ischis-public segment. If the joint of the upper and lower ends is interrupted, then migration and fluctuation can occur between the three points, which no doubt makes them non-support points. Thus, the importance of the anterior and posterior columns of the acetabulum is self-evident, as they are the link between the iliac segment and the ischial-public segment, as well as the structure that connects the top and bottom.

As long as one of them is intact, the three points are considered stable. With sufficient bone mass in the three points, it is considered supportable. The acetabulum turns from a ring to a "C" shape if the fracture occurs in one of the columns, more press fit, such as 3–4 mm, is required based on the final reaming to achieve ideal initial stability.

In comparison, the integrity of the posterior column is more important than that of the anterior column. When the posterior column is fractured and the anterior column is intact, the upper and lower three points are still stable. However, because most human activities are conducted under hip flexion, in which the lower extremities transfer stress to the posterior and superoposterior acetabulum through the femoral head and neck, the cup shifts posteriorly. Therefore, it is not ideal to ignore posterior column interruption completely. There are of course many options for the treatment of posterior column interruption, but it is generally believed that relying only on the existing three-point fixation is not enough. One of the commonly used methods is to apply extended fixation with buttress and other non-cement augments. The length and surface area of the buttress augment are used to extend the non-cement fixation length to the posterosuperior iliac crest. The distal part of the buttress augment extends down the posterosuperior acetabular bone, providing support for the hemispherical cup. This reconstruction method can be considered as follows: (1) The upward extended fixation improves the supportiveness of the posterosuperior point of the acetabulum to resist more posterosuperior stress and prevent the migration of the cup on the vector. (2) The distal part of the buttress augment can be extended to 1/3~1/2 over the posterior column, which can be regarded as a partial reconstruction of the posterior column. This partially reconstructed posterior column can naturally resist the posterior stress in hip flexion and provides pinch fixation to a certain extent.

1.4.1.5 The Function and Reconstruction of Medial Wall

The function of the acetabular floor or wall is to provide dome fixation of the external cup to prevent invagination and deflection of the acetabular cup, which is an important auxiliary and supplement of "circle fixation" and "three-point fixation."

It is not difficult to understand that the dome of the external cup has good contact or osseointegration with the acetabular floor. It greatly helps structures in acetabular periphery fixation (both rims fit and three-point fixation are periphery fixation) control torque against the oblique rotation of the cup. Moreover, the medial wall is reconstructed using disk augments, the curvature radius of which is significantly greater than that of the cup itself. Therefore, the left surface area of bone contact on the acetabular floor is much larger than that of the cup dome, so the snowshoe effect can be achieved to prevent the cup from migrating inward after loading and to increase the contact between the non-cement porous metal surface and the bone.

It seems that insufficient attention has been paid to medial wall fixation. For shallow acetabulum such as stunting ones, there have even been cases when the acetabular floor was purposely reamed through to move the rotation center inward and increase the bone covering of the lateral cup. Now that the integrity of the cup is good, "protrusion" like this is feasible. According to the results of medical wall reconstruction conducted by the author in recent years, bone remodeling and trabecular rearrangement around the medial wall reconstructed with porous metal have indeed been observed (see Fig. D.3). This can be strong evidence of medial wall reconstruction being an effective supplement for three-point fixation and cup fixation.

In summary, the initial stability of non-cement acetabular reconstruction relies on rim fixation or three-point fixation. The integrity of the anterior and posterior columns, especially the posterior column, is an important factor in the supportiveness of fixation points. This is the RPC theory of acetabular reconstruction. The medial wall reconstruction can be performed as a supplementary fixation of rim fixation or three-point fixation. A mathematician once proposed that "the cosmos is constructed out of triangles." Just as the saying, the reconstruction of the acetabulum, from a geometric point of view, also takes advantage of the stability of triangles by reconstructing a number of interconnected triangles to form a stable three-dimensional structure.

Recommended Reading

1. Zhou Y. Cementless fixation and reconstruction of acetabulum based on RPC theory. J Clin Orthop Res (in Chinese). 2019;4(1):1–2.
2. Zhou B, Zhou Y, Yang D, Tang H, Shao H, Huang Y. The utilization of metal augments allows better biomechanical reconstruction of the hip in revision total hip arthroplasty with severe acetabular defects: a comparative study. J Arthroplasty. 2018;33(12):3724–33.
3. Baghdadi YM, Larson AN, Sierra RJ. Restoration of the hip center during THA perfoimed for protrusio acetabuli is associated with better implant survival. Clin Orthop Relat Res. 2013;471(10):3251–9.
4. Pagnano W, Hanssen AD, Lewallen DC, Shaughnessy WJ. The effect of superior

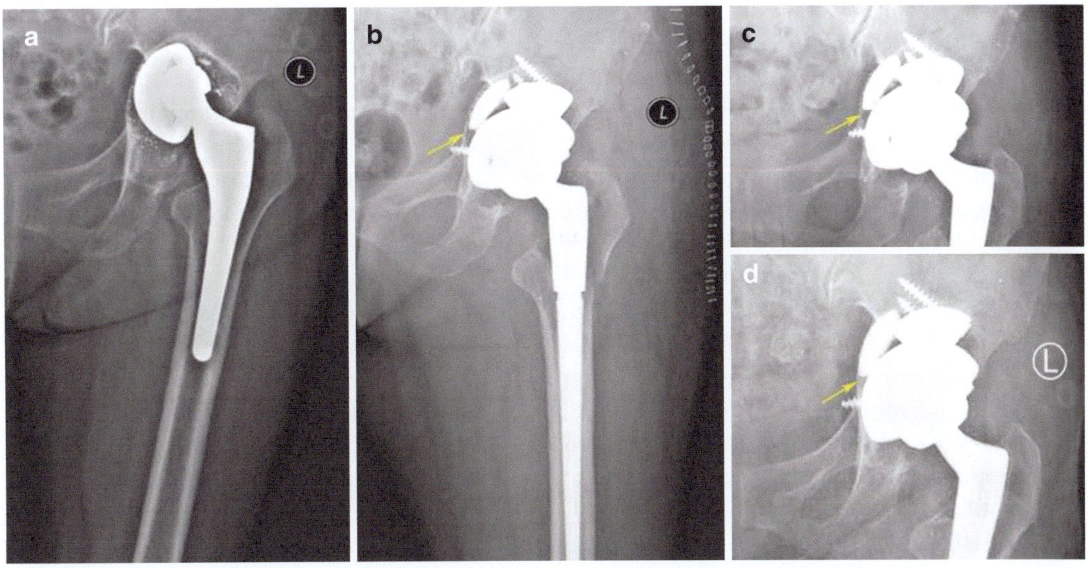

Fig. D.3 Case of porous metal reconstruction. (**a**) Preoperative AP view of the left hip. (**b**) Postoperative AP view of the left hip (disc augment was applied to reconstruct the medial wall). (**c**) Postoperative X-ray 3 months after left revision THA (yellow arrow shows bone ingrowth around disc augment). (**d**) Postoperative X-ray 1 year after left revision (yellow arrow shows bone ingrowth around disc augment, which significantly increased compared with the previous one)

placement of the acetabular component on the rate of loosening after total hip arthroplasty: long-term results in patients who have Crowe Type-U congenital dysplasia of the hip. J Bone Joint Surg Am. 1996;78(7):1004–14.
5. Tang H, Zhou B, Huang Y, Zhou Y, Chen B, Li X. Inferior extended fixation utilizing porous titanium augments improves primary anti-rotational stability of the acetabular component. Clin Biomech. 2019;70:158–63.
6. Guo S, Huang Y, Tang H, et al. Early outcomes of reconstruction of Paprosky III acetabular bone defects using tantalum trabecular metal cup combined with tantalum augment. Chin J Orthop (in Chinese). 2016;36(23):1479–86.
7. Huang Y, Zhou Y, Guo S, et al. Reconstruction of severe acetabular bone defect by tantalum trabecular metal cup combining tantalum augment. Chin J Joint Surg (Electronic Edition) (in Chinese). 2015;9(6):732–9.

1.5 Appendix E: Academic Publications on Revision Hip Arthroplasty of the Team

Recommended Reading

1. Zhou B, Zhou Y, Yang D, et al. The utilization of metal augments allows better biomechanical reconstruction of the hip in revision total hip arthroplasty with severe acetabular defects: a comparative study. J Arthroplasty. 2018;33(12):3724–33.
2. Bian T, Shao H, Zhou Y, et al. Tests for predicting reimplantation success of two-stage revision for periprosthetic joint infection: a systematic review and meta-analysis. Orthop Traumatol Surg Res. 2018;104(7):1115–23.
3. Zheng H, Gu H, Shao H, et al. Treatment and outcomes of Vancouver type B periprosthetic femoral fractures. Bone Joint J. 2020;102-B(3):293–300.
4. Huang Y, Shao H, Zhou Y, et al. Femoral bone remodeling in revision total hip arthroplasty with use of modular compared with monoblock tapered fluted titanium stems: the role of stem length and stiffness. J Bone Joint Surg Am. 2019;101(6): 531–8.
5. Yin X, Zhou Y, Tang Q, et al. Screw-hole clusters in acetabular cups a morphological study of optimal positioning of screw-holes. Hip Int. 2017;27(4):382–8.
6. Dou Y, Zhou Y, Tang Q, et al. Leg-lengtli discrepancy after revision hip arthroplasty: are modular stems superior? J Arthroplasty. 2013;28:676–9.
7. Huang Y, Zhou Y, Shao H, et al. What is the difference between modular and nomnodular tapered fluted titanium stems ill revision total hip artliroplasty. J Arthroplasty. 2017;(32):3108–13.
8. Tang H, Zhou B, Huang Y, et al. Inferior extended fixation utilizing porous titaiiimn augments improves primary anti-rotational stability of the acetabular component. Cliii Biomech (Bristol, Avon). 2019;70:158.
9. Zhou Y. Cementless fixation and reconstruction of acetabulum based on RPC theory. J Clin Orthop Res (in Chinese). 2019;4(1):1–2.
10. Dou Y, Zhou Y, Chu Y, et al. Analysis of risk factors relative to intraoperative fracture of the femur in revision of hip arthroplasty. Orthop J China (in Chinese). 2012;20(19):1749–53.
11. Gu J, Feng X, Gong L, et al. Correlation between serum cobalt chromium ion concentration and local histopathological ALVAL score of patients after revision total hip arthroplasty. J Clin Orthop Res (in Chinese). 2019;4(1):9–14.
12. Gu J, Huang Y, Du H, et al. Clinical outcomes of femoral revision using restoration modular stem. Chin J Orthop (in Chinese). 2017;37(23):1458–65.
13. Guo S, Huang Y, Tang H, et al. Early outcomes of reconstruction of Paprosky III acetabular bone defects using tantalum trabecular metal cup combined with tantalum augment. Chin J Orthop (in Chinese). 2016;36(23):1479–86.
14. Huang Y, Zhou Y, Guo S, et al. Reconstruction of severe acetabular bone defect by tantalum trabecular metal cup combining

tantalum augment. Chin J Joint Surg (Electronic Edition) (in Chinese). 2015;9(6):732–9.
15. Li W, Zhou Y, Wu J, et al. Radiographic appraisal between metal and bone interosculate backfill after total hip arthroplasty with trabecular metal cup. Chin J Surg (in Chinese). 2009;47(4):297–300.
16. Zhang L, Zhou Y. Progress in diagnosis and treatment of infection after joint replacement. Chin J Orthop (in Chinese). 2009;29(2):164–7.
17. Zhang L, Zhou Y, Li Y, et al. Treatment of infected total hip arthroplasty. Chin J Orthop (in Chinese). 2009;29(10):924–8.
18. Zhang L, Zhou Y, Zhou X, et al. Analysis of the failure mechanisms of the revision hip arthroplasties. Chin J Surg (in Chinese). 2009;47(3):164–7.
19. Zheng H, Huang Y, Shao H, et al. Uncemented modular stems used for Vancouver B2 and B3 periprosthetic femoral fractures. Chin J Orthop (in Chinese). 2017;37(15):914–20.
20. Zhou B, Zhou Y. Application of custom triflange acetabular components in complex revision total hip arthroplasty. J Clin Orthop Res (in Chinese). 2019;4(1):18–21.
21. Huang D, Zhang L, Jiang Y, et al. Trabecular metal cup combined with allograft implantation for severe defects in hip revision arthroplasty. Orthop J China (in Chinese). 2016;24(12):1057–61.
22. Huang D, Zhang H, Zhou Y, et al. Preliminary application of antibiotics impregnated bone cement spacer in two-stage revision surgery for infected total hip arthroplasty. Chin J Traumatol (in Chinese). 2007;23(6):403–6.
23. Li Y, Huang D, Zhang H, et al. The application of bone cement spacer on the treatment of infections following artificial hip replacement. Chin J Orthop (in Chinese). 2009;29(8):749–53.
24. Shao H, Song Y, Bian T, et al. Two-staged revision for hip periprosthetic infection. Orthop J China (in Chinese). 2018;26(17):1544–8.
25. Deng W, Wu T, Wang Z, et al. Medial wall reconstruction using metal disc augments in revision total hip arthroplasty. Int Orthop (SICOT). 2023;47(5):1203–12. https://doi.org/10.1007/s00264-023-05723-y.
26. Chen L, Zhou Y, Zhang L, et al. Revision total hip arthroplasty in patients with ankylosing spondylitis: mid-term results. Orthop Traumatol Surg Res. 2023;109(7):103504.
27. Huang Y, Zhou Y, Shao H, et al. Total hip arthroplasties for hartofilakidis type C1 and C2 high hip dislocations demonstrate similar survivorship and clinical function at minimum 10-year follow-up with cementless implants. J Arthroplasty. 2022;37(12):2374–80.
28. Huang Y, Tang H, Zhou Y, et al. Extended ischiopubic fixation using porous metal augments in cementless acetabular reconstruction during revision total hip arthroplasty. Orthop Surg. 2022;14(10):2480–8.
29. Guo S, Tang H, Ma Z, et al. Clinical and radiological outcomes of revision total hip arthroplasty for patients with prior hartofilakidis type C hip dysplasia. Orthop Surg. 2022;14(10):2571–9.
30. Zhang J, Huang Y, Zhou B, et al. Mid-term follow-up of acetabular revision arthroplasty using jumbo cups. Orthop Surg. 2019;11(5):811–8.
31. Zhou Y, Shao H, Huang Y, et al. Does robotic assisted technology improve the accuracy of acetabular component positioning in patients with DDH? J Orthop Surg (Hong Kong). 2021;29(2):23094990211025325.
32. Huang Y, Zhou Y, Tian H, et al. Minimum 7-year follow-up of a porous coated trabecular titanium cup manufactured with electron beam melting technique in primary total hip arthroplasty. Orthop Surg. 2021;13(3):817–24.
33. Guo S-J, Shao H, Huang Y, et al. Retrospective cohort study comparing complications, readmission, transfusion, and length of stay of patients undergoing simultaneous and staged bilateral total hip arthroplasty. Orthop Surg. 2020;12(1):233–40.

34. Zhou Y, Huang Y, He R, et al. Long-term effectiveness of total hip arthroplasty for Crowe type IV developmental dysplasia of the hip. Chin J Reparat Reconstr Surg (in Chinese). 2021;35(12):1531–6.
35. Guo S, Tang H, Zhou Y, et al. Accuracy of digital tomosynthesis with metal artifact reduction for detecting osteointegration in cementless hip arthroplasty. J Arthroplasty. 2018;33(5):1579–87.
36. Tang H, Huang X, Cheng X, et al. Evaluation of peri-prosthetic radiolucent lines surrounding the cementless femoral stem using digital tomosynthesis with metal artifact reduction: a cadaveric study in comparison with radiography and computed tomography. Quant Imaging Med Surg. 2020;10(9):1786–800.
37. Huang D, Zhang L, Zhou Y, et al. Total hip arthroplasty using modular trabecular metal acetabular components for failed treatment of acetabular fractures: a mid-term follow-up study. Chin Med J (English). 2016;129(8):903–8.
38. Tang H, Huang Y, Zhou Y, et al. Extended fixation for Paprosky Type III acetabular defects in revision total hip arthroplasty with a minimum follow-up of 2 years. Orthop Surg. 2023;15(1):205–13.
39. Huang Y, Zhou Y, Shao H, et al. A novel endosteal reconstruction of the femur from distal femoral remnant using 3D-printed titanium rings: a two-case report. JBJS Case Connect. 2021;11(3).
40. Gu J, Feng X, Zhou Y, et al. Results of revision total hip arthroplasty by using trabecular metal acetabular cup and restoration modular stem protheses in patients with severe bone defects. Chin J Bone Jt Surg (in Chinese). 2022,15(1):31–7.
41. Gu J, Feng X, Zhou Y, et al. Causes of revision total hip arthroplasty: an analysis of 1422 patients.Chin J Bone Jt Surg (in Chinese). 2021;14(4):267–71.
42. Gu J, Feng X, Du H, et al. Analysis of abnormally elevated serum cobalt concentration in patients undergoing revision hip arthroplasty with cobalt-containing materials. Chin J Bone Jt Surg (in Chinese). 2021;14(3):161–7.
43. Chu Y, Huang Y, Zhou Y, et al. Mid-term follow-up of non-modular tapered fluted titanium stems in revision total hip arthroplasty. Chin J Med (in Chinese). 2020;55(12):1327–31.
44. Gong L, Chen X, Gu J, et al. The correlation analysis of serum metal ion concentration and metal particles with histopathological features in patients with revision total hip arthroplasty. J Clin Orthop Res (in Chinese). 2020;5(3):176–82.
45. Peng H, Wang L, Chen J, et al. Revision burden due to periprothetic joint infection after total hip or knee arthroplasty of 9 hospitals in Beijing between 2014 and 2016: a multi-center survey.Chin J Bone Jt Surg (in Chinese). 2020;13(4):277–83.

Postscript

I still recall the sentence carved on a stone slab and placed on the roadside on Benjamin Franklin Avenue when I studied in Philadelphia a few years ago: "If you want somebody remember you, do something worth writing or write something worth reading." Every time I passed through, I always wondered, as an orthopedic surgeon of Jishuitan Hospital, Beijing, whether I should do something, or write something, so that our work can be inherited and passed on.

How time flies. By this day, I have been working in the Orthopaedics Department of Jishuitan Hospital for nearly 20 years. I have grown from an inexperienced resident to a qualified surgeon who can work independently. In the meantime, countless patients who had full trust in us have provided plenty of valuable clinical data. It was also the patient guidance of predecessors, fellow practitioners, and even international fellows, especially my professor Zhou Yixin who has led us in clinical practice, that allowed us to make continuous pioneering and innovation.

As is known to all, THA has been performed in China for nearly half a century. This technique has gradually matured and popularized. However, revision THA has been showing an increasing trend year by year alongside. Compared with the initial THA, revision THA requires higher technical skills and is more difficult to operate, which often needs the cooperation of various departments and team members.

Accurate diagnosis, careful surgical procedures, and good intraoperative teamwork are critical to the successful revision THA. A case of prosthesis loosening could be either with or without infection. The treatment options for the two situations are completely different. Therefore, how to accurately diagnose the condition is significant for surgical planning. How to determine if the patients requiring revision THA have an infection when their preoperative CRP is elevated? How to differentiate infection from metallosis? These are often confusing to most surgeons. I hope that through the cases presented in this book and the discussion after each of them, I have briefly covered the topics that are of interest. Revision THA often involves massive bone defects, which is a Gordian Knot in clinical operation, and also a hot topic that triggers discussion and attention in orthopedic surgeon meetings.

Through years of practice, Professor Zhou Yixin proposed the RPC theory for the acetabular side and the valid fixation length theory for the femoral side, which are of great clinical significance for all types of bone defect cases. A good number of cases in this book have illustrated the practice of them. These theories guide our daily operation work; hopefully, they are as helpful to other orthopedic surgeons. Indeed, some of these cases are not very common, but as an arthroplasty surgeon of Jishuitan Hospital, Beijing, I also wish to help the readers understand the diagnosis and treatment process of revision THA through the presentation of cases, even how to prevent failure after THA.

I sincerely hope that the publication of this book provides a little more information and help. For any inadvertent mistakes or inappropriate writing in this book, we humbly welcome your criticism and suggestions.

Hongyi Shao, Jishuitan Hospital, Beijing
01/01/2022

Y. Zhou (ed.), *Revision Total Hip Arthroplasty*, https://doi.org/10.1007/978-981-97-9804-9

MIX
Papier aus verantwortungsvollen Quellen
Paper from responsible sources
FSC® C105338

If you have any concerns about our products,
you can contact us on
ProductSafety@springernature.com

In case Publisher is established outside the EU,
the EU authorized representative is:
Springer Nature Customer Service Center GmbH
Europaplatz 3, 69115 Heidelberg, Germany

Printed by Libri Plureos GmbH
in Hamburg, Germany